**Everything you need to know, from buying
your first bike to riding your best**

THE
BIG
BOOK
OF
Bicycling

EMILY FURIA
and the Editors of
Bicycling

RODALE

Portions of this book previously appeared in *Bicycling* magazine. List of additional credits appears on pages 281–282.

© 2011 by Rodale Inc.
Photographs and illustrations were supplied by the following: pages 15–17, 80, 82–84, 120, 124–126, 157–159, 193, 259, (c) Charlie Layton; pages 38–39, 91–95, 219 (c) Thomas MacDonald; pages 99–100, 160–165, 238 (c) Jason Lee; page 87 (c) Matthew Vincent; page 56 (c) Renee Alejandro Hernandez; page 50 (c) Troy Doolittle.

Rodale books may be purchased for business or promotional use or for special sales. For information, please write to: Special Markets Department, Rodale, Inc., 733 Third Avenue, New York, NY 10017

Bicycling is a registered trademark of Rodale Inc.

Printed in the United States of America
Rodale Inc. makes every effort to use acid-free ♾, recycled paper ♻.

Book design by Chris Rhoads
Cover design by David Speranza
Cover photograph by Michael Darter

Library of Congress Cataloging-in-Publication Data

The big book of bicycling : everything you need to know, from buying your first bike to riding your best / by Emily Furia and the editors of Bicycling.
    p.   cm.
  ISBN 978–1–60529–282–3   paperback
  1. Cycling.   2. Cycling—Training.   3. Cycling—Equipment and supplies.   4. Bicycles.   5. Bicycle racing.   I. Furia, Emily. II. Bicycling.
  GV1041 .B536 2011
  796.6—dc22
                                         2010040295

Distributed to the trade by Macmillan

2 4 6 8 10 9 7 5 3   paperback

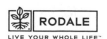

RODALE
LIVE YOUR WHOLE LIFE™

We inspire and enable people to improve their lives and the world around them.

Contents

PART IV

Bike Maintenance

PART V

Riding for Transportation

PART VI

Fitness, Training, and Racing

PART VII

Centuries and Cause Rides

PART VIII

Nutrition for Cyclists

PART IX

Touring and Travel

PART X

Getting Dirty: Riding Off-Road

PART XI

How to Raise a Cyclist

Introduction

LET'S RIDE

You know the old saying: "It's as easy as riding a bike." And the crazy thing is, it's true. Bicycling is a supremely accessible activity—just ask any 7-year-old. Grab a bike and a helmet, and start pedaling. No matter your age or fitness level, you too will feel that childlike joy of being out there, free, legs spinning, the wind on your face. That feeling that you're going somewhere. It's one of the simple joys of the sport.

At the same time, cycling is full of beautiful complexity. As you learn more about the sport, you realize how much more is waiting to be discovered. It doesn't matter why you ride—whether it's for fitness, fun, competition, transportation, or weight loss—the sport just keeps getting more interesting and more rewarding. The best part? Sometimes getting the right nugget of information at the right moment can literally transform a ride. I did not know how to fix a flat (not quickly, at least) or ride in a paceline or what the heck to do with chamois cream until other, more experienced cyclists showed me the ropes. Eventually, I knew enough to truly join the pack.

The *Big Book of Bicycling* can make that process a little bit simpler. Here, we invite you to ride with us and learn from the best. For the first time, all of our top advice is in one handy place, with our trusted experts (you'll meet them on page ix), staff editors and writers sharing the basic concepts, tips, and tricks that will just plain make biking more enjoyable and also help you reach your goals, whatever they may be. Before you know it, you'll be cruising.

See you out on the road.

Peter Flax
Editor-in-Chief
Bicycling magazine

Meet the Experts

Some of Bicycling *magazine's expert columnists and contributors appear regularly in these pages.*

Former Olympic and Tour de France cyclist **Chris Carmichael** is Lance Armstrong's personal coach and the founder of Carmichael Training Systems (trainright.com). He writes the Coach column for *Bicycling* and is also the author of *The Time-Crunched Cyclist: Fit, Fast, and Powerful in 6 Hours a Week*.

Bicycling's Road Rights columnist **Bob Mionske** is a former Olympic and professional cyclist, and a lawyer who specializes in cyclists' rights. His book *Bicycling and the Law* was published in 2007.

Alex Stieda was the first North American to wear the yellow jersey in the Tour de France in 1986. Today he leads tours and skills camps, and he recently released *The Smooth Ride*, an instructional road cycling DVD (stiedacycling.com).

Selene Yeager is a USA Cycling certified coach, elite mountain bike racer for Team CF (teamcf.org), and the author of *Every Woman's Guide to Cycling* and *Ride Your Way Lean: The Ultimate Plan for Burning Fat and Getting Fit on a Bike*. In 2008, she competed in her first Ironman triathlon, winning her age group and earning a spot at the world championships in Hawaii. Read her blog at bicycling.com/fitchick.

You'll also be hearing from some people we call our **BikeTowners.**

In 2003, *Bicycling* conducted an experiment to find out how the gift of a bicycle could change someone's life, by giving away 50 bikes to residents of Portland, Maine. Since then, nearly 3,000 people have received bicycles through *Bicycling's* BikeTown program. Many BikeTowners have gone on to become seasoned cyclists; nearly all report that riding has had a positive impact on their lives.

I

Getting Started and Motivated

THE LIST OF ALL THE WONDERFUL BENEFITS A BIKE CAN give you (more sleep! better sex!) is almost endless. We give you a multitude of reasons to get in the saddle. Already got the cycling bug? Congratulations: You'll find plenty of tips to keep you pedaling.

CHAPTER 1

The Greatest Sport in the World

You've probably heard that cycling is good for your body—it burns tons of calories, strengthens your heart and lungs, goes easy on your joints, and so on. But that's not all. Read on to find out about some lesser-known perks.

IT KEEPS YOU SHARP

Forget the dumb jock stereotype—aerobic exercise is exactly what your brain needs. Here are some of the cognitive benefits associated with cycling.

CONCENTRATION. Activities that require balance, quick reactions and decision-making skills—like martial arts, gymnastics and cycling—best control Attention Deficit Hyperactivity Disorder (ADHD) in children, says psychiatrist David Conant-Norville, MD. A Vanderbilt University study shows that these activities may help adults with focus and concentration, too. Participants who performed a short but complex exercise were 40 percent more likely to solve a puzzle than idle participants. The takeaway: If you're stuck on a problem, go for a ride.

MEMORY. For the hippocampus—a region of the brain that controls long-term and spatial memory—bigger is better. And as with the rest of your body's muscles, exercise makes the hippocampus grow. A University of Illinois and University of Pittsburgh joint study found that physically fit participants had larger hippocampi and performed 40 percent better on memory tests. Other reports show that exercise helps older adults retain cognitive function and avoid disorders like Alzheimer's and dementia.

IT REDUCES STRESS

Research has shown that vigorous exercise is so effective at quelling anxiety and depression that some patients have been able to reduce or eliminate the use of medications such as Prozac and Zoloft. In a study at the University of Southern Mississippi, participants who suffered from generalized anxiety disorder and exercised at 60 to 90 percent of their maximum heart rates for three 20-minute sessions per week saw significant decreases in anxiety, sensitivity and fear after just two workouts. Further research has shown that people who get regular vigorous exercise are less likely to develop anxiety disorders and depression.

Why I Ride

"I love to ride on a quiet road in the trees, climbing hills and coming down the other side. Cycling's not just a sport; it's who I am."—AMERICAN PRO CYCLIST LEVI LEIPHEIMER

IT MAKES YOU HAPPIER

LESS ANGER. Exposure to plants and the outdoors has been linked to reduced aggression in inner-city residents. Choose the right terrain and riding buddies, and you can comfortably spend all day in nature on two wheels—good luck lasting that long in running shorts.

MORE *AMOUR*. A German study discovered something that cyclists have known for a long time: Cycling gets us high. Exercise increases your body's production of endorphins—and sends them to the same parts of the brain that are activated when we fall in love.

IT BOOSTS SELF-ESTEEM—SERIOUSLY

According to psychology types, mastering a task that we find difficult—upgrading to clipless pedals, scoring a point in the Tuesday-night crit, truing a wheel for the first time—makes us feel better about ourselves. Of course, negative experiences reverse the process—all the more reason to get back in the saddle as soon as possible after a bad day. The President's Council on Physical Fitness and Sports concurs: "Aerobic exercise seems to be beneficial in enhancing self-esteem."

IT HELPS YOU HAVE MORE (AND BETTER) SEX

It's true: Here are five ways that time in the saddle helps you in the sack.

KEEPS YOU LEAN. According to the Centers for Disease Control and Prevention, overweight people are at increased risk for high blood pressure, diabetes, heart disease, cancer and more—any of which can ruin your sex life faster than seeing your grandparents in the altogether. The National Institutes of Health confirms what we all know: Exercise, such as spinning pedals, is inversely related to body weight and the rate of weight gain with age. Another tidbit to spur along male slackers: Abdominal fat can add up around the base of the penis, making it appear smaller. You can "lose" an inch of penis for every extra 35 pounds you carry.

IMPROVES ENDURANCE. The aerobic conditioning gained from regular riding translates to greater stamina in other activities, including sweet romance, says Steve Owens, exercise physiologist and a coach with Colorado Premier Training. A study conducted by the Harvard School of Public Health showed that men over 50 who kept physically active were 30 percent less likely to suffer from erectile dysfunction than men who were inactive. In fact, according to the researchers, the most physically active

Why I Ride

"It seems like cycling has become cool in the U.S. When I started, it was an outsider thing. Growing up in Queens, New York, I was the only person riding my bike, and everyone else was playing normal sports. Nobody knew what cycling was. But now everywhere you go people know what's going on, and they watch the Tour."—GEORGE HINCAPIE, WHO'S RIDDEN IN MORE TOURS DE FRANCE THAN ANY OTHER AMERICAN

men seemed to have the sexual ability of men two to five years younger. Schwing!

GETS YOU IN THE MOOD. A University of Texas at Austin researcher found that vigorous exercise—specifically, cycling—helped increase sexual arousal in women, both subjectively (the women reported being more aroused from an X-rated movie after a brief ride than they were without the ride) and objectively (blood flow to the genitals was significantly increased).

AMPS YOUR SEX DRIVE. Testosterone is directly related to sex drive in both men and women, making us want to have sex, pursue sex, initiate sex, and perhaps dominate the lovemaking. A 2002 study at Britain's University of Newcastle upon Tyne found that older men who exercise regularly produce more growth hormone and

testosterone than those who lead an inactive life. Regular exercise can boost testosterone levels in women, as well—proof that regular rides will make you want to ride regularly.

HELPS YOU GET MORE. Riding on a regular basis increases the frequency of coupling. In an *Archives of Sexual Behavior* study, 78 sedentary but healthy men (average age 48 years) participated in a moderate aerobic exercise program— mainly cycling and jogging—three to four days a week for nine months. At the end of the study, the men reported a significant increase in their sexual arousal, activity, function and satisfaction. One inspiring example: Their frequency of intercourse went up by 30 percent.

Fun **Fact**

Seven percent of readers polled by *Bicycling* admitted to wearing a heart rate monitor during sex.

OKAY, YOU'VE CONVINCED ME . . . BUT WHERE DO I FIND THE TIME?

Funny you should ask—that's one of the most common questions *Bicycling* gets from readers. The truth is, riders of all levels struggle to fit riding into a busy schedule. Here's how to make it happen.

→If you think ride time will simply appear during your day, you might as well put your bike on Craigslist. Schedule it on the family calendar, in your datebook, on your work schedule—wherever you can to be sure others will know you're busy.

→Log every ride. It could be a total data dump or just the date and route in a notebook. There are multiple training benefits to this, but also the thought of a blank space on the calendar often strengthens the urge to squeeze in a ride.

→When ride time rolls around, go for the ride; postponing it sets a negative precedent. Cycling is a sport of momentum: The more you ride, the more you'll ride.

→Boldly suggest to colleagues or clients that your next meeting should take place on a ride.

Or buy a couple of cruisers for your office—they'll be easier on your expense report than a month of greens fees, and even noncyclists can experience the beauty of doing business on the roll.

→When all else fails, pay someone so you can ride. Hire a babysitter, a cleaning service, a lawn-care company. It's an investment in your health. It's worth the money.

→Look at your daily routine in terms of how much riding time you lose, and you'll find ways to prune. If cooking dinner takes 45 minutes each night, that's more than four hours over the workweek. Spend an hour or two on Sunday cooking a chicken, prepping salad greens and stocking the fridge with a few nights' healthy meals. Things like watching television and posting on web forums will feel even more expendable.

But Don't Just Take Our Word for It . . .

See what some of our BikeTowners have to say about taking up cycling.

"I tell my patients that cycling is 'sneaky exercise.' You don't realize how good it is for you."—*family practitioner Tom Del Giorno, BikeTown Philadelphia 2006*

"I've gotten rid of all my fat clothes. For the first time in my life, I feel like a woman."—*Lynda Thomas, BikeTown Denver 2005*

"It seems like the more you ride, the more energy you have—you don't want to come back in. Maybe next I'll train for . . . what's that bike race? The Tour de France? I know I'm exaggerating, but that's how confident I feel."—*Robert Dickerson, BikeTown Boston 2006*

"I want to be someone who people can look at and say, 'Look what he did. Look at the results he got—and it wasn't that hard.'"—*Michael Freeman, BikeTown Los Angeles 2006*

"It's like, wow—all of this comes from a bike?"—*Karen Phillips, BikeTown Boston 2006, who credits cycling with helping her quit smoking*

Why I Ride

"Now I spend my days thinking about my next adventure instead of my next meal."—FORMER *BIGGEST LOSER* CONTESTANT JERRY LISENBY, WHO NOW BIKES FOR CHARITY

→To give yourself a fighting chance in winter, invest in a quality light, such as the helmet-mounted Stella from Light & Motion (lightandmotion.com).

→The lunch ride rules. You're not shortchanging work by skipping out for an hour; you're improving your focus. In a U.K. study, 75 percent of workers credited flex time with helping them increase their ability to concentrate, and therefore boost their productivity.

→If you can carve out only 20 minutes, give your bike a loving caress and then go do squats, crunches, pull-ups and planks, which will make your time on the bike even more enjoyable.

→Make repairs or adjustments when you finish a ride so little fix-its don't stall you when you want to leave for your next one.

Pro **Tip**

"I BELIEVE THAT BALANCE MAKES YOU SUCCESSFUL. IF ALL YOU DO IS WORK AND ANSWER HUNDREDS OF E-MAILS A DAY, YOU'RE GOING TO DRIVE YOURSELF INTO THE GROUND. SAME THING IF ALL YOU DO IS RIDE. YOU HAVE TO HAVE MORE THAN ONE THING IN YOUR LIFE."—KRISTIN ARMSTRONG, 2008 OLYMPIC TIME TRIAL GOLD MEDALIST

→Next family outing, meet your loved ones by bike. You'll get your day's ride in on the way and have more time to spend with them when you get there.

BUT I'M SO TIRED . . .

Ride anyway—chances are you'll end up with more energy, not less. But because that's easier said than done, here are some tricks to get motivated.

→The number-one way to guarantee that butt meets saddle: Map out a 30-minute loop for those occasions when you're short on time or can-do attitude. More often than not, you'll ride longer than planned; the rest of the time, hey, you rode half an hour.

→Guilt is a strong motivator. Set up a riding group with one or two friends, at most, just small enough that your skipping the ride spoils it. Large groups go off whether you show up or not.

→Your stomach is a motivator, too. Pick a delicious destination at least as far away as half the total distance you want to ride. Maintain an honest pace there, enjoy your treat, and pedal back.

→A big ride, like having a mortgage or raising kids, can be overwhelming when considered in its entirety. Focus on small intermediate goals, or if that doesn't work, distract yourself: During the final, hallucinogenic miles of an epic, dedicate each mile to someone: your spouse, your neighbor with cancer, your pet, your secret celebrity crush, your other bike at home.

→Tension slows you down. Keep facial muscles relaxed, and the rest of your body will follow. The easiest way to do this? Smile.

→Volunteer at a junior race or clinic. Kids have an unbridled enthusiasm for riding bikes that is contagious, and the bad teenager haircuts will quickly dispel any notions you had about wanting to be 16 again.

RIDER **RESOURCES**

Pick the brains of riders of all levels on *Bicycling's* forums (forums.bicycling.com).

Find more time to ride with tips from organizing expert Julie Morgenstern, author of *Never Check E-mail in the Morning,* at juliemorgenstern.com/blog.

II

Gearing Up

THERE'S NO QUESTION THAT GEAR IS AN INTEGRAL part of bicycling. When faced with this truth, people generally fall into one of two camps—wildly excited or just plain scared. While it pays to acquire the basics, you can enjoy the sport without spending a fortune. That said, there are plenty of fancy cycling goodies to be had if you choose to indulge—and don't be surprised if you find your thirst for new technology growing along with your riding ability. Here's our guide to navigating the maze.

CHAPTER 2

How to Buy a Bike

While purchasing a bike is less daunting than, say, buying a new car, it's still a sizeable investment. But spending a little extra time to get just the right bike will inspire you to ride even more than you thought you would—a worthy reason if ever there was one. Here's all you need to know to be a savvy shopper.

THE BURNING QUESTIONS

Walk into a bike shop, and you're confronted with a dizzying number of options. That's a good thing—once you know the one that's best for you. We get bike-buying questions from hundreds of people each year—readers, family members, friends, friends of friends, complete strangers who call us out of the blue. Here we answer some of the most common queries to help you find the right bike.

Which is a better bike, a Trek or a Specialized?

Or Cannondale or Orbea or Scott or Schwinn or Cervélo? We're asked "Which brand is better?" almost daily. While each brand has its diehard fans, we can't answer the question. It's not because of any political reason, but because it's not the right question to ask—

you're buying a bicycle, not a brand. If you shop by brand first, then you're making a style decision, not a performance one. When deciding which bike is better suited to you, it's the model that counts. To find the best bike, pick your price range, identify the ride feel and features you're after, and then look for models from various brands that meet those criteria. From there, a winner will emerge.

What about custom bikes? We get this one, too: Which is best, a Serotta, Parlee or Seven? The answer: Write the names on a note card, blindfold yourself and throw a dart—you'll end up with a bike you adore. The United States is home to the best custom builders in the world. An established custom builder has the knowledge and experience to build a bike that suits you as long as you fully communicate what you want. Still, every custom house has its flavor. Give the same data to two companies, and the fit and ride quality of the bikes will differ. To find the taste that's best for you, interview the builders, asking about the theories they use to interpret fit, handling and ride-feel requests. From here, you'll learn a builder's tendencies and be able to choose.

When do bike shops have sales?

Bikes are like cars: New models arrive on the bike-shop sales floor each year, typically in the fall as the riding season winds down. This is the best time to look for deals, because shops don't want soon-to-be-year-old inventory lingering through the slower winter months. While hot models in popular sizes will sell out over the summer, you may get lucky and find last year's model at a discount, but do your homework before buying: A model typically gets a dramatic redesign only every few years, so if the new model has only different paint and minor parts tweaks, you'll save on last year's bike. But if the new model has big frame changes or parts upgrades, then it can be worth paying for the new model. Beware of bikes that are more than a few seasons old. Advances in carbon fiber and component technology happen quickly, so a seemingly great deal may be only an average one.

Can I haggle with the shop over price?

You can try, but don't expect dealers to be flexible on current-year models. Profit margins on bike sales are razor thin. It's not uncommon for a shop to net more money on the extras—

helmet, pedals, computer and so on—than on the bike sale itself. For this reason, dealers are often more willing to throw in a free seat bag or bottle cage than to give a deal on the bike. If you're buying an expensive bike, more than one bike, a model left over from last year or a package including a helmet, tools, shoes, pedals, shorts and more, there's no harm in asking for a small discount. The worst you'll hear is no, but you may hear yes. Service is an area where you can seek out value: It's common for shops to provide a year of free basic adjustments on your new bike, so it's worth asking for this if your shop offers less.

If you don't like the deal offered by a shop, then quietly go elsewhere. You may find a better price in a nearby town, but it's not worth driving an hour to save a few bucks. Having a good local bike shop will save you time and money in the end with service and any warranty issues. Shops tend to go the extra mile for you if they know you bought the bike there.

Should I buy a carbon-fiber bike?

Absolutely. Maybe. Unless you shouldn't. Carbon is generally lighter than other materials, can be constructed to provide specific ride qualities in ways that metal tubes can't, and offers unlimited tube shapes—aero or just freaky cool. If you race and want a superstiff frame, carbon offers the best mix of low weight, aerodynamics and drivetrain stiffness without a buckboard ride. But it's also expensive. And not all carbon is equal: Less expensive frames use lower grades of fiber, which are heavier and less stiff, and often have a dead ride quality when compared with higher-grade carbon.

If you're on a budget, there are many racy bikes made of high-tech aluminum or a mix of alloy and carbon, which are stiff and light but will ride a bit more harshly than their all-carbon brethren. If you prize a smooth, refined ride feel, carbon can deliver—but so can steel and titanium, both of which continue to advance as frame materials. Ultimately, you should decide based on what you're willing to spend and whether you're a carbon person. Did you stand in line to buy the iPad? Carbon's cutting-edge tech will appeal to you. But if you're restoring a 1952 MGTD in your garage, then a ti or steel bike from a small builder may be just right. For more info on frame construction, see "This Is Your Frame," page 15.

I'm a woman; do I need a women's bike?

Standard bikes are built based on male physiology. Women's bikes are proportioned to suit the general female population, and most have components to suit women's anatomical needs, such as shorter-reach levers for smaller hands. A few companies even tune frame tubing to suit women's generally lighter bodies. All of this leads to a significant if obvious benefit—improved fit—but it also makes you a better, more confident rider.

The longer cockpit of a standard bike often causes female riders to stretch their torsos and arms, as well as move forward on the saddle.

This makes getting a secure grip on the levers more difficult, but it also moves a rider's center of gravity too far forward, compromising balance, mitigating power output and removing some rear-wheel traction. None of this is good.

To find out if you're better off on a women's bike, visit a shop with a selection of women's models. Take a test ride on a women's bike, then on a comparable men's model; go fast, brake hard, sit up, get aero—make all the moves you make when riding. Chances are you'll feel more in control on the women's bike.

Should I go for plush or race positioning?

An upright or plush position on the bike—when the angle between your back and the top tube is greater than 45 degrees, generally—causes less stress on your arms, neck and lower back, while providing good slow-speed control and an easy view of surroundings—ideal for in-town riding, or for those interested in the experience, not the clock. A more stretched-out, racy position—less than a 45-degree angle—makes you more aerodynamic and helps get more power to the pedals, perfect for fast road rides. In addition to geometry tweaks, a more plush ride uses a stem with a rise that puts the handlebar even with or above the saddle. A bike with a flat stem and a bar lower than the saddle? It's built for speed.

What components are best— Shimano, Campagnolo or SRAM?

All three companies make several tiers of well-functioning, dependable component groups.

(A group is typically defined to include brake and shift levers, brakes, derailleurs, crankset, bottom bracket, cassette and chain.) Among similarly priced groups, shifting and braking performance as well as weight are close enough that the real deciding factors are style and ergonomics. Be sure to put your hands on all three brands before buying.

Shimano shifts with a lever nestled inside a swinging brake lever. Shifting action feels smooth on your first ride, with uniformly positive and distinct ratchets. Its cassette bodies and wheels are compatible with SRAM (and vice versa), which gives you a greater choice when buying new wheels. Shimano is the most available, too, if you're ever stuck needing replacement parts, and its 105 group more or less rules midpriced bikes.

Campagnolo uses a swing lever and a thumb button to shift. Shifting feels stiff initially, then wears in and operates so smoothly that some find the minimal action disconcerting. Of all the groups, it's the easiest to repair. While top groups from all three companies allow multiple shifts with a single action, Campy's high-end Record and Chorus let you dump the chain—shift it all the way down the cassette with a single punch of the button.

SRAM accomplishes shifts with either a single- or double-length tap of a swing lever nestled against the brake lever. Its levers are praised for their ergonomics and tend to be the most accommodating for small hands. Shifting action lies somewhere between Campy's fluidity and Shimano's precision. Its Rival group is fast becoming popular on mid-range bikes.

Is it worth the money to go the next level up in components?

In terms of performance, the gap between Shimano Dura-Ace and Ultegra is smallest, followed by that of SRAM Red to Force and then Campagnolo Record to Chorus. Top-level parts use bearings instead of bushings and have better finishing and materials. Dura-Ace, Red and Record offer lighter weight and fractionally faster shifts, with better feel at the lever.

Often in a company's line of bikes the price difference between the top two or even three models reflects upgraded components, wheels and other parts—the frame may be exactly the same. Because parts wear out before frames, we generally advise investing in a quality frame first, and then picking a component level. Will you be putting in 300 miles a week? Then spend to have the best components. But if saving scratch is a priority, go with the nice frame and second-tier parts. Ultegra, Force and Chorus will last as long and work almost as well as top-shelf parts.

The gap between second- and third-tier groups is more substantial. Shimano 105, SRAM Rival and Apex and Campy Centaur are solid and reliable for recreational riding but lack the performance of top-level parts. Below that, Shimano's Tiagra and Sora and Campy's Veloce are a big step down, aimed at the occasional rider. Compared with even 105 and Centaur, they shift slowly and feel notchy.

Should I get a flat or a drop road handlebar?

A bike with a flat handlebar combines the easy speed of a road machine with the upright position and maneuverability of a mountain bike— perfect for commuters and casual fitness riders. Extend your time in the saddle, and you'll quickly notice the flat bar's main drawback: a lack of alternative hand positions. Drop bars offer several hand positions, and allow you to grab the drops and hunker low for greater speed and efficiency.

Do I need standard, compact or triple gearing on my road bike?

Gearing is a small choice that has a big impact. There are three typical options: standard (often chainrings with 53 and 39 teeth up front, paired with a 12-25 tooth-range 10-gear cassette), triple (three chainrings, with granny gears, often 50/40/30 or 52/42/30) or the increasingly popular compact (50/36 or 50/34 chainrings).

Pro Tip

"TEST-RIDE A VARIETY OF BIKES. EVEN IF YOU'RE [LOOKING TO BUY] IN THE $1,000 RANGE, TRY A $5,000 BIKE. YOU'LL FEEL THE DIFFERENCES AND UNDERSTAND WHAT YOU'RE PAYING FOR. YOU'LL END UP FEELING BETTER ABOUT YOUR PURCHASE, AND THAT YOU'RE GETTING WHAT YOU REALLY WANT, NOT WHAT THE SALES GUY IS PUSHING. IT'S LIKE IF YOU'RE LOOKING AT LCD TVS—YOU LOOK AT THE BIG ONES AND THE SMALL ONES AND NARROW IT DOWN TO WHAT'S RIGHT FOR YOU."—ARMANDO ENRIQUEZ, SALES MANAGER, BICYCLES PLUS, FOLSOM, CA

Which is best depends on how you ride. If you ride only a few miles a week or live near killer hills, then a triple may be best. But if you ride regularly over varied terrain, we recommend a compact. The smaller gear ratios enable nearly the same climbing prowess as a triple, but without the weight and added mechanical complexity of the extra chainring. Compacts also tend to cross-chain well; you can stay in the big chainring and gear down to the easiest cog to power up rises. Standard gearing makes cross-chaining a challenge unless you're a racer or big-wattage masher. Choose a standard double if you're fast and fit, or ride mainly flat terrain.

What about my commuter bike— should I get internal or external gears?

On town and commuter bikes, internally geared hubs offer minimal maintenance and easy gear changes, even without pedaling, and with no protruding derailleurs. However, a traditional derailleur/cog combo is lighter, often less expensive, and gives you a greater range of gears, making it more versatile overall.

Should I buy a full-suspension mountain bike or a hardtail?

If you're not sure then you've just revealed yourself as a trail-riding newbie—what a wonderful thing. Go with the hardtail. Without a rear suspension the bike will be lighter and less forgiving, which will help you feel the bumps, pick lines and correct mistakes without the handholding of a shock. Think of it this way: Kids who learn to drive on a standard transmission can drive anything, but those who learn on an automatic are spoiled forever.

Then there's value. For $1,000, you can buy a quality hardtail with good spec. Full-suspension bikes in this range have low-quality parts. If your heart is set on full suspension, be ready to spend more than a grand for decent tech, and at least $2,500 for a true performance bike.

Can't I save a bundle buying online?

Just as with books, cat litter and everything else, bikes are sold online at reduced prices. But you might not get a bargain. Many reputable sellers offer new and used bikes online, but steer clear of ads that are vague or downright shady, like one we saw on eBay that read, "not recommended for the Pittsburgh area," presumably because that's where the bike had been stolen. When you venture online, you're on your own. If you know your preferred frame angles, top-tube length, and stem and handlebar sizes, you might find a barely used dream ride and save hundreds. We've seen it happen. But if those measurement terms mean nothing to you, visit a bike shop for help. Otherwise you'll get a bargain online but spend twice the savings trying to make the bike fit, and it may never feel right. We see that happen all the time.

THIS IS YOUR FRAME

The ride quality of a frame is an alchemy of its angles and manufacturing process. While the tech geeks and retro-grouches debate the merits of lugs, monocoques and other aspects of design, we present this simple primer on how frames are made, as well as the (arguable, of course) pros and cons of each construction method. One thing you can be sure of: Material and construction methods have some inherent limitations— but we continue to be astounded by how far builders push those limits year after year.

Tube Making
MITERING

For this technique, engineers design the cut ends of metal and carbon tubes to fit together like puzzle pieces.

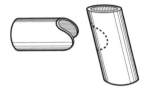

Advantage: The increased surface area creates a stronger joint without added weight; allows more variability in frame angles than other methods.

Disadvantage: Some argue that a mitered, welded or glued tube-to-tube construction isn't as strong over time as monocoque.

Wall Thickness/Butting

In the old days, we referred to butts, or distinct zones of a certain wall thickness. A triple-butted tube, for instance, would have three distinct wall-thickness variations along its length (see illustration on next page). Technology has all but eliminated the traditional concept of butting— though bike-makers still use the term "butted" liberally—because wall thickness can now be nearly infinitely variable along the length of a tube. The reason for varying wall thickness remains the same: to put more material where it's needed for strength and stiffness, and to eliminate material in less-stressed areas to save weight.

7 Valid Reasons to Buy a Custom Bike

1. YOU NEED CUSTOM GEOMETRY TO FIT YOUR BODY
You are exceptionally tall or short, or genetics or injury place you far enough out of the typical fit curve that no sane amount of jiggering with bar/saddle/cranks can lead to comfort on an off-the-shelf bike.

2. YOU WANT CUSTOM GEOMETRY TO FIT HOW YOU WANT TO RIDE
After time on many different bikes you know exactly what you want in terms of angles, tube lengths, bottom bracket drop, stiffness vs. compliance, maybe even specific types of tubing or materials.

3. YOU WANT SOMETHING WEIRD
You are puzzled that no big manufacturer builds a 29er rigid mountain bike you could race crits with after reassembling it with the couplers that allow you to fit it into your apartment, which you're subletting so you can fit the bike with panniers and do a transcontinental trip—and, by the way, you love Campy shifters but want disc brakes for your rainy commute, and you also might want to use the bike as the front end of a coupler tandem you'll have built some day.

4. YOU WANT A WORK OF ART
Breathtaking finishes, finial-like dropouts, hand-filed lugs with personalized cut-outs—you believe that, besides operating as a vehicle, a toy and an exercise machine, a bicycle can also be an aesthetic statement.

5. YOU WANT SOMETHING UNIQUE
Cyclists who just want to stand out from the local pack can find a rare brand from another country; you want your bike to be an idiosyncratic and personal expression with details and a back story no other bike on earth shares.

6. YOU ADMIRE THE BUILDER
Whether it's the ATMO of Richard Sachs or the classic-frames-meets-classic-rock vibe of Dario Pegoretti, you've identified a builder who embodies qualities you aspire to—and riding that person's bike brings you closer to what you believe.

7. YOU WANT TO BUY LOCAL
Getting a bike from a regional builder isn't simply an economic decision; it says that you love where you live, that your community is important and you are a part of the scene.

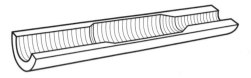

Advantage: Varying wall thickness allows frame makers to "tune" the strength, stiffness and ride qualities beyond the inherent properties of the material used.

Disadvantage: Adding a little material here and removing a little there requires a more intensive build process and costs more than does maintaining a constant thickness.

Bike Making
LUGGED
Premade intersections for the corners of the bike (at the junctions of the seat and head tubes, for instance) hold the frame tubes. This construction is used for both metal and carbon frames.

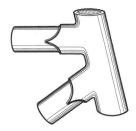

Advantages: This construction creates more load-bearing surface area; some think it's more durable; classic-frame snobs say it has the best ride quality; select carbon-lugged bikes may be more easily repaired.

Disadvantages: More material equals more weight; also, lugs predetermine viable angles, so customizing can become a challenge.

TUBE TO TUBE

Mitered tubes can either be welded (if they're metal) or glued (if they're carbon) together. In carbon frames, glued tubes are wrapped with carbon to reinforce the junction and soften the appearance of the joint.

Advantages: This is a simple, effective and comparably affordable process; it's lighter than lugged construction and sometimes monocoque. Also, size customization is easier than with either lugs or monocoque because it allows a small builder to make a carbon bike without expensive molds or forms.

Disadvantage: Some say tube-to-tube is less durable because it creates more stress on smaller joints than other processes.

MONOCOQUE

In this process, carbon layers are hand-laid over a form (following a specific pattern or "schedule"), placed in a heated mold, then pressed. The exact sequence of applying the resin, pressing, and so on is often proprietary and very much depends on the goals of the frame maker.

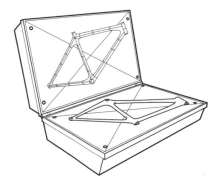

Advantage: A single frame can be designed to have precise properties, such as a somewhat forgiving ride that's exceptionally aero with a stiff pedaling platform and a very rigid head-tube junction for race-quick steering.

Disadvantages: The equipment, builder training and R+D don't come cheap, and some monocoque frames can be heavier than tube-to-tube models.

HYBRID

This is a blend of tube-to-tube and monocoque construction, often featuring a monocoque main triangle (top, down and seat tubes) and tubed rear.

Advantages: This construction sometimes shaves grams. Also, it's easier to ride-tune a size run by designing a more compliant rear triangle on smaller bikes and a less compliant one on larger sizes.

Disadvantage: Such frames are more costly and laborious than monocoque.

HOW TO BUY A BIKE

Once you've taken some time to ponder the information and questions above, follow the steps below to get the most out of your bike-buying adventure.

Before You Go

SKETCH YOURSELF. Grab a pencil, paper and some brutal honesty. Now make two lists. The first is an inventory of your current status as a cyclist or, for first-timers, your fitness level: how competitive you are, how much time you spend riding (or working out) each week, your highest achievements on a bike. The second is your ultimate vision of yourself as a cyclist: completing multiple charity rides each year, kicking butt on the local race circuit, riding to work every day and so on. Then, imagine a rider who fits between the two—the bike that's right for that middle-ground you is the minimum you should purchase. Buy below that level, and you won't have enough room to grow.

GET ON THE HORN. Look up the bike shops closest to you. Convenience isn't the deciding factor when choosing a shop, but the ideal shop is one that's easy to reach. Then call at least two or three of them. Note what brands the shop carries. Ask whether the shop specializes in a particular bike style—if you're looking for a road bike and the shop carries mostly mountain bikes, it's probably not a good fit. Also, ask what kind of service plan the shop offers on a new bike purchase; a year of free tune-ups is a good starting point.

CLICK AND READ. Hit the websites of your chosen brands, which tend to be organized so that it's easy to find the bikes that match your intended riding style. Study frame materials, components (wheels, derailleurs and cranks in particular—you can spot them right away on the bikes at the shop) and price, if it's listed. A model line will often have the same frame, with more expensive wheels and parts as the bike prices go up. Frames last longer than components, so we generally recommend investing in a higher-quality frame worthy of parts upgrades later, if need be.

TAP THE LOCALS. Ask your cyclist friends what they like and don't like about their current bikes; you can judge by their riding style whether you should have the same concerns. Also, ask for opinions on local shops or the bike models you found on the Internet. If you don't know many cyclists, e-mail a local cycling club. Bonus: You'll have people to ride with when you have your new bike.

At the Shop

STROLL THE FLOOR. Check out the models you've researched. Eyeball those easy-to-spot components, and note if they don't match the specs you saw online. Similar-level components from a different manufacturer shouldn't be a concern. If you see lower-level components than those stated on the web, with no corresponding drop in price, ask why.

CHOOSE YOUR CHAMPION. If a salesperson hasn't approached you, seek one out. Talk about what you're looking for and the models you've researched. The reaction should be along the lines of, "I can show those to you, and I have a couple of others you should look at."

If you feel like you're being pushed to look at a bike that doesn't suit you, a race bike when you don't race, or a cruiser when you plan to ride a serious commute, hold your ground or head to another shop. But if the salesperson listens to your goals and recommends a slightly different bike style than you were considering—say, one with a more upright position versus a more stretched-out ride—just ask why. There may be a good reason for the switch.

LOOK UP AND DOWN. Check out the bikes a step above and a step below the bike you like most. Ask your salesperson about the pros and cons of the frame material, components, rider position and intended use of each bike. If the bike you're considering still seems to be the best fit at the best price, you may have a winner.

TAKE A RIDE. A quick test spin around the block won't be enough to completely judge the bike's performance, but you'll be able to find any glaring fit problems. Be sure the saddle is set so that you have a slight bend to your knee at the bottom of the pedal stroke. Ask yourself these key questions: Does my upper body feel cramped, or too stretched out, when I'm on flat road? Does the bike feel unstable or twitchy when I turn? Is the reach to the brake levers comfortable? Is it awkward to go from sitting to standing on a hill?

GET A MAINTENANCE LESSON. Before you leave the shop, make sure you ask someone to teach you how to work the quick-releases to remove the wheels, and how to use the barrel adjusters to tweak the brakes or shifters. Also make sure you know how to inflate the tires, which will slowly lose air and go flat over time unless you intervene.

Pro **Tip**

"IF THE FIRST QUESTION THEY ASK AT THE SHOP IS, 'WHAT DO YOU WANT TO SPEND?' THAT'S NOT A GOOD SIGN. INSTEAD, THEY SHOULD BE ASKING, 'HOW DO YOU WANT TO RIDE?'"—*MIKE GROTZ, CO-OWNER, CYCLESPORT, PARK RIDGE, NJ*

Once You're Home

TAKE A BREAK-IN RIDE. Plan for your maiden ride to last about an hour, and leave time to stop to fiddle with your seat height or make other minor adjustments. The whole idea is to familiarize yourself with the shifting, braking and ride feel without going on an epic.

DO THE TWIST. If the shifting is off, or your brakes feel soft after your first ride, don't worry. It's because the cables have stretched or the housing has wiggled a little farther into position—common occurrences when a bike is first used. A careful counterclockwise twist of the barrel adjuster connected to the offending component should make things work smoothly again. While you're at it, check that the brake pads are still lined up so that they contact only the rim when you apply the brakes. Confused? No big deal. Just take your bike to the shop for your first free service call.

CALL. VISIT. UPGRADE. REPEAT. Your shop is your ally. Have a question about your bike? Give the shop a call. Something feel amiss on a ride? Stop by with your bike and chat with someone. A tune-up or a specific accessory could get things back in line and keep you riding. And that's the best deal around.

HOW TO NOT NOT BUY A BIKE

Been dreaming about a new ride, but can't bring yourself to take the plunge? Writer and cyclist Bill Gifford can help.

I have this friend, Roy, who needs a new bike. And I mean, badly. His Trek dates from a time before humans had tamed a substance called "carbon fiber." I think it's made of bronze. Possibly stone.

We talk about it a lot. He'll say, "I've been looking at this Cervélo." Sometimes it's a Scott. Or another Trek. Or, when he gets crazy, a tri bike. Sometimes he'll just open with the classic question: "What kind of bike should I get?"

And we'll be off to the races, yammering and jabbering about gruppos and wheelsets and frame angles and price points, until his wife and my girlfriend roll their eyes and wonder if we're secretly gay.

The thing is, Roy has needed a new bike for about five years, which is how long I've known him; he probably needed one before we met.

The other thing is, Roy is not just some weekend warrior who trundles his beer gut up and down the rail-trail on Saturday afternoons. Not

that there's anything wrong with that, but Roy is, shall we say, different. He doesn't just "ride." He crushes mofos. Friends, rivals, relatives—he grinds them to fine powder, smiling and chatting all the while. He competes in triathlons, placed in his age group in a half-Ironman, and rips through century rides without stopping for peanut-butter bagels. We did a summertime 50-miler once that left me feeling like a gutted deer. His body has been scientifically measured, and it turns out he is about 85 percent lung.

In other words: Roy doesn't just "want" a new bike; it's nearly a medical necessity. Even his wife agrees. But like a lot of us, he's stuck on the ride he bought several years ago. It was perfect, back then, for the rider he was. But he soon outgrew it, as inevitably as a 12-year-old will outgrow his first real bike. Now it's not nearly good enough for the rider he has become.

Lately he's been talking about a Felt something-or-other; it's carbon and aero and perfect, and I feel quite confident in predicting that Roy will not buy that bike, too.

But Roy is not merely paralyzed by indecision. In a weird way, he has mastered the most important step in buying a new bike. Which is: Not Buying a Bike.

Not Buying a Bike is a delicious state of longing, like being in love with that flaxen-haired beauty in comp-lit class, the one with the motorcycle-riding, soccer-playing boyfriend, who will never talk to you unless multiple laws of the universe are suspended simultaneously. Nevertheless, you sit there and your entire being is suffused with purpose and desire.

Luckily, Not Buying a Bike is less painful than that. But like love, it is a stage that must not be rushed. You must want and wait and research and compare; you test-ride bikes until every shop in town is sick of hearing you say you "want to think about it for a week." When you meet other bike people at parties or at work, you ask them: "What kind of bike should I get?"

And you pity the Type A "doers" who rush out and just get a bike, whatever bike. They read the reviews, find a shop, plunk down plastic, and bada-boom. They're missing a key part of the process. And their relationship with their custom Seven or their Trek Madone or whatever high-priced, flashy, well-recommended bike they read or heard about and simply bought will be much less satisfying. It's the difference between falling in love and paying for it.

When I was a kid in upstate New York, I used to flip through the Sears catalog, dreaming about what kind of Free Spirit I was going to buy with my snow-shoveling money. Wisely, I went to a real bike shop instead and got a Fuji 10-speed. But that catalog occupied many long winter evenings. And although the Fuji was a wonderful machine that I fell in love with at first sight, the long period of wanting it made having it all the sweeter.

Like Roy, I lived in a world of limitless possibilities. Unlike Roy, I managed not to talk myself out of buying the right bike at the right time.

"Say I get the bike," he explains, trying to rationalize his dithering. "If there's one single thing I don't like about it—I'll be crushed.

"This way," he goes on, "I can have all of them."

Or to put it more accurately: This way he can have none of them.

Because poor Roy has fallen victim to the little voice inside all of our heads, that sensible, maddening little voice that pipes up right about the time our "big" voice is about to say, "I'll take it!"

But you don't really need a new bike, the voice chirps.

And it's right, of course. None of us needs a new bike, given that kids are starving, and the economy, and blah-de-blah. But the voice is also wrong, and needs to be subdued, lest you end up like Roy. So, in a firm voice, try some of the following counter-arguments:

For real? To quote a T-shirt that was popular at mountain bike races in the '90s: Your bike sucks. Of course you need a new one. Because, let's face it, new bikes are better. They're like computers, almost, getting exponentially sleeker and faster and more wow every few years. Today's $2,500 "midrange" bike can burn doughnuts around anything you could have bought 10 years ago—just as Apple's cheapest current laptop is more powerful than HAL, the spaceship computer in 2001. Not to mention a lot more user-friendly.

You can't afford it right now, the little voice says.

Of course not. And you never will. Face it, most people don't have an extra few grand laying around, unless they're named Bill Gates. The car companies learned this long ago, which is why you can drive off the lot in a new Subaru without removing a dollar from your wallet. Buying things we can't afford is what made America great. And right now, with the recession still in full swing, America needs you. (As do Japan, Taiwan and everywhere else bikes are actually made.) It's why they invented credit cards.

But you don't race, the little voice says.

Oh, you don't? Easily remedied: Go to Active.com and find a triathlon or time trial or charity ride near you. Pick one about four months out, so you can train—and boom, you race!

Two grand (or five grand, or $900, whatever) is a lot of money.

No, it isn't. A thousand bucks is a Starbucks latte every workday. Two grand is less than you spent on gas last year. And try buying a new car for five grand. Think of it this way: On a relative scale, a $5K bike is about the same as a $50K car. So you're getting a Bimmer for the price of a used Jetta.

You won't ride it enough, the voice mopes.

Okay. Say the bike costs $3,000. If you ride it only once, then that ride will have cost you . . . $3,000. Yeah, that is a lot. But if you ride it again, your cost per ride just dropped by 50 percent. Four more rides, and you're down to $500 per. And it keeps going from

there. The more you ride, the cheaper it gets. And if you keep that bike for five years, it works out to $600 a year, or less than two bucks a day. You can't even take the bus for that anymore.

But then you'll be so poor that you'll have to ride the bus . . . .

Exactly! And taking the bus sucks, so you'll ride your new bike instead. See how it all works out?

Pro **Tip**

"I ALWAYS TELL CUSTOMERS THAT AFTER THE INITIAL INVESTMENT, BIKES ARE INCREDIBLY CHEAP. THE BIKE IS GOING TO LAST 10-PLUS YEARS AND YOU'LL REPLACE JUST A FEW PARTS SUCH AS TIRES AND CHAINS. PEOPLE KIND OF BREATHE A SIGH OF RELIEF WHEN THEY HEAR THAT."—*PETER MOONEY, CO-OWNER, BELMONT WHEELWORKS, BELMONT, MA*

CHAPTER 3

Find Your Perfect Fit

We can't stress this enough: The best bike for you is the one that fits. Dialing in the proper size, components and positioning takes some effort, but it's worth every minute—and penny.

MAKE YOUR BIKE FIT YOUR BODY

While there is no universal method for fitting a bicycle to the rider, fit theories do agree on most things, and proper training and equipment help bike-shop workers and fitters do their job consistently well. Bike fitting is part science and part art, and it's best accomplished by working with a fit specialist to mesh fit theories with your personal needs (for example, limited range of motion from an old injury).

That said, here are the seven areas to focus on to get yourself close to an ideal fit. You'll have an easier time shopping if you know a few benchmark measurements. Start with figuring your frame size and seat height, and then, when you have the bike, determine your proper cleat placement, saddle position and handlebar reach, in that order. See a fit specialist to fine-tune these or diagnose the origins of any lingering aches and pains.

Frame Size

In socks, place a thin hardcover book, spine up, between your legs with about the same upward pressure a saddle produces. Measure your inseam, from the book's spine to the floor, in centimeters. Multiply that number by 0.65; the result is your approximate road frame size. For example, 81cm x 0.65 = 52.65—a 52- or 53-cm frame (sizes are the seat-tube length). Note that compact sizing uses a virtual seat-tube length, so don't go by the stated size unless it has the same virtual size. To convert to inch sizing, divide by 2.54. For mountain bikes, subtract 10–12 cm from your road size.

Pro **Tip**

"I BELIEVE THAT THE NUMBER-ONE REASON PEOPLE DON'T RIDE MORE IS BECAUSE THEY'RE UNCOMFORTABLE, USUALLY DUE TO IMPROPER BIKE FIT."—*ALEX STIEDA*

Seat Height

Too high: Hips rock trying to extend to pedals; pain in back of knee

Too low: Can't fully extend leg; pain in front of knee

Just right: Slight bend in knee at full extension

Your knee should have a slight bend in it at the bottom of your pedal stroke. (The bottom is when the crankarm is parallel to the seat tube, not perpendicular to the ground.) To check this, wear cycling shoes and pedal unclipped with your heels on the pedals. You should barely maintain contact with the pedal at the bottom of the stroke, without rocking your pelvis. Measure the distance between the bottom bracket and the top of the seat. This is your seat height. It should be very close to the product of your inseam (in centimeters) multiplied by 0.883.

Cleat Placement

Too far forward: Feels like you're pedaling with your arch; foot pain, power loss

Too far back: Feels like you're pedaling with your toes; forefoot cramps, power loss

Just right: Start with the ball of the foot directly over the pedal spindle and move forward or back a few millimeters to the most comfortable position

Cleat Angle

Overly toed in: You may feel the cleat reach its float-range limit during the pedal stroke; pain on outside of knee

Overly toed out: Heel strikes crankarm, or cleat reaches float limit; pain on inside of knee

Just right: Cleat moves freely within float range

Mount your cleats on your shoes so that the ball of your foot is directly over the pedal spindle for maximum power transfer. Unless you have an unusual stride or stance (splayfoot, etc.), point the tips of the cleats at the tips of the shoes for a neutral pedaling stance to start out. Pay attention to your pedaling style on the first couple of rides and adjust as needed—this is one place where professional fit advice may be worth the cost to help avoid injury.

Saddle Position

Too far back: Can feel like seat is too high or reach to bar is too long

Too far forward: Can feel like seat is too low

Just right: Knee positioned over pedal spindle (move saddle slightly fore or aft to tune for comfort and power)

The front of your forward knee should be directly over the ball of your foot when the pedal is at the 3 o'clock position. Check this with a plumb line. If the line doesn't pass the front of the pedal axle, move your seat forward or back on the rails until it does. Your seat should be level, or point at most a couple of degrees up or down. Check it with a carpenter's level.

Reach to Handlebar

Too short: Hunched shoulders, possibly causing neck or shoulder pain

Too long: Arms fully extended, which affects handling and control

Just right: Slight bend in elbow when hands are on brake hoods or drops

This is the most variable of all measurements, as it depends greatly on your flexibility. You want a slight angle at the elbow when your hands are on the hoods or drops, but you shouldn't force yourself to bend double to get it.

Handlebar Height

Too high: Front end feels light or twitchy; saddle pain from too much weight on seat

Too low: Stiff arms, back and neck from too much weight on arms

Just right: For road bikes, aim for a 60 to 40 percent body weight distribution between the rear and front of the bike

On a new bike, ask the shop to leave the steerer tube long and add 2 inches of spacers under the stem. Move the spacers above or below the stem to fine-tune your fit, and have the shop cut the steerer later, if needed.

Pro Tip

"I AM AMAZED AT WHAT PEOPLE DO TO FIT THEMSELVES TO A BIKE THAT THEY HAVE NO BUSINESS BEING ON. FIT THE BIKE TO YOU, NOT YOURSELF TO THE BIKE." —*BERNARD CONDEVAUX, USA CYCLING PHYSICAL THERAPIST*

HELP YOUR SHOP FIT YOU RIGHT

A good shop helps you find the proper fit, even if you're not buying an expensive custom. Here's what to ask to ensure success.

WILL YOU BUILD ME A TEST RIDE? Always ride before you buy. If a shop doesn't have your size on display, ask to have a sample built up. Or test a similar model from that brand; product lines often share geometries, even whole frame designs.

WHAT ABOUT PARTS SWAPS? Not all saddles and stems work for everyone. A shop should be willing to swap a part here and there to ensure proper fit, and it may offer upgrades at a discount.

DO YOU USE A FIT SERVICE? A good shop uses a recognized fit service, like Fit Kit or the Serotta Size Cycle, which has a defined methodology and offers technician training. (Serotta requires it.) A fit session will cost between $40 and $200, depending on the complexity of service you want, but it can be a worthwhile investment.

IS THERE A FIT GUARANTEE? Some elements of bike fit, such as reach to the bar, bar height and cleat position, manifest themselves only over time. Is the shop prepared to help you dial in those issues as part of your bike-buying investment? Look for a written guarantee that lasts at least 30 days.

Warning Signs

Most bike shops are great, but beware if:

THEY SAY NO TEST RIDES. A few shops have stopped offering test rides for liability reasons. We recommend steering clear of them because it could lead to potential future headaches on fit issues.

YOUR OBJECTIONS ARE OVERRULED. If a salesperson insists a frame is the right size and you think it's not, seek a second opinion at another shop. The first shop may be trying to get rid of old inventory. A key tip-off here is low levels of floor stock, especially if you're considering a discounted model from last year.

YOU GET ATTITUDE, OR IGNORED. If the salesperson seems uninterested in you, go elsewhere.

Things to Know about Fit

John Brown, manager at Philadelphia-area shop High Road Cycles, began fitting cyclists about 10 years ago. "The old way of thinking about bike fit was, 'You'll get used to it,'" he says. Fortunately, times have changed. Here's Brown's advice on making bike and body work in harmony.

LEAVE THE STILETTOS AT HOME. It may seem obvious, but come to the shop ready to ride your bike. "I once had a customer show up dressed to go to dinner downtown," Brown says. Instead, wear (or bring) the shorts, shoes and pedals you usually ride with.

[TEST] RIDE LOTS. "We have customers who come in with a list of bikes they're interested in, and they might spend just five minutes in the shop—the rest of the time they're out riding," he says. "They even bring a lunch." Don't worry about taking up too much of the shop's time: "It's your job to be an educated consumer."

LADIES: YOU DON'T HAVE TO GET A CHICK BIKE. Women's bikes are a good option to consider, but not a necessity, says Brown, especially now that many companies make plush unisex bikes with taller head tubes. Each bike-maker approaches women-specific differently, so try a variety of bikes from several brands.

THINK FRAME SIZE FIRST. While you can use stem selection to fine-tune cockpit length, it's important to choose a frame that fits as well as possible in the first place, Brown says. A stem

Why My $450 Bike Fit Was a Bargain

"When I went to see Andy Pruitt at the Boulder Center for Sports Medicine, I had been riding pretty seriously for nearly two decades and, because of my job at *Bicycling*, had ridden more bikes in the past dozen years than most people will in a lifetime. I'd written numerous stories about bike fit and had been tuned by every major fit system in existence. I was confident my position was dialed in, and that I was just there to meet another deadline. When Pruitt administered his $450 "3-D Bike Fit," he praised the way I'd fused my imbalanced body with my bike—except for one detail. A motion-capture computer analysis of my pedal stroke showed that neither knee tracked in line with my ankles. This defect never bothered me and, in fact, I'd come to think of the way my knees ran so close to the top tube as a kind of signature style. But Pruitt persisted in installing two angled shims under my right cleat and one under my left. A quick follow-up analysis showed that I was producing 20 more watts at the same heart rate—and for me that turned out to be the priceless difference between leading the slow group and hanging onto the fast one."—*Bill Strickland,* Bicycling *editor at large* that's too long will require an exaggerated amount of upper body motion to turn the bar. If it's too short, "it might feel like the bike is steering you."

GET HAPPY FEET. For years, conventional wisdom held that the pedal axle should line up with the ball of the foot for optimum efficiency, Brown says. But if you experience hot spots in that position, fit experts now believe that moving the cleat back slightly can ease discomfort without decreasing power. Try it yourself: While wearing your cycling shoes, stand up straight and have a friend mark the widest points on either side of your forefoot with a pen (put electrical tape down first). The pedal axle should fall between those marks.

TAKE THE BAR EXAM. A bar that's too wide "forces you to lean further forward, so it effectively makes the frame longer," Brown says. "Plus, it side-loads your wrists." (Conversely, a bar that's too narrow can hinder breathing.) To find your ideal bar width, have a friend stand behind you and find the bony bump on the top of one of your shoulders. Then have her measure the distance between that bump and the corresponding spot on the other shoulder.

IT'S ALL CONNECTED. Replacing or adjusting one component might necessitate tweaking or even swapping another. For example, says Brown, rotating the handlebar to bring the brake hoods closer to you can push the brake levers farther away, which can make them hard to reach while riding in the drops. You may need short-reach brake levers or a bar with a shal-

lower drop. Similarly, moving the saddle forward effectively lowers your seat height.

COMFORT IS FAST. "You may be able to hold an aggressive position for 10 miles, but after 40 or 50 miles it won't feel comfortable, and you'll get fatigued," Brown says. He points out that aerodynamics are less important on road bikes than they are on tri bikes because you can draft on a road ride.

YOU MAY BE A RACER. If the highlight of your Saturday ride was being the first to the top of the hill, that carbon superbike may be worth it even if you never pin a number on. "If you're trying to keep up with people faster than you, then you're racing," Brown says. "And if it's your bike that's holding you back, and not you, then that sucks." Sound like a sales pitch? Well, sure. But we agree with him.

Pro **Tip**

"EVEN IF YOUR FRIEND IS THE SAME HEIGHT, WEIGHT AND OVERALL BUILD AS YOU, DON'T ASSUME HIS BIKE SETTINGS ARE THE SETTINGS YOU SHOULD USE. IT'S SIMPLY NOT ALWAYS THE CASE. HIS BIKE MAY RIDE LIKE A DREAM TO HIM WHILE IT RIDES HORRIBLY FOR YOU—AND VICE VERSA. ALSO, FITTINGS ARE FLUID AND DYNAMIC AND CHANGE OVER TIME. WHAT WORKS TODAY MAY NOT WORK, SAY, TWO YEARS FROM NOW. WHETHER IT'S FROM YOUR BODY CHANGING—YOU MAY LOSE OR GAIN WEIGHT, OR BECOME MORE OR LESS FIT—OR FROM GETTING OLDER, YOUR BIKE FIT WILL MOST LIKELY CHANGE."—*MATT LODDER, SEROTTA-CERTIFIED FITTER AND OWNER OF THE CYCLE SURGEON, CARY, NC*

D.I.Y. AERO

On a flat road, as much as 95 percent of a rider's energy is used to overcome wind resistance, says Todd Carver, who runs Retul, a bike-fitting company in Boulder, Colorado. Just 20 percent of that drag comes from the bike—80 percent of it is from you. At the same time, Scott Holz, an instructor for Specialized's BG Fit program, says that he sees more mis-fit triathletes than any other group of cyclists. Here's how to tweak your road bike for fit and efficiency.

Attach Clip-On Aero Bars

Don't worry about the position at this point—you'll tweak it later.

Move the Saddle Forward and/or Swap Your Seatpost

One of the most common conversion fit mistakes: slapping on aero bars but leaving the saddle where it is. If you're effectively moving the handlebar forward, you need to move your body, too. Think of it as rotating yourself forward around the bottom bracket, like hands on a clock. Your elbows should be 2 to 3 cm behind the rear edge of the aero bar pads, with a roughly 110-degree angle at the elbow. For road bike fit, a plumb line dropped from the rider's forward knee (with crankarms level) should pass just in front of the pedal spindle. For ideal tri fit, you want your knee farther forward, 1 additional centimeter in front of the pedal spindle for every centimeter of height difference between the saddle and the aero pads. You may need a two-position seatpost, depending on how much adjustment your seat rails offer.

Correct Saddle Height and Angle

Moving a seat forward also effectively lowers it. You want about a 30-degree bend in your knee when the crankarms are perpendicular to the ground. (Note: This is a different measure than the one used for road bike fit.) A normal road position has a level seat, but for a multisport fit, you should rotate the saddle downward one degree for every centimeter of drop between the seat and the aero bar pads, up to 8 degrees. This will allow you to roll your hips forward and open up your hip angle for a more natural pedaling style.

Make these adjustments at the same time you move the saddle forward and/or swap the seatpost, as one measurement affects the other.

Dial in Your Back Angle

If the aero extensions are too high, move a steerer-tube spacer or two above the stem, or flip a positive-angle stem upside down, or both. Ideally, your back will be flat, but spinal flexibility may limit you. If the bars are too low, consider a higher-rise stem.

Tweak Your Bars

The key here is to decrease frontal area as much as comfortably possible. Align the elbow pads so your elbows sit directly in line with your hands. It's fine to create a wider "stance" on the bar by increasing the distance between the extensions; just keep your forearms pointing straight, not angled inward, which increases drag.

If, after some break-in time, you can't stay in your tuck over the distance of your goal race (cornering, climbing and tricky descents excepted), then your position is too aggressive, says Specialized's Holz. For sprint tris or time trials that last less than an hour, your position should be as aggressive as you can tolerate. For Olympic-distance events or a 40-kilometer time trial, increase your torso angle five degrees. For a half-Ironman, add five to 10 degrees, and for a full Ironman, 10 or more degrees.

When in doubt, choose comfort over aerodynamics. You'll go faster in a less aerodynamic position if you can reliably produce lots of power over a longer period of time. That said, with any aero position you will probably give up some amount of power compared with your road position, but that's okay. "Cyclists are macho and like to focus on power," says University of Utah researcher Jim Martin, who consults on aerodynamic efficiency with the Australian Institute of Sport. "If you give up a few percentage points in power output, but gain that same amount in aerodynamic efficiency, you'll still go faster."

CHAPTER 4

Everything but the Bike

To get the most enjoyment out of your bike, you'll need to budget for some accessories. Here's our guide to the essentials. We give extra space to two of the most important components: the saddle—your potentially most problematic contact point with the bike—and tires, which are your bike's only contact point (you hope) with the road.

FIRST THINGS FIRST: THE GEAR YOU NEED

Buy a helmet, and use it every time you ride. Beyond that, you should strongly consider purchasing:

FLAT FIXERS, such as tire levers, a spare tube and a minipump for midride flat repairs. Have the salesperson show you how to use them.

LUBE keeps your chain rolling smoothly. Ditto on the lesson in use.

CYCLING SHORTS make your life much better. And relax—nobody thinks he or she looks good in bike shorts.

A JERSEY provides comfort and ventilation, and the rear pockets hold your tire levers, tube and minipump.

GLOVES add hand protection, a good idea.

BOTTLES AND CAGES hold your favorite beverage—you'll get thirsty out there.

WHEN TO SAVE, WHEN TO SPLURGE

The countless miles that *Bicycling* has spent testing clothing and equipment have led us to an undeniable conclusion: The pleasure payback from your gear investment can vary widely. With some items, spending a little more yields tremendous increases in speed or comfort, while in other spots improvement comes in tiny, expensive increments. Here are the five best ways to spend your gear dollars.

Save on: Pedals

Pricey pedals are a bit lighter thanks to techy materials such as carbon and titanium. But you'll notice little or no performance bump compared with midrange models of chromoly and glass fiber. Quality, workhorse pedals cost

$100 to $150, half that of feathery ones. And generic pedals compatible with Shimano SPD or Look Delta cleats go for as little as $35.

CLIPLESS OR FLAT PEDALS? Flat pedals make sense at both ends of the spectrum. Pedaling to the ice cream stand in loafers? Flat pedals. Launching a no-footer off a monster dirt jump? Flat, too, for the same reason: quick, straightforward dismounts. For everyone else, there are the vastly more efficient clipless pedals (skip the toeclips—to find out why, see page 46).

SINGLE- OR DOUBLE-SIDED PEDALS? Single-sided pedals often have a broad platform that feels solid underfoot for stability and comfort on long rides. Double-sided pedals have advantages, particularly for mountain bikers—no flipping the pedal to engage the proper side, and should one side get gummed up, there's always the other.

Splurge on: Shoes

Inexpensive shoes disappoint, with poor closure systems that won't cinch your feet comfortably, and flimsy uppers that wear quickly. Quality footwear includes features such as ratcheting buckles and stiff carbon soles. Spend what it takes to find the proverbial shoe that fits, and don't order online just to save $5. Buy from a shop so you can try multiple models and sizes.

ROAD OR MOUNTAIN SHOES? Road shoes are lighter and have a stiffer sole for better power transfer; however, doing anything besides riding in them is like walking on ice with buttered feet. Softer-soled mountain bike shoes can be more flexible and have bottoms with treads for easier walking. Are you a high-mileage, road-only rider looking for the ultimate in weight and efficiency? Opt for road-specific shoes. Like to linger at stops? Choose the convenience and comfort of mountain shoes.

Save on: Jersey

The fit and feel of a finely made jersey is a worthy treat for long, special days in the saddle. But for everyday squeak-in-an-hour-after-work rides, most any synthetic, snug-fitting top with back pockets will suffice. One way to get a high-end jersey for cheap: Look for replica jerseys of now-defunct pro teams, which often populate the closeout racks at shops.

Splurge on: Shorts and Bibs

The best shorts are constructed with multiple panels—look for eight or more—for a more conforming fit. And they use vastly superior padded inserts. Spend $100 or more (they start getting really good in the $150 range) for shorts that boast multilayer or multi-density, stretchable, smooth-seamed, gender-specific padding. Your bum will thank you every ride.

Save on: Tubes

A generic, $5 innertube is all that your bike ever needs. Spending more gets you either special thin, lightweight tubes, which are less weighty but more prone to punctures, or a brand-name box that contains a $5 tube.

Splurge on: Tires

Better tires have superior puncture resistance and wear, and reduced weight and rolling resistance, so you go faster. Look for supple casings—sidewalls flexible like a leather glove, not rigid like a car tire—and thread counts of 60-plus threads per inch. Tires with folding beads, rather than wire, are often lighter and easier to mount.

Save on: Helmet

All helmets sold in the United States meet CPSC safety standards, so a $30 lid is equally as good at protecting your head as a $200 one. Also, keep in mind that you'll need to buy a new helmet every time you crash, although many manufacturers have replacement programs. Many under-$60 helmets offer fit systems similar to pricier models, often head straps with buckles or dials for easy adjustment. They just lack flashy styling and extra vent holes.

Pro Tip

"THE MOST IMPORTANT PIECE OF CYCLING GEAR IS A GOOD PAIR OF SHORTS. IF YOU CAN AVOID SADDLE SORES, PAIN AND NUMBNESS, YOU'LL BE MORE COMFORTABLE. IF YOU'RE MORE COMFORTABLE, YOU'LL RIDE LONGER. IF YOU RIDE LONGER, YOUR FITNESS AND SELF-ESTEEM WILL IMPROVE. IT ALL STARTS WITH THE SHORTS."—*SHEILA MOON, CYCLOCROSS RACER AND CYCLING FASHION DESIGNER*

Splurge on: Sunglasses

Quality glasses offer the 100 percent UV protection claimed (drugstore cheapies often don't), and they're more scratch-resistant. Sport glasses also have pliable ear- and nosepieces that keep them stuck to your face, even on descents or choppy trails. And many offer interchangeable lenses or prescription options.

Save on: Rain Jacket

Except for hardcore commuters or racers, and maybe Northwest dwellers, few of us really ride in the rain much. For the rare occasions you do get caught in a shower, a $200 waterproof and breathable shell is nice, but you'll get wet eventually. And a simple $20 clear plastic jacket, still the choice of countless pros, does the job, too.

Splurge on: Vest and Base Layer

The vest allows more versatility than any other piece of cycling clothing. In cold and windy conditions, it protects your core, and it packs small to stow in your pocket. A quality base layer, which fits like a second skin and wicks sweat, will keep you cooler in summer and warmer in winter.

PICK THE RIGHT TIRE

To make sure the rubber meets the road, choose the tire that best fits the conditions in which you'll be riding.

Make the Lid Fit

A 2006 New York City report on a decade's worth of crashes found that 74 percent of fatalities involved a head injury, and 97 percent of those killed weren't wearing a helmet. But if yours doesn't fit properly, it won't work as intended. Here's how to ensure a perfect fit:

1. Sit the helmet on your head with the strap undone. The front of the helmet should be just visible when you look up. Yes, that means your hair might get messed up.

2. Adjust the rear occipital strap to be snug against your skull. You should be able to drop your head forward without the helmet sliding.

3. The helmet buckles should rest just below each ear. Gently pull down on them and adjust as necessary so there is equal tension on each "Y" strap.

4. Finally, adjust the chin fastener; it should be tight enough for only a finger's width of slack between the strap and your chin.

RAIN RIDING. The points of contact on rain tires have two purposes. They break the surface plane of the water so that the tire can make contact with the road, and they enhance the grip of the tire once it does. To accomplish this, good rain tires are typically outfitted with a diamond or file tread pattern. Rain tires also use soft compounds that grip the road better but wear out faster. In wet conditions, run your tires 5–10 psi lower than normal, which increases the contact patch—the surface area of the tire touching the road.

RACING. In the tire casing, a high number of threads per inch leads to a supple and controlled road feel. When you roll across uneven pavement, supple tires absorb impact and maintain grip with the road, minimizing vibration and maximizing control. The high-tpi casings are teamed with flexible belts to add some measure of durability, but the downside to all light, sup-

ple racing tires is that they cost the most and wear out the fastest.

ROUGH ROADS. Rubber is the heaviest substance in tires (there are also threads and layers of nylon, cotton, silk, Kevlar and other substances), and it's also resistant to punctures. So adding rubber to low-tpi tires to fill in the spaces between threads results in an inexpensive, flat-resistant tire. For further protection, durable, nearly bulletproof belts are sometimes laid over the casing. The downside of these sturdy belts is that they detract from rolling efficiency and road feel.

WINTER TRAINING. A hybrid of flat-resistant and rain tires, off-season tires are made with tread compounds that maximize the surface area of the contact patch and maintain grip. Because the road is typically more cluttered with debris, the treads are also tougher to guard against cuts, making them stiffer and slightly less grippy than rain tires. A good way to counteract the loss of traction is to increase surface area: If you ride 21 or 23c, switch to 25c to gain more control in turns.

THE HARD TRUTH ABOUT SADDLES

The good news: The medical firestorm linking cycling to impotence has been doused. The better news: Research sparked by the furor led to more comfortable seats.

The link between bike seats and erectile dysfunction arose in 1997, in two stories published by *Bicycling*. In one, a former executive editor reported on research by a then-unknown urologist, Irwin Goldstein, MD, who believed he'd established a causal relationship between pedaling and impotence. The story was accompanied by a personal essay written by an editor who was experiencing impotence—after averaging 14,000 miles annually for the previous seven years and, at age 50, training for and riding the Race Across America. The mainstream media picked up the story, and the most sensational aspects took center stage. The general public's take: Cycling causes impotence.

Goldstein's conclusions—that a bike saddle can compress the perineal region, restricting blood flow and leading, ultimately, to impotence—weren't universally accepted by the scientific community. In 2001, two urologists—heads of well-known university departments—publicly challenged Goldstein's contentions in reports published by the *Washington Post*. Goldstein's studies, they said, had small sample sizes, questionable methodologies and were never peer-reviewed. Cyclists were also assured by anecdotal evidence; while all of us had experienced or knew someone who'd experienced numbness while riding, outright impotence seemed rare—especially if riders followed a few simple rules.

The one unequivocally beneficial result: Saddle-makers began redesigning seats to increase comfort and minimize reduced blood flow. While testing continues to find saddle designs with the least compression, there are five simple ways you can avoid numbness and, potentially, more serious maladies:

1. Position your seat so that it's level or just a few degrees down in front. Roger Minkow, MD, who designed the Body Geometry saddle for Specialized, says even the best seats instantly compress arteries when pointed upward.

2. Make sure your knees aren't fully extended at the bottom of your pedal stroke, which puts more weight on your crotch.

Fun **Fact**

Lance Armstrong rode the Selle San Marco Concor Light saddle, introduced in 1985, to all of his Tour de France victories.

The Path to Saddle Nirvana

Three tips for buying that little perch that supports more than half your body weight.

TRY IT ON FOR SIZE

Saddles need to match your shape—what feels good to your riding buddy might not feel good to you. Luckily, there's a variety of widths and styles to choose from. Some have cutouts to relieve pressure. Women-specific saddles are wider across the back than men's to accommodate wider sit bones. There's no magic formula for finding the right saddle other than trying a few out. Keep in mind that overall bike fit impacts how your bottom feels, so the perfect saddle may be only one part of the puzzle.

GET JUST ENOUGH SQUISH

Padding helps disperse pressure points over a larger area. Beware of too much of a good thing, though: Thick padding may feel good to the touch, but under your butt it can migrate to off-limits areas, creating a saddle-wedgie. The right combination of padding, shell flex and shape makes a saddle work for you, and an extra helping of gel can't make up for the wrong shape.

PRO TIP

"Even minor changes in handlebar reach and drop can make a huge difference in weight distribution and saddle comfort. I can't tell you how many fits I've done where the cyclist comes in with saddle complaints and leaves with a new stem and a smile."—*Ward Griffiths, fit specialist, River City Bicycles, Portland, OR*

3. Firm saddles are generally better; they support the sit bones without pushing into the arteries in the perineal region.

4. Saddles with flat or concave centers seem to perform better, says Minkow; padding that continues to arch over the saddle's curve can push up into the perineal region.

5. And finally, the simplest cure: Stand up every 10 minutes or so. In hilly areas, this is probably automatic. Flatlanders and those riding stationary bikes might want to incorporate cues to stand: Get out of the saddle whenever someone else does, or after you take a drink or pass a town sign, for instance.

MAKE YOUR MOVE TO MULTISPORT

If there's a time trial or triathlon on your calendar, but you're not ready to commit to a full-on tri bike, these components can give you an edge.

Triathlon Saddle

Most of an aero rider's weight rests on the front third of the saddle. A tri saddle such as Vision's Trigel Elite (visiontechusa.com) has a broader, more supportive nose.

Setback Seatposts

Profile Design's Fast Forward Carbon (profiledesign.com) has 38mm of forward offset.

Thomson's Elite (lhthomson.com) can be reversed for 16mm of forward offset (flip the hardware) if you want one post for road and tri.

Seatpost Shim

If your seatpost is too narrow, USE's shims (use1.com) can help. For example, Profile's Fast Forward is 27.2mm, but the shim lets it adapt to clamps as big as 32.8mm.

Moderate Race Wheels

Aero wheels reduce drag significantly, but ultra deep-section wheels handle poorly in cross-winds. Blackwell Research 50mm Clinchers (blackwellresearch.com) have moderately deep rims and are a decent value.

Clip-On Aero Bars

Profile Design's alloy T2+ has adjustable reach, width and pad position. It weighs just 512 grams and costs less than some comparable carbon bars.

HOW TO WASH YOUR CYCLING DUDS

Good cycling clothes are an investment—one that rubs right up against your most treasured body parts. Though care instructions from manufacturers seem to vary from the extreme "hand wash in our proprietary soap and dry with a soft lint-free towel" to the lackadaisical "machine wash, tumble dry," the truth is out there. Or, rather, it's here, in our guide to the smart way to care for your clothes and keep smelling fresh.

ADD SOAP. Use the most basic detergent you can find, without dyes, perfumes or softeners. Cycling clothes are made of high-performance fabrics meant to channel moisture away from your skin. Any residue from fancy soaps or fabric softeners will clog up the works, keeping the fabric from doing its job well.

Some manufacturers recommend against using liquid detergents—straight, concentrated detergent is potent stuff—but as long as you run water into the washer first, add the detergent, then the clothes, you'll get gentler, easier-to-rinse cleaning. A note on wool: Treat it like you would any other wool garment, using a wool-specific soap and machine washing only if the tag says it's okay.

SEAL UP. Zip zippers and close hook-and-loop fasteners before washing—both can chew up clothes faster than skidding on loose gravel. Also, turn screenprinted or sublimated clothing inside out to protect the graphics. Before you wash, sort your clothes—your cycling gear shouldn't be mashed in with your hard-tumbling jeans or a mess of heavy towels. They're "delicates" and should be treated as such. Use the delicate cycle on your washing machine, too.

WASH, RINSE, SNIFF. Wash in cold or lukewarm water. If your clothes still smell like detergent at the end of the cycle, run them through for an extra rinse.

3 Tips for Laundry Idiots

HOW OFTEN MUST I WASH MY STUFF?

As often as you want, provided you follow the recommended care instructions. If you tend to sweat like a pig, wash your gear after every ride. But if your clothes still smell okay and you're all about conserving water, wash them when you feel it's necessary.

WHAT IF I DON'T WASH MY CLOTHES THE WAY THE TAG SAYS?

It's always best—though not always convenient—to follow the tag instructions. If you decide to ignore the manufacturer (or us) and go your own way, your clothes will still be okay. Probably. For a while. But they won't last as long or work as well as they could if you wash them with extra care.

UM, WHEN IT COMES TO WASHING MY CHAMOIS, IS THERE SOMETHING I SHOULD KNOW?

Most chamois don't require special cleaning, unless you have an exceptionally old-fashioned pair of shorts with a real leather chamois. If you line-dry your shorts, be sure to hang them chamois-side out; the high-end Swiss clothing company Assos recommends washing shorts inside out as well.

DRY. Heat is used in the finishing process of most stretch fabrics, so a little hot air can give clothing a boost (unless it's wool, in which case it's best to avoid the dryer; lay the damp clothes on a towel to dry). But high heat, or drying in a Laundromat-type commercial dryer, will lead to shrinkage—and not the temporary *Seinfeld* kind—that will damage the elastics. It could also bake in any lingering funk. Stick with low heat, and only for a little while, as high-performance fabrics dry quickly. And remember to skip the fabric-softener dryer sheets.

Line-drying nonwool clothing is fine, too, as long as the clothes are out of direct sunlight—the added UV exposure can cause fabrics to break down prematurely.

CHAPTER 5

Cycle in Style

Some might say "cycling style" is an oxymoron, in part because the sport has so many subcultures, each with its own unique look. If you want to ride with a rubber chicken on your handlebar, or adorn your bike with anodized components from the '80s, or wear matching outfits as you and your significant other cruise around on your tandem, you're sure to find others like you.

That said, if you want to fit in with the serious roadies who take their style cues from professional racing, or channel your inner hipster commuter, the tips here will help you make it happen. Remember, many style rules exist for a purpose—not only do they prevent us from becoming fodder for ridicule among the group, they function to make us safer, faster, more efficient and more comfortable.

Pro **Tip**

"I GOT THE IDEA, WHY DON'T I GET SOME SNOW-BOARDING PANTS? I CUT THEM TO THREE-QUARTER LENGTH—THEY'RE WATERPROOF AND WARM. MY BUTT DIDN'T GET WET. IT WAS SO PERFECT, IT WAS RIDICULOUS."—*NFL LINEBACKER AND BIKE COMMUTER DHANI JONES*

THE 10 MOST COMMON STYLE FAUX PAS

Aside from the team presentation at the Tour de France, cycling doesn't have the equivalent of a red carpet. But there are still some serious fashion felonies. Here is a display of the most egregious style disasters, with simple solutions to preserve your panache.

Arm Warmers with a Sleeveless Jersey

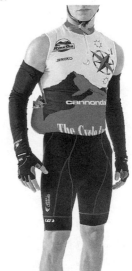

Fix: Yes, Allen Iverson popularized this look. The key here? Remember that you'll never be an NBA all-star.

Lopsided Jersey

Fix: Evenly distribute your necessities in the jersey pockets by weight rather than bulk. This pattern is best: If you don't have much stuff, use the center pocket. More stuff, use the two outer pockets. Lots of stuff, use all three.

Jersey Tucked into Shorts

Fix: Remember this rule—tuck in only when you're wearing a belt. Fanny packs don't count, though if you're wearing one, nothing you do with your jersey can make you look any worse.

Exposed Skin Between Shorts and Jersey When You Bend at the Waist

Fix: Wear a longer jersey or one with rubber grippers at the waist—or wear bibs.

Seatbag Swings and Bounces as You Ride

Fix: When it comes to rear ends, you want your bike to be more like Alberto Contador than Jan Ullrich. Keep it light—and cinch it tight.

Four to Six Inches of Excess Helmet Strap Dangling Below Your Chin

Fix: After you properly adjust your helmet for fit, cut the strap so only about 2 inches protrude from the buckle. (The extra lets you loosen the strap to accommodate a winter hat.) Singe the cut with a match, or glue the ends, to keep the fabric from unraveling.

Salt-Stained Helmet Straps

Fix: When you clean your bike, rinse the helmet straps under the faucet or dunk them into the bucket of soapy water (before you attack the drivetrain).

Panty Lines or Underwear Beneath Cycling Shorts

Fix: Do a hundred-miler with your skivvies on, then contemplate the swamp that is your crotch. Now you know—and will never forget— why nothing comes between chamois and skin.

Shorts So Well Worn They Are See-Through in Spots

Fix: Just buy new ones—or ride past the local elementary school until you're arrested.

Straps of Bib Shorts over Jersey

Fix: Bib straps under your jersey, of course. If you like the external-strap method because it makes answering the call of nature easier, switch to a full-zip jersey, which you don't have to pull over your head to slip off.

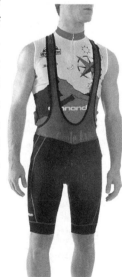

FUNCTIONAL AND FASHIONABLE

Here are six situations when it's practical to ride with panache.

Sunglasses

Wear them over, not under, your helmet straps.

Fashion: Spend upward of $100 on eyewear, and it's key to keep the hinge logos visible. Otherwise, who's to say you're not sporting truck-stop specials?

Function: Tucking the arms of your eyewear under your helmet straps can push the earpieces into the sides of your head, creating unwanted pressure. Wearing your shades over your straps lets you quickly and easily pop them off or prop them up on your helmet if they get fogged or splattered with sweat.

Knickers

They're just the right length for commuters.

Fashion: A staple of bike messengers, knickers (cycling specific or homemade, hacked-off Dickies) have become the essence of townie cool. Only dorks wear spandex or khakis when cruising around town.

Function: Getting a pant leg stuck in your chainring is dirty and dangerous. Knickers are short enough to not get caught in the drivetrain and long enough to keep you from getting arrested for indecent exposure.

Embrocation

Look shiny and chiseled, not chapped and cracked.

Fashion: Legs lathered in warming cream look glossy and toned—and make you appear fast, even if you're not.

Function: Besides keeping your legs warm, the deep-heating effect of embrocation soothes muscles and stimulates circulation. On rainy days, cover the warm base layer with a water- and wind-proof gel.

Spandex

Sport it form-fitting, not ill-fitting.

Fashion: Your jersey should stop just above your hipbones, and the leg bands on your shorts should never be loose or too long at your thighs. Both should fit your body's contours like a second skin. Pros often get their gear tailored.

Function: High-tech, ergonomically cut cycling clothing is designed to breathe, wick moisture and feel comfortable against your body. If it's flapping in the breeze, it's not serving its purpose.

Bibs

One-piece design keeps your middle from oozing out.

Fashion: Bibs are every serious rider's secret for a polished look; you're not in the club otherwise.

Function: They fit better, are more comfortable around your midsection and keep your shorts from drooping, so your chamois stays in place and you never reveal the top of your butt crack.

Tire Hot Patch

Take the extra second to align it with the valve stem.

Fashion: Aligning your tire's label with your wheel's valve stem proves that you pay attention to even the smallest details. Skip this simple step and you may as well be walking around with your fly open.

Function: The valve and label act as reference so you can easily locate the debris that punctured your tube. If you need to fix your flat fast, you'll save valuable seconds not having to look for the valve stem.

FOR THE FELLAS: LEG SHAVING 101

Among the many rites peculiar to the tribe known as the cyclists, none elicits more comment than the shaving of the legs. Anthropologists studying the tribe in its well-dispersed homelands (Italy, France, the western United States, New York City's Central Park, the southern tip of Africa, numerous viticultural areas) have long noted that many riders remove the hair from their legs in time-consuming and often painful rituals conducted with bars of soap and single-use razors in showers. The rite is said to aid in the application of soothing emollients known as embrocation and bandages, to facilitate massage and to serve as an act of self-worship when the bare legs are flexed in front of full-length mirrors.

Should you wish to join this tribe, consider these nine tips from a shaving veteran:

→Do a pre-mow with electric clippers or a depilatory such as Nair. And if you're really bushy, do it in a motel. Order in champagne.

→Do it in or after a shower, so your legs are warm and moist.

→Don't do it the day before a race, or when you want to get a lot of sleep—the sheets will drive your freshly nude legs wild with sensual awakenings.

→Shave with the grain, then against on the quads (front and back) to get the really thick hair. (You should only need to shave one way on calves.)

→Go as high as you feel you must so as not to give the appearance of wearing black cycling shorts when nude.

→If your hairy feet and toes look out of place, do them, too.

→Don't expect perfection—you can remove stragglers when you do the maintenance shave in the future.

→Rub on baby oil or lotion afterward—men traditionally don't moisturize, and their legs look like dandruff sticks.

→A couple times a week works for most guys.

Pro **Tip**

"I SAY NO ON THE SHAVING LEGS. STRAIGHT UP, WHATEVER'S THERE IS THERE."—*JOE MADDON, CYCLIST AND MANAGER OF THE TAMPA BAY RAYS BASEBALL TEAM*

RIDER **RESOURCES**

Read thousands of bike and gear reviews with *Bicycling's* Gear and Bike Review Finder (bicycling.com/gear).

Learn way, way more than you ever wanted to know about blood flow to the genitals in Joshua Cohen's book, *Finding the Perfect Bicycle Seat* (roadbikerider.com).

Watch custom builder Richard Sachs make a bike—and live his ideals—in the DVD documentary *Imperfection Is Perfection* (richardsachs.com).

Bike Snob NYC (bikesnobnyc.blogspot.com) serves up hilarious critiques of all facets of cycling style.

III

Road Skills

ONE OF THE GREAT TRUTHS ABOUT CYCLING IS THAT there's always something new to learn, and each new skill you pick up makes your riding more enjoyable. Whether you're riding alone or with a group, on freshly paved rolling hills or twisty gravel roads, knowing the proper tactics will add to the fun—and could even save your life.

CHAPTER 6

The Fundamentals

Once we learn to ride a bike, the act of pedaling is pretty easy. But becoming truly confident on two wheels is an ongoing process. The advice here will help you build a foundation for better bike handling and smoother riding. And by learning to get comfortable with clipless pedals, you'll be ready to take your cycling to the next level.

BASIC BALANCE

We asked Alison Dunlap, a former mountain bike world champion and Olympian who also competed in the 1996 Olympic road race and completed four women's Tours de France, for her best tips.

→ If you remember only one thing, remember to keep your upper body relaxed. Think of your arms as shock absorbers—not just on a mountain bike, but on a road bike, too. You want to keep them soft and slightly bent.

→ The number-one thing you should be able to do without swerving: Look over your shoulder. This comes only with relaxed arms and shoulders. Even though you try to twist only your head, your upper torso will shift naturally when you turn. If you're stiff-armed, this will pull your handlebar out of line. Practice in a field or empty parking lot, turning your head for only a second, two at the most. If you didn't catch what was behind you, wait, and then turn your head again. Even if you have to look five times, it's better than looking so long that you swerve out of line or miss something happening in front of you.

→ Number two: Take a drink. It's very important to grab the bottle without looking at it. First, practice riding one-handed as you look ahead. When you can ride in a straight line, practice reaching down and touching the bottle, then removing it, then drinking, then replacing it, mastering each step before adding the next. Then do it with the other hand.

Fun **Fact**

Scientists estimate that 20 percent of the fibers in your optic nerve are connected directly to balance centers in the brain. This means that what you see influences your sense of equilibrium: In the same way that staring at the horizon makes your body feel still so you don't get carsick, looking ahead on your bike will help you feel balanced, while staring down at your wheel or an obstacle right in front of you bombards the brain with motion.

Advanced Balance: The Trackstand

Small occurrences—a traffic light turning red, someone falling on the trail in front of you—set into motion the most annoying series of events in cycling: the unclip, the dismount and the fumble to remount. Forget it. The trackstand, named for the ability of velodrome racers to balance their fixed-gear bikes on the track, can help you stay upright without unclipping, and it lets you take off quickly. Beyond smooth starts and stops, practicing this move will also help you improve your overall balance on the bike. Much as when you first learned to ride a bike, your first trackstands will be wobbly and uncertain, but after your sense of equilibrium clicks, you'll stand perfectly and turn heads wherever you stop.

THE SETTING. In an area free of cars and hecklers, find a spot with a slight grade, which will give you some resistance and speed up your learning curve. Most roadways slope about two degrees at the shoulder, and that's perfect, but if the road has regular traffic, find a yard or driveway with equal slope.

Because of their upright position and wide tires, mountain bikes are easiest to learn on. Unless you can unclip in an instant, use flat pedals. Choose a gear you can turn easily, but that won't launch you forward if you happen to sneeze. The perfect gear is one you'd use to cruise on flat ground.

THE ACTION. Good general bike balancing technique is key: Keep your grip light, your body weight centered, and look ahead. Clenching the handlebar tightly tenses your entire upper body. Having too much body weight forward, over your handlebar, throws off your center of gravity; concentrate on keeping your weight over the bottom bracket of your bike. Also, looking down at your front wheel—which is especially tempting at slow speeds or when practicing your trackstand—disrupts your equilibrium.

Approach your balancing point perpendicular to the slope, with the rise going upward to your left. Stand on the pedals, legs slightly bent, with your left, or uphill, foot in front so that it won't hit the back of your front tire.

Come to a gradual stop at your spot. As your momentum ebbs, gently but sharply turn your front wheel into the slope. Press your front pedal just hard enough to hold your position. It may be tempting to grab the brakes to still yourself, but resist anything more than an occasional light feathering; let the slope do the work.

At first, don't try to be perfectly still. Gently ratchet your left pedal back a few degrees to release pressure and let your bike roll back about a foot, then push down again so your bike rolls up to the left. Try one back-and-forth, and dismount. Then try the move with more back-and-forths before stepping off. As you gain confidence, you'll be able to swing your bike like a pendulum.

THE NEXT LEVEL. Now that you can balance with some movement, try to minimize it. Staying relaxed is key. Apply light pressure to your front pedal to keep yourself still. If you feel like you're falling to the left, push harder. If you feel like you're falling to the right, ease the pressure. At some point you'll feel perfect, motionless equilibrium.

For a how-to video, visit bicycling.com/trackstand.

CONVERTING TO CLIPLESS PEDALS

It's time to become one with your bike. Most cyclists start out with flat pedals, sometimes with metal toeclips attached. But for optimum efficiency, speed, comfort and safety, eventually you're going to want to get clipless pedals and cycling-specific shoes, with cleats that clip into the pedals. (Yes, we know it makes no sense that you clip into "clipless" pedals. Just go with it.) Here, *Bicycling* editor Jennifer Sherry explains why she decided to make the switch, and gives you tips for making the conversion as smooth as possible:

I remember my mounting frustration as my pedals spun on the cranks while my sneakered toes chased those strappy contraptions until they finally caught up and worked their way in—just in time to yank them back out when fear got the best of me. When I grew weary of the battle of the toeclip, I flipped the pedals cage-side down and rode with the clips and straps dragging along the trail, smacking rocks and chipmunks in their path. If I loosened the clips, my feet slid in and out with ease, but I lost pedal power. If I tightened them, I could zip up hills, but I spent more time lying on the road—still attached to my bike. It was then that I knew the time had come to retire my medieval foot-jails and go clipless.

At first, I fell—sometimes because I wasn't used to the new system, others because I simply forgot I was attached to it. But after a few embarrassing and painful tumbles, I got the hang of it. Now I can't imagine riding anything but clipless. And when I meet other riders who fear what I feared, I always tell them the same thing: "Once you get used to it, you'll never go back."

The Benefits of Clipless

EFFICIENCY. With your feet attached to the pedals and your body attached to your feet, you become one with your bike, which means more of your energy makes its way to each pedal stroke, giving you more juice to climb and accelerate.

POWER. Clipless pedals let you pull on the upstroke as efficiently as you push down, creating a smooth and constant application of power through each crank rotation. The only way to achieve this with toeclips is to snug them dangerously tight, and even then you won't have as smooth and steady a cadence as with clipless pedals.

CONFIDENCE. When clipping in and out becomes second nature, you'll begin to notice that your skills will improve, and you'll take more chances, knowing that you're only a quick foot-twist away from detaching yourself from a doomed bike.

CONTROL. Clipless pedals let you pull your bike up off the ground to bunnyhop logs, curbs and potholes, and let you safely swerve around roadkill. And when you're rolling over a jagged rock garden, you can easily pop out a foot to dab. Plus, when you ditch the toeclips and straps, you lose the hassle of snagging debris on the trail or catching sticks between your pedal and shoe.

FREEDOM. Nearly all clipless pedal systems have float and tension adjustment. Float allows your foot to swivel a few degrees laterally to ensure that you don't injure your knees by having them locked into one position. Tension adjustment lets you control how hard or easy it is to get in and out of the pedal.

Practice Makes Clipless

SETUP. Follow your pedal manufacturer's instructions to set your cleat tension so entry and exit are as easy as they can be. Some brands and models have no release-tension adjustability, so ask before you buy.

TWIST. Stand over your bike and practice getting one foot in and out of the pedal by twisting your heel outward. Do this until it feels natural—50 times if you have to. Switch sides.

CRUISE. When you feel comfortable clipping in and out, go for a spin around your neighborhood or on a patch of grass. Practice clipping in and out as you roll.

STOP. Try coming to a complete stop as if you were riding in traffic. As you slow to a stop, clip one foot out and use it like a kickstand. Not feeling that confident yet? Stop next to a tree or telephone pole so you can grab it if you have to.

RIDE. Once you feel comfortable cruising your 'hood, clipping in and out, and stopping on a dime, show up at the next group ride looking like an old pro.

THREE COMMON BEGINNER QUESTIONS

They may sound basic—but we get asked all the time. Fortunately, Alex Stieda has the answers.

How do I know when it's time to shift gears?

Your bike's gears are designed to help you keep a consistent cadence (usually in the 90-rpm range), allowing you to pedal at maximum efficiency. Riding conditions such as wind resistance, terrain and group dynamics are constantly changing, and you should adjust your gear ratio accordingly. A cadence meter can provide a steady gauge of how fast you're pedaling.

The first tip I offer at my camps is to anticipate conditions that will affect your effort level so you can shift before you actually need a smaller or bigger gear. Changing gears when there is less pressure on the pedals allows for a much smoother shift and less wear on your drivetrain, especially when you're shifting the front derailleur.

Reader Tip

FOR BEGINNERS WHO HAVE A TOUGH TIME REMEMBERING WHICH WAY TO SHIFT FOR EASIER PEDALING AND WHICH WAY FOR HARDER PEDALING, STICK COLORED DOTS ON THE BAR— GREEN FOR EASIER, RED FOR HARDER. IN TIME, THE STICKERS CAN BE REMOVED.

—*DEAN ROBBINS, MARYLAND*

When should I be riding in the drops?

Any time you need greater control of your bike. With your hands in the drops of the handlebar, you put more weight on your front wheel, which stabilizes the bike and increases your braking power. On long descents, move your hands down before your speed rises above your comfort level. For some new cyclists, riding in the drops can cause hand, neck and shoulder discomfort. Correct handlebar selection and brake-lever adjustment and proper bike fit should allow most people to comfortably ride in this position.

How can I stand up on my bike without falling over?

The key to staying balanced is a smooth pedal stroke. To practice this, ride indoors on a trainer at least once a week, spending 20 to 30 minutes of an hour's session out of the saddle. Wrap your thumbs around the brake hoods before standing up. Your arms should be slightly bent and your hands and shoulders relaxed. Start with a cadence in the 50- to 60-rpm range. Your pedal stroke should feel like a walking motion. Focus on one foot at a time until you are moving smoothly. Switch to an easier resistance and increase your cadence until you're comfortable pedaling out of the saddle in the 90-rpm range.

CHAPTER 7

Up, Down, and All Around— Climbing, Descending, and Everything in Between

Consider this chapter your guide to free speed: By improving your pedaling and shifting, and your prowess on corners and hills, you'll become a more efficient cyclist.

THE PERFECT PEDAL STROKE

Pedaling in a simple circle is a complex thing, but mastering it can save energy, says Todd Carver, owner of bike-fitting company Retül, and formerly a biomechanist at Colorado's Boulder Center for Sports Medicine. He says that with proper technique, riders can churn out the same amount of power at a heart rate as many as five beats per minute lower. This stroke is for flat terrain at threshold, or time trial, intensity.

HIP-KNEE-ANKLE ALIGNMENT. Viewed from the front, your hip, knee and ankle should line up throughout the pedal stroke. "You don't want knee wobble," says Carver. "Just think pistons, straight up and down." If you can't cor-rect this, or if you experience knee pain when you try to restrict lateral movement, you may need orthotics or another type of biomechani-cal adjustment.

SADDLE POSITION. Proper bike fit, especially saddle height and fore-aft adjustment, is a prerequisite for a smooth pedal stroke. With-out it, says Carver, you won't be even remotely as efficient as you could be. "If your saddle is too high, you're not going to be able to drive your heel effectively," he says. "If it's too low, you'll have knee pain." In the right posi-tion (knee over the ball of your foot with the pedal at 3 o'clock; knee slightly bent with the pedal at 6 o'clock), you'll maximize your energy output and also be able to adapt your technique to different terrain, cadence and effort levels.

ZONE 1. Known as the power phase, the portion of the pedal stroke from 12 o'clock to about 5 o'clock is the period of greatest muscle activity. "A lot of people think hamstrings are used only on the upstroke," says Carver, "but a good cyclist uses a lot of hamstring in the downstroke, because it extends the hip." The key to accessing the large muscles in the back of your leg is dropping your heel as you come over the top of the stroke, says Carver. "At 12 o'clock, your toes should be pointed down about 20 degrees, but as you come over the top, start dropping that heel so that it's parallel to the ground or even 10 degrees past parallel by the time you get to 3 o'clock." The biggest mistake Carver sees in novice riders: not dropping the heel enough in Zone 1.

ZONE 2. Using the same muscles as in the power phase, but to a lesser degree, this phase acts as a transition to the backstroke. "As you enter Zone 2, think about firing the calf muscles to point your toe," Carver says. As you come through the bottom of the stroke, the toe should be pointed down 20 degrees. "This technique transfers some of the energy developed in Zone 1 by the bigger muscles to the crank," Carver says. He uses the advice popularized by Greg LeMond: "Act like you're scraping mud off the bottom of your shoe."

ZONE 3. Even though you feel like you're pulling your foot through the back of the stroke, you're not. "When you look at even the best cyclists, they're losing power on the upstroke," says Carver. "The pedal is actually pushing your leg up, so the goal is to lose as little power as possible and get that foot out of the way." One fun way to improve the efficiency of your upstroke: mountain biking. "The terrain keeps you honest," Carver says. "If you're focusing only on the downstroke, you'll lose traction and fall off your bike in steep sections." As for other exercises, Carver advises against single-leg pedal drills—"for recreation-level riders, they injure more people than they help"—but recommends hamstring- and glute-strengthening lifts, as well as squats, "done correctly, in a squat rack with someone showing you how."

ZONE 4. As you enter the second half of the upstroke phase, think about initiating your downstroke. "Many riders don't initiate early enough," says Carver, who often sees riders wait until 3 o'clock—but they should be starting before 12 o'clock. A tip: As you begin to come across the top of the stroke, think about pushing your knee forward, toward the bar. But only your knee, says Carver: "Your pelvis should

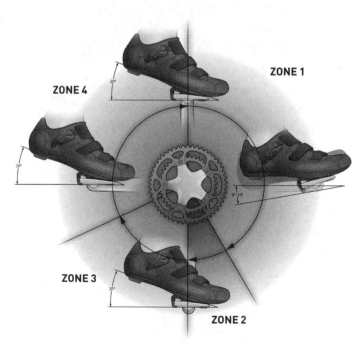

ZONE 4

ZONE 1

ZONE 3

ZONE 2

remain a stable platform, not sinking down and not moving forward." As the knee comes forward, you should feel your hamstrings and glutes engage, and your hip extend.

SMART SHIFTING

Cyclists are weak. No, we're not singling anyone out—even the mighty Lance has a maximum power output that's roughly the equivalent, in horsepower, to a Go-Ped scooter. Gears let us maximize our low-power motors on the bike; specifically, being able to choose a gear that keeps us in our cadence comfort zone, the point at which we can pedal seemingly indefinitely without flailing around or succumbing to a muscle-scorching slow grind.

If you really want to rock the gears, though, you need to know when to shift outside your comfort zone, into a slightly higher (harder) or lower (easier) gear, even momentarily, to suit what you hope to accomplish on the bike. This takes practice and timing, says 1996 mountain bike Olympian and five-time Canadian cross-country champion Andreas Hestler. Know what you're doing, he says, and you'll ride faster and extend the life of your drivetrain. Here are his best tips.

THE CROSS-CHAIN DILEMMA. Cross-chaining—riding in a combination of the big chainring and big cog, or the small ring/small cog—can at times provide the ideal gear, but it can lead to clumsy shifts. If you're on the inner chainring in the front and the small cog in the back, chances are if you shift into the big ring the chain will fall off. Conversely, shifting from the big ring/big cog is often slow.

DON'T GET CAUGHT. "The key to proper shifting is thinking ahead," says Hestler. "Anticipate what gear you need, and anticipate when to accelerate." Shifting after the terrain changes slows you down and robs you of energy. The same idea holds true when approaching traffic on the road or a sand or water crossing while mountain biking. Look ahead and be in the right gear before you get there.

THINK ON YOUR FEET. When you want to get a jump on someone in a group ride or race, don't telegraph your attack with noisy shifts, Hestler says. Instead, use your feet to unload the drivetrain, so you can "butter up or down into the gear you need," he says. Done correctly, this decreases your wattage for just a moment, so you can quietly shift into your attacking gear and pounce.

REMEMBER THE CHAIN. If your chain is shot, shifting suffers. "Change the chain more frequently, and you won't have to replace your cogs and rings as often," Hestler says. He often changes his chain after spring training camps or after he's been riding in wet weather because, he says, constant wet-dry riding can weaken the chain. If your chain is in good condition, and a cable adjustment doesn't fix your shifting issues, inspect your chainrings and cassette for burrs and nicks.

BE KIND. When he does a crit and can walk back to the car if something breaks, Hestler slams shifts and stands on the gears hard. On long rides that take him away from civilization, though, such as the TransRockies Challenge, a weeklong epic, he is a bit more gentle. "I don't want to break something and throw away a good finish, or worse," he says. "If you love your bike it'll love you—shift lightly and carefully."

CLIMBING

Every climb contains one fundamental element: effort. But there are other ingredients that can make or break a successful ascent. Here are six essentials that Andy Applegate, climbing specialist and coach with Carmichael Training Systems, swears by. They'll help you reach the top faster, easier and with less pain.

PACE YOURSELF. If you go above threshold too soon, you'll blow up and slow down before you reach the top. Keep your breathing deep and comfortable and your heart rate below threshold at the start of the climb. As you fall into a rhythm, gradually increase your effort until you're climbing at threshold. The final 200 meters is the perfect place to take it to the max and attack. If you start smart, you'll have the energy to finish strong.

SIT—MOST OF THE TIME. Unless you're a 120-pound Spanish climbing specialist, your rear end should be planted on your saddle for most of the climb. You use about 5 percent more energy when you stand during a climb than when you sit. Shift your weight back slightly for maximum leverage on the pedals. Stand only when your body needs a break from the seated position or when you have to jump and accelerate to attack or chase. When you stand, keep your butt back so the nose of your saddle brushes the backs of your thighs and your weight is over the crank. Shifting your weight too far forward will cause you to overweight the front tire and lose traction in the back.

Shifting Situations

Here's how to handle two common scenarios.

A LONG, GRADUAL ROAD CLIMB
The Shift: This is usually the easiest shifting situation, after flat terrain. At the base of the climb, you should be in your comfort-zone gear—it varies from rider to rider, but for most of us it's in the 90-revolutions-per-minute range. When your cadence starts to slip, ease the pressure off the pedals slightly and shift into an easier gear. Remember, shifting in the front means a big resistance change; rear shifts are for fine-tuning your cadence. If you need to stand, shift up a cog or two in the rear; the slightly harder gear will allow a smooth transition. Shift between these sitting and standing gears as you make your way up the climb.

A GROUP ROAD RIDE THAT'S HEADING INTO A SPRINT-FINISH AREA
The Shift: The biggest mistake most of us make in just-for-fun sprints is telegraphing our move—we suddenly (and noisily) shift into much higher gears, alerting everyone to our intentions. Surreptitious presprint shifting is partially done in advance (with the front chainring) and partially on the fly—you need to be in only a slightly harder gear to start, as upshifts in the rear can be managed after you jump. Move up one gear at a time, spinning out each gear (meaning faster than your comfort zone) before shifting again.

LOOSEN YOUR UPPER BODY. Your entire upper body should be relaxed so you don't waste energy. A good marker for a loose torso is slightly flared elbows. "Your elbows should be outside your knuckles," says Applegate. "This allows you to remain relaxed. If your elbows are in, your lats are stretched tight, which can restrict breathing."

USE THE RIGHT GEARING. Don't be afraid to use your easiest gear. "Riders want to use their big gears, but the goal is to gear down and keep the cadence in a comfortable range," says Applegate. Try to keep your cadence above 70 rpm.

INCREASE YOUR POWER-TO-WEIGHT RATIO. The number of watts you can crank out per kilogram (2.2 pounds) of body weight is the key to climbing success. The Alberto Contadors in the crowd are known to produce an amazing 6 to 7 watts per kg. "If you can hit 5, that's awesome," says Applegate. Through high-intensity training, you can raise your wattage by 5 to 7 percent over the course of a season. One surefire strategy: Climb for 10 to 30 minutes at or near lactate threshold heart rate (about an 8 on a 1 to 10 scale of perceived exertion) twice a week. If you want to improve your ratio, work at lowering the weight part of the equation. (For more tips on increasing power and losing weight, see Chapters 19 and 26).

BREATHE DEEPLY. "Riders often use just the top half of their lungs, taking shallow, jagged breaths as they climb," says Applegate. This limits how quickly and efficiently you can get fresh oxygen to your working muscles. "Practice breathing deep into your belly, filling your lungs entirely," he says. As a bonus, deep breaths help keep you calm under the stress of the climb.

DESCENDING

Few things in cycling are as blissful as a long, winding descent, but if you want to maximize speed, you need to do more than kick back to admire the scenery. Not many cyclists are born descenders, a fact visible even in the pro ranks, says downhill scorcher and former national criterium champion Antonio Cruz. "Some guys may be super climbers, but they get squirrelly on descents," he says. They, and you, can improve downhill form. Here is Cruz's advice on finding the mix of speed, stability and maneuverability that results in the fastest safe way down.

FIND YOUR BALANCE. The straight-on downhill stance is, of course, low and aerodynamic: hands on the drops of the handlebar, elbows bent and tucked in, and, if you aren't pedaling, pedals level, knees slightly bent and tucked in, and butt slightly out of the saddle for balance and mobility. You'll need to experiment to find the right front-to-back position for your body. "You want your weight balanced on the bike," says Cruz. "If you're too far back or your upper body is too high, the front wheel will feel loose and you'll be afraid to push it in the corners; if you're too far forward or too low, the rear wheel will feel unstable." The trick is to notice how subtle shifts in body position affect stability as you descend. When both wheels feel glued to the ground, you've hit the jackpot: This is your basic descending position.

STOP THE CYCLE. Relaxation is key. Any tension in your body will be transferred to the bike, which creates a vicious circle, says Cruz. Body stiffness makes the bike harder to control, which makes you even more tense, which then makes the bike even harder to control. So, along with bending your knees and elbows, focus on keeping your shoulders relaxed and maintaining a loose grip on the handlebar. "When your shoulders are tense, it's hard even to steer," he says. "You're basically all locked up."

THINK DOWN THE ROAD. Don't focus on what's happening beside you or directly in front of you, because it's too late to do anything about it anyway. Instead, look at least four or five riders ahead so you have time to react to potholes, gravel or other obstacles. If you're not riding in a pack, just remember that the faster you're descending, the farther ahead you should look. A good basic rule is to "double down." If you're going 25 mph, look 50 feet down the road. Along with this anticipation comes one of the

6 Things to Know About Descending

Start with a neutral body position: hands in the arc of the drops (not on the flat ends) with index and middle fingers on the brake levers, and butt slightly rearward on the saddle.

TO GO FASTER
Drop your head lower and farther forward, and draw your knees and elbows in.

TO INCREASE STABILITY
Shift your weight back, raise your chest, and pedal or, if coasting, bring your thighs in against the top tube.

TUCK AND COAST WHEN PEDALING NO LONGER BENEFITS YOU
According to *Bicycling's* calculations, that's about 25 mph on a 5 percent grade, or 40 mph on a 10 percent grade, for a 155-pound cyclist.

TO SLOW DOWN
Shift your weight rearward as you apply both brakes, gradually squeezing the left lever harder to engage more front brake, which supplies most of your stopping power.

IT'S FINE TO SIT WHILE DESCENDING, BUT IF YOU HIT A ROUGH STRETCH OF PAVEMENT OR A PATCH OF GRAVEL
Lift your butt off the saddle. "If you're sitting, you're reacting to what happens—you're on defense," says 2001 world mountain bike champion Alison Dunlap. "But you want to be on offense."

TO GO DANGEROUSLY FAST
Pros used to drop their butts so far off the back that their chests lay atop the saddle. Now the technique is to move so far forward that your chest rests atop the handlebar, and your head acts as a wedge to part the air. Keeping your hands in the drops gives you a slight chance of being able to brake, but to do the full tuck, put your hands atop the flats, under your chest. This is ridiculously unstable, ill-advised—and fast.

hardest lessons for any would-be high-speed descender to learn: Use the brakes less. "As soon as you hit the brakes, your weight pitches forward and you can't react as quickly," Cruz explains. "Sometimes not using the brakes is the safest way to get down." Look far enough ahead, and you could avoid trouble without resorting to braking.

WORK THE CORNERS. "A lot of people will dive into a turn full throttle, and then scrub speed as they exit," explains Cruz, "but that's the opposite of what you want to do." For a demonstration of efficient cornering, Cruz recommends watching a MotoGP motorcycle race the next time you're channel surfing. Moto racers start wide and sit up to slow down before entering the turn, then get down on the bike and lean hard into the corner, and accelerate out of the turn as the bike comes upright. Keep that "slow early, exit fast" image in mind on your next descent. Plant your weight on your outside pedal to keep control as you lean the bike through the turn, and you'll be carving turns in no time.

PUSH IT. "Riding at your limit is a sure way to improve," says Cruz, who suggests trying to hang with riders who are better descenders than you are. Remember, though, that you want them to push you to the edge, not over it. If you start to feel uncomfortable, back off by sitting up slightly or lifting your head to let wind resistance slow you down.

PLAY IT SMART. Always descend according to the situation. If you're off the front of a group and want to stay there, or you're off the back and trying to catch back up, get into a tuck on straight descents, and pedal hard out of corners for more speed. If you're in a group, don't make sudden or unpredictable moves to gain minor bursts of speed—it's not worth risking the safety of everyone else. And if you're in the middle of a three-hour solo spin or totally blown from the effort of your ride, don't try to pin it. Instead, study the downhill for another day.

CORNERING

Turning a bicycle can be scary—especially if you're trying to maximize speed at the same time. But with proper technique, you can go faster and tilt your bike farther than you think is possible. Alex Stieda, the first North American to wear the yellow jersey, claims he once leaned so far his glove got a burn mark from rubbing against the top of someone's rear wheel. Here's what he has to say about changing directions:

"As a pro cyclist, I worked to improve my cornering skills. During a stage of the Tour of Britain, I remembered there was a turn 400 meters before the line. I attacked early, railed the corner and opened a gap. I raised my arms in victory at the finish, only to be told that this gesture was against the rules. I was relegated to last in the break, but relished the fact that my strategy had worked.

Once you feel the power and control of a properly carved turn, there is nothing better. It takes practice, so be patient. Find an empty parking lot and mark off a corner with water bottles or cones. Here are some techniques that helped me."

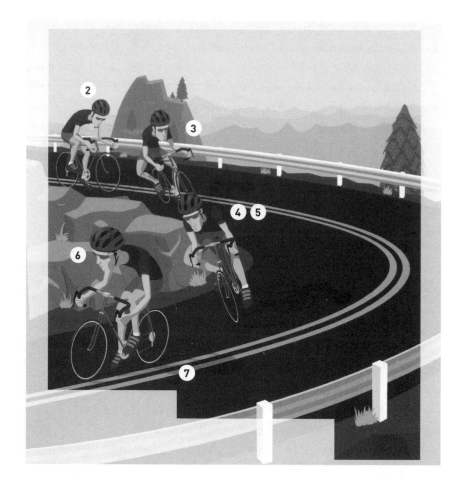

1. MIND THE TERRAIN. Look for and avoid sand, rocks or cracks that could cause you to slip. After you know what the riding conditions are in a particular corner, you can slowly increase your speed each time.

2. APPLY PRESSURE. Do all your braking before the turn. Weight distribution is critical: To keep from sliding out, weight the front wheel by putting your hands in the drops of the handlebar with your elbows bent. Next, exert pressure with your outside hand and foot, creating angulation like you would in a ski turn. Don't try to pedal in a corner.

3. LEAN THE MACHINE. Release the brakes and start the turn by leaning the bike—not your body—into the turn. This can be accomplished by pushing lightly with your inside hand; some call this counter-steering. If the turn is tight or your speed increases, lean the bike farther in, and vice versa.

Two Great Cornering Tips

REFINE YOUR MOTOR SKILLS

Swimmers practice their pulls and kicks. Runners do strides and form drills. But cyclists rarely practice specific skills, and that's a mistake, says coaching veteran Carl Cantrell of Alamogordo, New Mexico (coachcarl.com). Cantrell has his racers do circle drills and figure 8s once a week to refine the motor skills needed for cornering so those reflexes are automatic when they hit the real thing: Shift into a low gear and ride in slow left-hand circles, gradually picking up speed and bringing the circle tighter until you feel the rear wheel lose traction and skid slightly. That's your tipping point. Get a feel for that point and you'll feel comfortable riding within it. Practice in both directions. Graduate to figure 8s, which force you to change directions quickly and maintain control.

REGAIN LOST CONTROL

Losing control in a corner can be terrifying. But nearly every rider has an "oops" episode when misjudging a curve and carrying too much speed. The right response can save your hide. When you feel yourself losing control, Cantrell says, kick your hips to the outside to shift your center of gravity. This will stop the bike from cornering, set the bike up, and bring you back on top of the bike with the wheels down. Then shift your weight back and hit the brakes, bringing the bike back under control so you can slowly bring it through the curve without sliding across the road into the line of traffic or other riders.

4. AIM FOR THE INSIDE. Carve a smooth arc through the apex of the turn: Start at the outside of the corner, near the center line. Aim toward the inside of the turn, then exit as far to the outside as possible. Do not cross the double yellow line.

5. KEEP LOOKING. . . in the direction you want to go. This will help you maintain a smooth line.

6. MAKE YOUR EXIT. As you come out of the turn, gradually straighten the bike until it's upright, then start to pedal again.

7. MIND THE RAIN. Painted lines, manhole covers and oily pavement become slippery in wet conditions. Wet roads exaggerate everything you do: Braking while the bike is leaning will cause you to skid more easily, and sudden turning can make your wheels slip. So slow down.

CHAPTER 8

The Art of Group Riding

Riding as part of a pack is the utopian ideal of cycling: You go faster and farther with less effort, and colorful commentary from your riding buddies on monster hills or nasty roadkill or too-tight cycling shorts always makes the harder sections seem less grueling.

But initiation into a cycling group doesn't always come easy. There are hand signals, code words and seemingly bizarre rules that were largely created for safety reasons. New riders usually pick up pack skills on the fly, through observing, trying, getting cussed at and eventually catching on.

The best way to become more comfortable riding in a group is (not surprisingly) riding in a group. That said, there are a number of skills and tricks you can practice to speed the process along—and ensure that you don't end up with a nickname like "Swerve."

JOIN THE PACK— SAFELY

Alex Stieda shares five key skills to master before jumping into a group.

PEDAL SMOOTHLY. First, you need to learn to ride steady on your own. Many beginners use too low a cadence, which makes the bike surge forward with every pedal stroke—annoying and even dangerous in a group. I recommend riding at least at 90 rpm on every ride. Keeping your cadence high will also allow you to adjust to speed changes in small increments, rather than braking or all-out acceleration. To keep your rpm constant, change gears frequently to match the terrain and wind conditions. Remember: Don't look down at your bike's drivetrain as you shift. Practice solo until you can do it by feel.

GET CLOSE AND BE PREDICTABLE. Packs are most often formed of one or two lines of riders to maximize the wind-breaking benefits. To feel the draft, go with one or two other riders to a quiet, flat road and practice riding single file. Gently move laterally a foot or so to find the space where there is the least wind resistance. That's the sweet spot. This position will vary depending on where you are relative to the wind, much like sailing.

KNOW WHEN TO PULL OFF. In general, the higher the wind resistance, the shorter your time leading the pack should be. In stiff headwinds you may see the front for only a second or two. On a gradual downhill, you may spend two minutes leading before you pull off. The length of a pull also depends on the ability of the rider; if you find yourself struggling to maintain the group's speed, it's time to drop to the back. If you're feeling strong, you can stay up front longer—just save something for the trip home. When you're ready to pull off the front, let the rider behind know with a hand or voice signal, check over your shoulder for cars, gradually pull out of line and then ease up just enough to drift slowly to the back of the group.

DOUBLE UP. Next, ride two by two, trying to get within an arm's reach of the shoulder next to you. You should be riding near enough to carry on a conversation without those behind you hearing what you are saying—really, that close. Build to a group of four to six riders before you join a larger pack.

LOOK AHEAD. No matter where you are in the pack, it is essential that you watch the road surface in front of the group. Those at the front should be pointing out dangerous objects coming up—holes, rocks, dogs and the like—but everyone is responsible for sharing this awareness. Gaining confidence in lifting your gaze from the wheel in front of you takes time, but you can jump-start it by going to a grass field with a friend and riding single file to practice. You'll find it's not so hard if you both ride steadily and predictably.

Don't Be Shy

When riding in a group, communication is key to keeping everyone rolling along safely. Here are four situations where you need to speak up.

CARS
When you hear a car behind you waiting to pass, alert the other riders by calling "Car back." If you're the first to reach an intersection, survey the scene and call out "Car right," "Car left," or "Clear" before stopping or rolling through.

SLOWING OR STOPPING
Extend your right arm toward the ground, palm facing back—or call "Stopping" if you'd rather keep both hands on the brakes.

POTHOLES AND GRAVEL
Point these out to other riders, either verbally or by gesturing.

ROADSIDE OBSTACLES
When you encounter a pedestrian, parked car, or wayward garbage can blocking the right edge of the road, it's time for the Butt Tap: pat your right glute before drifting over to the left and weaving around the obstacle.

DO I HAVE TO RIDE SINGLE FILE?

For many cyclists, riding with others, whether on an outing with a friend or an organized ride, is one of the fundamental pleasures of our sport. But if legally bikes are vehicles, like cars, the question arises: Is side-by-side riding legal? Here, cycling lawyer Bob Mionske examines the legality of riding two up. The laws on two-abreast pedaling vary by state, but can be classified into three general types:

EXPLICITLY ALLOWED. In 39 states, the law specifically allows cyclists to ride two abreast. In 21 of these states, cyclists may ride two up only if they are not impeding traffic. Three states—Massachusetts, New York and Virginia—specifically require cyclists to roll single file when being overtaken by a passing vehicle. Even if your state allows riding two abreast, be aware that there may be nuances to the law, and that local and state laws might differ: Some cities or municipalities prohibit two-up riding, even though it is legal elsewhere in the state. And if your ride takes you through an Indian reservation, tribal law trumps state law. Be sure to check the laws in your area before heading out.

GENERALLY PROHIBITED. A few states still restrict riding two abreast, generally prohibiting the practice but allowing some exceptions. In Nebraska, cyclists must ride single file, except when on the shoulder. In Hawaii, you must ride single file except when a bicycle lane is wide enough to permit riding two abreast and traffic flow is unimpeded. In Montana, you can ride two abreast in a single lane, but only if there are at least two lanes in each direction, and only if

Fun Fact

Behold the power of the paceline: In the 2005 Tour de France, Lance Armstrong finished second in the 12-mile Stage 1 time trial with an average speed of about 34 mph. Three days later, his Discovery Channel team won the 42-mile team time trial with an average speed of about 36 mph, approximately five percent faster.

you are not impeding the normal and reasonable movement of traffic any more than you would be if you were riding single file.

IMPLICITLY ALLOWED. Finally, eight states neither explicitly prohibit nor permit riding side by side. Because the activity is not prohibited by law, and because the vehicle codes of these states contemplate that cyclists will be sharing lanes when it is safe to do so, riding two (or more) abreast is implicitly allowed by these states. Sometimes, law enforcement officers in these states will cite two-abreast riders because one of the cyclists is not riding as close to the right as is practicable. However, when officers do so, they are misinterpreting the law.

If you ride solo, the legalities of riding two abreast will not be an issue for you, even if you are involved in a pass with another cyclist—passing is legal everywhere when it is safe to do so. And, legal considerations aside, when contemplating riding side-by-side it is important to remember common courtesy. Helping motorists safely pass your group by singling up when you can will go a long way to improving cyclist-motorist relations. It's a small courtesy worth extending.

RULES OF THE PACELINE

When carried out properly, a paceline enables cyclists to share the work of pushing through the wind. When performed poorly, the formation becomes counterproductive. "Most people are never taught the proper way to ride a paceline," says Ray Ignosh, a USA Cycling expert coach based in Pennsylvania's Lehigh Valley. "So they make the same common mistakes that eventually become habits." Whether you're riding in a single or double formation, try these tips for keeping your group together and in good formation.

KEEP THE PACE. The number-one mistake riders make is picking up speed when they get to the front, says Ignosh. "Some people just want to show off; others are well-intentioned—they just aren't in tune with their effort and feel like they're supposed to take a pull, so they pull." As you're riding through the line, pay attention to the group's average speed and effort. When you get to the front, do your best to maintain those levels. The goal is to keep the pack together, not blow it apart or shell riders off the back.

MICROADJUST. It's nearly impossible for everyone to put forth equal amounts of effort, especially on undulating terrain. You need to make adjustments along the way to prevent what Ignosh calls the Slinky effect, where the line alternately bunches together and becomes strung out, with big gaps. "It's better to make two small undercorrections than one big overcorrection," he says.

"Think of it like driving: You don't slam on the brakes, then hit the gas; you moderate your speed." To do that in a paceline, try one of these techniques:

Soft pedal: If you feel like you're getting sucked into the rider in front of you, take a light pedal stroke or two to adjust your speed accordingly.

Air brake: An easy (and safe) way to trim speed is to sit up and catch some wind. It'll slow you down a notch without disrupting the rhythm of the line.

Feather brake: Gently squeeze the brakes while continuing to pedal. You can scrub speed while shifting up or down as needed to alter your pace.

DON'T STARE. Focusing on the wheel directly in front of you is a natural instinct when riding in a line, but it gives you zero time to react should something go awry. "Keep your head up and check about 10 meters down the road," says Ignosh. "Look through holes in the leading rider—over his shoulder, under his arm or through his legs—and ride proactively instead of reactively. This will help keep the line moving smoothly."

EASE OFF THE GAS. Rather than accelerating when you pull, try to ride in the line at a steady pace and decelerate as you pull off and drift to the back. "This provides the right work-to-recovery ratio without all the punchy surges that tend to blow the weaker riders off the back," says Ignosh.

SHARE AND SHARE ALIKE. Pacelines are designed to share the workload, so limit your pulls to a few minutes to stay fresh and give other riders a chance.

CONSERVE ENERGY. If you feel tired, sit out a few turns until you're ready to take another pull. Simply open a spot for riders to rejoin the

Don't Worry, Be Happy

Three ways to stress less about getting dropped.

→Don't panic if the first couple of miles of a group ride feel too fast. The excitement of rolling out with the pack can cause your heart rate and breathing to increase before you're properly warmed up, but your body should settle down within 10 minutes or so.

→Carry your charged cell phone—the 21st century's security blanket—on every ride, and make sure you have the digits of several people in your group.

→Riding with a group is fun, but if you're finding that keeping up with the pack is causing you a lot of mental distress, ride alone. You can set your own pace, rediscover your strengths—and practice the skills that you need for pack rides.

line in front of you, or come to the front and immediately pull off and drift to the back. You'll do the pack a favor by staying with them rather than working yourself into the red and falling off the back, which makes the group slow down to let you catch up.

ALL TOGETHER NOW

It's tough to achieve harmony on a group ride when speed demons pedal alongside up-and-comers—but you can learn to reap the benefits of chasing the faster riders or leading the slower ones. Here, writer Dimity McDowell talks to experts, coaches and everyday riders to help you make the most out of a group outing, no matter what your speed.

How to Hang On

Jenni Gaertner could lead almost any pack if she wanted to. But the Cat 2 road cyclist, expert mountain bike racer, elite cyclocross racer and coach with Portland, Oregon–based Wenzel

Coaching is also aware that, as she says, "Getting my butt kicked makes me a better racer." So in 2007, the 32-year-old decided to jump into the weekly group ride and race with the Category 1 and 2 men who leave from Vertical Earth, a bike shop she owns with her husband in Coeur d'Alene, Idaho. "I knew I wouldn't stay with them for the full time on the first ride," she says. "But I wanted to go as long as I could." Now, a year after her first ride, she can stay on the wheels of the testosterone train for the entire route some days. "I become the picture of stealthiness," she says. "I stay out of the wind at all times. I know the route, so I can anticipate the attacks." Her strategies aren't always foolproof, though. "Some days, I know I'm going to be dropped. I'm mentally prepared for that," she says. "When it happens, I just put my head down and work on time-trialing."

Stay with a group that would normally scream past you by employing these tactics:

PICK YOUR PACK POSITION WISELY. Stay in the front third of the group. Think of the slipstream as an inverted V: Riding directly behind the front riders gives you the maximum advantage, while farther back, the pull-you-along effect is diluted. Also, riding toward the front allows quicker reactions when somebody surges. "Attacks have a yo-yo effect, like a red light turning green," Gaertner says. "The first car takes off quickly, but it takes a while for the 10th car back to get through the light. You don't want to be the 10th car." Unless, of course, you're new to group riding. Toward the back, you have a little more mental breathing room and space to maneuver. "You can get a feel for the group without feeling pressured to take pulls at the front," says Daniel Hart, a former member of the American University cycling team in Washington, D.C., a veteran bike-shop employee and compassionate rider who happily pedals casually with his girlfriend.

ATTACK THE HILLS. In fact, try to lead. If you begin in the back third on an uphill (not as draft-friendly as the flats), the stronger riders book up it and gain distance down the other side by the time you crest. If you start close to the front, you may still be passed, but you're more likely to see the top before the last rider rockets away.

ATTACK THE HILLS, PART II. On downhills, shift into a big gear and pedal so you can be in the heart of the group when things even out. You can rest after you return to the safety of the draft. Often after a hard effort, the group will chill on the descent and for a few more minutes postclimb to give everybody a chance to catch their breath.

HANG ON, HANG ON. "If you get dropped, shift into a hard gear, get as aero as you can and give it everything you have," says Abby Ruby, a senior coach at Carmichael Training Systems, based in Colorado Springs. "You typically have one or two superhard efforts like that in you per ride, so pick your blastoff point wisely." Look for times when the group is slow, such as in a town or on a stretch of road with many stoplights. If the pack continues to disappear into the horizon, don't burn out your legs. Shift to plan B: Ride alone.

EAT IN STAGES. Eating and drinking tend to become afterthoughts when you're hanging on for dear life—which is a mistake. "If you don't take in calories and fluids, you'll be off the back, with plenty of time to eat and drink," says Ruby. Smooth the hand-to-mouth process by tucking a gel or two into your shorts legs for easy access, and open wrappers and bottles before your ride. "Never rush to open containers and eat at the same time," says Hart. "You'll lose speed and get flustered." Instead, if you're at the front, grab a bite or sip when you peel off to the back.

FLATTEN YOUR RPMS. While drafting on flat terrain, shift into a slightly bigger gear, slow your cadence and pedal minimally. Your muscles will provide enough power to pull you along, but your heart rate won't rocket.

ADMIT TO BEING THE WEAKEST LINK. If you can't hold onto the wheel in front of you any longer, don't make the group behind you pay. "Yell 'gap' and move over," says Ruby. Let the person behind you catch the wheel while you integrate yourself back into the group.

ROLL OVER A PIECE OF GLASS TO GET A FLAT. You can catch your breath while changing the tube. Kidding—sort of.

LEAVE THE SUPERMAN CAPE AT HOME. "Be completely willing to do as little work as possible," says Hart. "Everybody knows what it feels like to be the slowest, so no one will give you a hard time for not taking a turn up front." If you do end up leading, do so for only a short bit—25 to 50 pedal strokes is fine—and exit gracefully by saying something like "That's all my legs have today."

BUT WEAR THE REST OF YOUR SUPERHERO DUDS. "If there's a little voice in you saying, 'You can't hang on,' you probably won't," says Kristen Dieffenbach, PhD, an assistant professor of athletic coaching education at West Virginia University, in Morgantown. "Negative self-talk poisons any chance of success." Instead, she suggests, embrace the challenge. "When it gets tough, tell yourself you're going to hold on until you count to 10. By the time you get there, the group may have slowed or your body may have adapted."

BE PREPARED TO HURT. "People tend to have a distorted sense of how much their bodies can handle," says Dieffenbach. Don't redline for an entire ride, but realize that going fast has some pain associated with it. The more you hurt now, the faster you'll be on future rides.

DON'T TAKE IT PERSONALLY. When, not if, you do lose the group, don't start calling yourself a loser or a slacker. "Every cyclist has been dropped at some point," says Dieffenbach, "and if they tell you otherwise, they're lying." After you're spit out, process the ride positively. "Ask yourself, 'Why didn't it work today?' Maybe it's because you didn't eat a good dinner last night, or that work this week demanded 60 hours of your time. It's not always your legs," says Dieffenbach.

How to Hang Out

Until recently, the only two-wheeled place Scott and Andrea Myers, top age-group triathletes from Wellston, Ohio, found marital peace was on their tandem. When they rode on separate bikes, Andrea, 34, would easily become frustrated. "I'd try to hang onto him, but couldn't. So then I'd get mad and just have an awful workout," she says. But the two, who both finished fifth in their age groups at the 2007 Louisville Ironman, continued to work toward finding a riding rhythm. They've settled into a four-wheeled groove, provided Scott, 35, is deliberate and thoughtful. "I aim for steady power and am careful about accelerating," he says. "And I spend more time sitting up, not using my aero bars, to let Andrea maximize the draft." On descents, though, he pushes the power and doesn't worry about losing his caboose because of the slipstream he creates. The end result? Andrea isn't always bringing up the rear—and Scott gets a solid training session. "I ride close to the redline for an hour, which is exactly how you want to race in a triathlon: consistently, but still pushing the pace," he says.

With these tips, slowing down doesn't mean working less:

BE THE ENGINE. Take extra-long turns up front or lead the entire way—just keep your speed in check—and point out the best place for your companions to ride behind you to maximize efficiency. You'll get a good workout while they enjoy the fruits of your labor.

SHIFT UP. On a hilly route, use a bigger gear as you climb so that you slow to 50 to 65 rpm. "You'll develop power in your legs without adding significant speed," Gaertner says.

SCHEDULE WISELY. Use rides with beginners for active recovery. Have no expectations except to help them discover the sport. "People often train too hard," says Ralph Frazier, a USA Cycling–certified coach. "Slower days force you to hit both ends of the training spectrum, which actually makes you faster because you give your muscles a chance to recover." If your legs must get their ya-yas out, crush them for an hour on a solo ride, then meet the group and cruise.

TACKLE THE HILLS. Make a plan to ride hills at your own pace, says Ruby. "Then go as hard as you can and wait for the group at the top." After you regroup, don't take off immediately. Remember: The cyclist who came up the hill last needs some rest, too.

INSTITUTE A NO-DROP POLICY. Frazier likes leave-no-cyclist-behind rides; out of the nine rides his Suwanee, Georgia–based company hosts weekly, seven are no-drop. "You cut out snobbery, and build teamwork and spirit," he says. "Slower cyclists become confident and faster cyclists become leaders."

PICK A BEGINNER-FRIENDLY ROUTE. If the pack isn't going to stay together, two options work well: a short loop course where you pass each other repeatedly, and an out-and-back—when faster riders heading home pass the slower ones still on their way out, the slower ones turn around. And bike paths, conducive to conversation and not to racing tactics, are always a good call.

Group Snot-Blowing Etiquette

Three ways to clear your blowhole without smearing your friends.

MID-PACK VOID
As long as you're on the left edge of the pack, and the group decorum allows it, signal with a left-pointing finger, then swing out of the paceline, blow to the left and resume your position.

BACK-OF-THE-PACK SHOOT
If you've just finished a pull and are drifting back, you can rocket your nasal effluvia with abandon.

EVERYWHERE-ELSE BLOW
Rather than hurl snot over your shoulder, shoot it down between your bent arm and thigh. At speeds above 25 mph, or on windy days when the discharge is more likely to kite and plaster the riders behind you, try slipping it between your pumping thigh and the top tube. You'll likely splatter your quad but, at least in terms of etiquette, better you than the rider behind you.

DON'T BE A JERK. It's obvious, but it bears repeating: If you're trying to help somebody become a better cyclist, don't make him or her feel ashamed or inferior. Some actions hurt more than words, like not giving slower riders enough time to take a drink and regain composure after catching up on a climb.

BE THE CABOOSE. By bringing up the rear, you'll get a new perspective. But don't turn into an annoying cheerleader. "Somebody struggling up a hill, possibly dying a thousand deaths, doesn't want to hear you riding beside him, yelling encouragement and not breathing hard," says Hart. Pick your words, and the time you say them, wisely. "Saying specific things like, 'Nice job keeping your shoulders relaxed,' or 'Maybe shift down one' are helpful," says Dieffenbach. Constantly saying "Good job, good job"—even if you're sincere—can ring hollow to someone in oxygen debt.

WEAR YOUR PATIENCE HELMET OR DON'T GO. "Nobody wants to be the slowest rider," says Gaertner. "If you can't go out with a good attitude, don't go out."

CHAPTER 9

Stopping—Intentionally or Otherwise

Learning how to brake properly can help you avoid many crashes. But if all else fails, we'll also teach you how to fall as safely as possible—and offer tips on getting back in the saddle.

BETTER BRAKING

Braking is one of those things that seems so easy—you squeeze the levers, the pads hit the rims, you slow down and eventually the bike stops—that, like breathing, we tend not to think about it unless we're forced to. But just as controlled breathing can ease tension and stress, controlled braking can not only get you out of hairy situations safely, it can actually improve your overall speed. The following stopping advice comes from *Bicycling* columnist Alex Stieda as well as former pro cyclist Chris Wherry, owner of Hub Training Center in Durango, Colorado.

FINGERS READY. Any time there's a wheel in front of you (i.e., you're drafting), rest your fingers on the brake levers. This way, you'll be able to brake quickly and minor slowdowns won't develop into emergency-stop situations while your hands find the brakes.

KEEP IT EQUAL. In 99 percent of braking situations, you want to apply pressure evenly to each brake lever so that both tires share the load. This helps maintain stability and control. Practice on a grass field, sprinting up to speed then slowing as fast as you can without skidding. You'll need to modulate finger pressure on each brake lever, much like ABS on a car, to stop individual tires from skidding.

TURN SMART. Always brake before a turn. As you near the curve, apply equal pressure to the brakes to reach a manageable speed, and then release the levers before you begin the turn to let your speed carry you through. Braking in a turn wreaks havoc on momentum, but if it's necessary for safety, then use the rear brake only—remember "right rear" to keep them straight in your mind, unless you've reversed the cables—because a front-tire skid guarantees a crash. Skidding the rear may raise your heart rate, but it will allow you to steer out of trouble.

LEARN TO STOP HARD. When you master the emergency stop, you'll have greater overall stopping confidence because you'll know this move is there when you need it. For more braking power, put your hands in the drops. Then, for added stability, push your weight back behind the saddle by shifting your butt and straightening your arms. With your weight back, you can hit the front brake harder than you can the rear—just short of locking it up—without getting pitched over the bar. Hard braking pushes your weight forward, which gives the front tire plenty of traction—and thus, stopping power—while unweighting the rear, making it more likely to slide. If your back wheel does start to slide, let up on the brakes for a millisecond to let it regain traction. Practice on the grass, with a goal of not skidding. Remember: Fresh brake pads greatly increase stopping performance—replace them regularly, consulting with your bike shop if you're not sure when.

SIT UP AND DRIFT. If you flat in the middle of a pack, don't panic. Simply stop pedaling—stay off the brakes, sit up and coast to a stop. And try to keep your bike going in as straight a line as possible. Any time you turn with a flat, your chances of going down are high.

After you master these skills, you'll be able to anticipate—a key skill for every cyclist from beginner to Tour de France champion. When you anticipate that the rider in front of you is going to swerve, for example, you won't have to overreact by slamming on the brakes. In many scenarios, continuing to pedal while braking lightly will get you out of trouble. The overall effect: You won't be a yo-yo, that person who brakes hard, then accelerates to regain momentum and wastes energy in the process.

Pro **Tip**

"I DON'T KNOW IF BRAKING HAS HELPED ME WIN A RACE, BUT IT HAS SAVED MY LIFE A COUPLE OF TIMES."—*CHRIS WHERRY, FORMER US PRO ROAD CHAMPION*

TAKE A DIVE

You can't skirt the big crash—but you can minimize the damage with proper technique. For the basics behind any kind of fall, we turned to Dave Hines, a karate black belt and instructor in California. Hines says there are three major principles in falling; the first is particularly important for cyclists.

GO WITH THE ENERGY. Cycling, as with most action sports, results in forward or front falls, and our natural reaction is to throw out our arms for protection. Though it seems like the best way to protect the head and upper body, it's not. When your arms go up you risk breaking a wrist, fracturing a collarbone or lacerating your chin because these three points will ultimately absorb the force of the fall and in the process snap back at unnatural angles. The safest way to handle a high- or low-speed get-off is to tuck and roll. By utilizing what's known as a judo or karate roll, you'll tuck your chin to your chest, pull your arms in and let your body roll through the fall on your shoulder. This neutralizes the energy and prevents neck and back injuries that result from your body coming to a sudden, limb-burying stop.

TAKE AWAY THE ENERGY. For a backwards fall, take away the force of the impact by throwing your hands back toward the ground to prevent the most common results of this fall, a head injury or whiplash. To properly execute, tuck your chin tight to your chest and, as you land on your back, extend your arms back and slap the ground with your hands—it's a slap to stop momentum, not an attempt to brace with your arms, which could break a wrist. This keeps the momentum from going to your torso and head.

LOWER YOUR CENTER OF GRAVITY. By moving your hips as close to the ground as possible, you'll reduce inertia and force of impact. Take snowboarders, for instance: They might be in a prone position at speed but as soon as they start to fall they buckle their knees and get close to the ground. While cyclists may be limited to how low they can go because of that pesky bike beneath them, it's still helpful to keep in mind. To lessen impact, get as low as possible when you feel yourself going down.

PUT IT TO PRACTICE. The only way to make falling second nature is to practice, says Hines, who recommends simply rolling and tumbling to get the idea into your brain. Regular somersaults are good, he says, but after you tuck your chin to your chest, let your body roll on your shoulder, not your head. Also consider taking a judo or karate class, which will show you a lot of ways to fall properly.

ROAD RASH RX

Sooner or later, all cyclists hit the deck, and the almost inevitable result is road rash. Such abrasions usually require only basic care. Wyoming-based Helen Iams, MD, developed a preferred course of treatment as the staff doctor for the Jelly Belly Pro cycling team. She has also served as the medical director for races such as the U. S. Pro Criterium Championships. "Pro riders give me lots of practice with road rash," says Iams. Here's her prescription for fast healing after a close encounter with the pavement.

FIRST RESPONSE. Before sizing up skin loss, evaluate the injured person's whole self. "I've had riders come into the medical tent with cracked-open helmets, but no idea they had hit their head," says Iams. If you're with a group and the injured rider has slowed or slurred speech, call for medical assistance. Solo? That's a good reason to carry a cell phone. Got a gash that's more than a scrape? Iams's rule: If you can't stop the bleeding by applying pressure for 15 minutes, you need stitches.

FIELD DRESSING. Postcrash, a cyclist often sprays the wound with his water bottle. "That's not a bad idea to get rid of dirt," Iams says. "But the bacteria on the bottle valve are bad." Antiseptic wipes are Iams's top pick. Or try her secret remedy: Preparation H wipes, which include witch hazel and a little soap.

GET THE GRIT OUT. Wash the rash as soon as you get home. To clean it well, says Iams, you should begin with painkillers. She starts by blanketing the wound with 4x4-inch gauze pads saturated with nonprescription Band-Aid antiseptic wash.

Back in the Pack

Chris Carmichael helps you get your mojo back after a crash.

Once you've hit the deck, it's natural to be nervous about riding again. But getting over your fear is essential to staying safe. When you're scared, you hesitate or change your mind midstream and become even more likely to crash again. If you have recently fallen or had a frightening close call, try these strategies.

CRASHED IN A CORNER
Go to an empty parking lot and practice cornering. Start by focusing on technique at low to moderate speeds. Get comfortable moving around atop the bike, relax and have fun.

CRASHED MIDPACK
Bring two friends to a field or empty road. Have them ride side by side with just enough space for you in between. Practice going through that hole, rubbing shoulders, hips and elbows on your way through. As you gain confidence, your friends can try to box you out.

CROSSED WHEELS
Grab a buddy, head to a field and practice tapping his rear wheel with your front at low speeds. Progress to riding 10 feet with wheels overlapped and rubbing. Focus on being agile, staying over your bike so you can use hips, shoulders and hands to pull back off the wheel or stay upright when the wheel accelerates off your front.

"The antiseptic wash has lidocaine, a local anesthetic," she says. "I let the gauze soak in for a few minutes until the nerves are numbed." (Iams cautions that large quantities of lidocaine can cause an irregular heartbeat, so avoid overuse.) Then Iams gently wipes the grime from the scrape using soap and water. "You need to get all the grit, bits of asphalt—everything," she says.

Stay clear of iodine, alcohol and hydrogen peroxide. "Those damage skin cells," she says. "The less damage there is to the skin, the faster it heals." For stubborn, sticky contaminants like road tar, Iams recommends baby oil or Dawn dish soap. "Either will dissolve the tar, and you won't need to scrub."

LET THE HEALING BEGIN. After you wash the area, cover the abrasion to keep it clean and moist. Iams applies Bacitracin, which kills bacteria and prevents the wound from drying or sticking to the bandage. Then she uses generic, nonstick, gauze-type bandages, secured with silk tape. "I use cheap dressings until the oozing slows down, maybe a few days," she says. Then it's time for advanced hydrocolloid bandages like Tegaderm—precious stuff for road-rash victims. "Put them on, and just leave them for a week until they fall off," she says. "They keep bacteria out, but let water come through and evaporate." Iams's other days-after tips: Ice the afflicted area to reduce swelling, and use acetaminophen for pain—not ibuprofen, which thins blood and can increase bruising. If you have any concerns, hotfoot it to your doctor.

CHAPTER 10

The Real World—From Wind and Rain to Rutted Roads

Cycling magazines and catalogs depict riding at its best: The sun is shining, the pavement is smooth, and the rider is all smiles. But this section is about how to deal when conditions are less than perfect—whether you're being chased by a farmer's dog, or it's raining cats and dogs.

BREAK WIND

The wind is an equal-opportunity element: It batters everyone, from tough old pros to weekend warriors. Consider a rider pedaling along at a brisk, 20-mph pace in calm conditions. If a headwind of only 10 mph kicks up, the rider's speed drops to 16 mph for the same effort. Forces of nature may be beyond our control, but there are ways to minimize the breeze's smackdown. Here are a few pointers for punching through the wind, plus advice from Dominique Rollin, the Cervélo Test Team pro who won an infamously blustery stage of the 2008 Tour of California.

TUCK. It sounds obvious enough: If you duck down on the bike, you're less exposed to the wind. But there's more to it than just improved aerodynamics. "By crouching, you get more compact on the bike," says Rollin. "But with your hands on the drops you also have more control when a gust blows at you." In other words, you have a better chance of keeping your bike pointed forward and out of roadside ditches.

STREAMLINE. The more formfitting your clothing, the less energy the wind will sap from you, which is why bike-specific clothing is a wiser choice than general outdoor garb. To prevent your jersey or jacket from filling up with air, pull zippers up to your chin.

DRAFT. The stronger the headwind, the more it helps to tuck in behind another rider. Sticking as close as safely possible to the wheel in front of you dramatically cuts the number of watts required to maintain your speed. Energy savings of 10 to 30 percent are possible, depending on variables such as the size of each rider and the direction and magnitude of the

Chris Carmichael's Top Aero Tips

Don't have access to a wind tunnel? Here are three tips for improving your aerodynamics on any road ride.

→**Lead with your chin.** Not all the time, but when you're focusing on being aero, lower your head by bringing your chin down and forward, toward your stem.

→**Maximize your horizontals.** Any part of your body that's horizontal should present only its leading edge to the wind. Lower your elbows so your forearms are parallel to the ground. This may mean that riding on the hoods might be better than moving down to the drops.

→**Coast downhill with your cranks level.** Analysis of descending positions from Discovery Channel riders in 2005 showed their drag numbers were lower when their pedals were level compared with having one pedal down.

wind. Of course, you need to share the work. Take a 30-second pull on the front before swinging off and letting the next rider in line move through. The quick turnover ensures that fresh legs are doing the grunt work.

SALUTE. Look for flags and weather vanes— they'll show you what direction the wind is blowing. Often, you're not pedaling straight into a headwind, but rather encountering a breeze from one side. In a group, use the wind direction to your advantage: When it's blowing from the right, position yourself behind and a little to the left of the rider in front of you. For maximum shelter, fine-tune your position by feel. Watch the pros in a spring Classic, and you might see a staggered row of riders spread gutter-to-gutter clear across the road (yes, closed to traffic)—that's an echelon, one of the sport's most beautiful sights.

PERSEVERE. Just making the effort to suit up and head out into a whipping wind takes willpower, so start with something forgiving. "Don't head straight into the wind—you'll just want to go home," says Rollin. "Start on sheltered roads, then return on open roads where you can feel the wind at your back." Rollin also advises staying conservative. "Wind is like a climb: You hit the lower slopes and you get all excited," he says. "If you suddenly turn into the wind, you may feel faster by pushing a bigger gear, but your muscles will fatigue more quickly and you'll end up going slower. To stay efficient, use a smaller gear." And keep it fun, he says: "Ride with friends. You can echelon and play with the wind."

NEITHER RAIN, NOR SLEET. . .

Roads and weather aren't always cycling friendly, especially in late fall and early spring. That doesn't mean you should sit on the sidelines. After all, if you want to boost your performance, putting some miles in during those months can give you a jump-start on the rest of the season. With these basics, you can turn any soggy outing into an enjoyable, fitness-boosting spin and emerge unscathed.

USE COMMON SENSE. If a storm recently spread a quarter-inch of ice on the roads, put the bike back on the trainer until conditions improve. Obvious advice, we know. We also know that most cyclists have at some point, despite knowing better, found themselves on dangerously slick roads asking, "What was I thinking?"

GET KNOBBY. Slap cyclocross tires on your road bike for extra traction and additional protection against punctures. The added rolling resistance means you'll go slower for a given effort, which in turn cuts down on your self-made windchill and makes you less likely to career into obstacles or debris patches in your path. Plus, when you switch back to your regular tires you'll feel like a superhero.

DON'T BE A JERK. Sudden movements, such as grabbing a handful of brake or being aggressive in corners, especially in iffy conditions, will surely land you on your butt. Instead, stay centered on the bike and look far enough ahead that you have plenty of time to slow down for corners or react to slick patches. If you do encounter sand or ice, level your pedals, point your bike straight ahead, relax your upper body and exhale as you cross. If you have to pedal over a larger patch, keep your stroke extra smooth with steady, even pressure on the pedals—no quick stabs.

DEHUMIDIFY YOURSELF. Nothing sucks the life out of a ride more than being wet and cold. The right clothing varies with the temperature, but, in a nutshell, you want a base layer that wicks moisture away from your skin (crucial, as the chill from sweat often sneaks up on you so you're cold before you can react to it), a midlayer for insulation, and a shell with a windproof front to block the breeze. Layers should be easy to shed so you can stash them in a pocket. On your lower body, windproof crotch and knee panels are essential when weather is truly foul.

MIND YOUR MACHINE. Mix road salt and grit with a little water and you get a crunchy solution that chews through bike parts faster than a seven-year-old can gorge on his Easter basket haul. To minimize damage, clean and lube your chain after every ride. Remember the last step in the clean-and-lube: Thoroughly wipe down the chain. Clean any stuck-in gunk from the chainrings, cassette and pedal bodies, as well as any exposed cables. Then check your brake pads: Grit can become trapped on and in them and grind down your rims when you brake. Even if you use a spare set of wheels as your beater hoops, you can save them from an early demise by inspecting your brake pads frequently and replacing them if they're full of embedded grit (you can pick out smaller amounts) or if they're approaching the wear-indicator mark.

DOG FIGHTING

When a blur of teeth and slobber gives chase, most cyclists instinctively sprint, reach for the pump to nail the dog in the head, unclip to kick him in the gut, or scream profanities—all exactly the wrong responses, according to experts.

"I wouldn't suggest being aggressive at all," says Suzanne Hetts, PhD, a certified applied animal behaviorist. "There's so much potential for that to backfire and arouse the dog even more." Most dogs aren't out to hurt you, she says—they think you're just a big ball to chase, or a rude invader who needs a verbal spanking.

The key to safely riding away is to rein in your fear and act with confidence, says Steve Schmitt, a licensed certified instructor for the League of American Bicyclists. Trying to hit or kick a dog is just as likely to cause you to crash as it is to repel the beast, says Schmitt. Chemical sprays can blow back into your face (then you'll be blind, gagging and crashing). Shouting can incite dogs rather than scare them, and if you try to outrun dogs you risk colliding with them when they intercept you.

Here are 7 tactics our experts recommend:

→Stop. If you're not moving, you're less exciting, and the dog might lose interest.

→Impersonate the owner, says Schmitt. Look at the pooch and use a strong, steady "bad dog" voice.

→If your routes are routinely plagued by problem dogs, or you're canine-phobic, carry an air horn. It's the best deterrent, say both Schmitt and Hetts.

→Use only a nontoxic spray such as Direct Stop. Dogs don't like the citrus odor but you won't be bothered if it accidentally blows into your face.

→Toss treats or tennis balls. This will distract or surprise the friendly dogs just looking to play, says Hetts.

→With a dog that's out for blood, sprinting could make things worse. Get off, and put the bike between you.

→If you do fall and are attacked, get into the fetal position with your hands clasped over your neck. Stay still. You'll be bitten more if you struggle.

A GOOD RIDE ON BAD ROADS

Former Olympian and current USA Cycling coach David Brinton rides bikes for a living—and he used to get paid to crash them, too. "I was a professional stuntman," he says. "So I know how to take a fall." In the event you prefer to stay upright, Brinton tells how he handles his bike in eight common road hazards.

GRAVELLY OR CHIP-SEALED ROADS. "It's better to pedal through than to coast," says Brinton. Propulsion provides stability. There is such a thing as too much speed, though. If you start sliding, back off the power (without braking) while staying in the saddle to keep your bike planted.

GRAVELLED CORNERS. Take the turn wide and lean your bike more than normal at the beginning. Straighten the bike as you approach the gravel, then, once on clear road, resume leaning. "It's pretty much the opposite of how I recommend taking turns in normal conditions," says Brinton.

WET ROADS. The first minutes of a rainfall are the most dangerous, Brinton says. "Before the oil residue from cars is washed away it creates

Don't Beat 'Em, Join 'Em

Tips for riding with Rover

Dogs are always eager to get out the door, follow you up a sick grade or get lost on a new trail. And your dog will respect you no matter how much wind you suck. But remember, your canine buddy will do anything to stick with you—including running itself to death. Just like ours, their muscles and bones need to be conditioned, as does their cardiorespiratory system, says Craig Angle, a certified coach and a research associate at the veterinary sports medicine program at Alabama's Auburn University. And, he says, "The dog doesn't have the luxury of coasting."

Angle and other experts recommend that before you take your pooch pedaling, you should have a vet perform a checkup for general health, then ease into the long distances with a training program that builds gradually. Be extra watchful in hot weather (paved surfaces can get hot enough to burn a dog's paws). If your dog won't drink out of a water bottle, carry a portable dish. And check for thorns or tears in the dog's pads at every rest break.

The best dogs for cycling have long legs, a long snout and short hair, says Angle. Sprint dogs such as greyhounds will blow up; short-legged dogs and squashed-nose dogs are built for walking. Here are five dogs that are friendly—and athletic enough to maintain a 7- to 12-mile-per-hour pace for up to 10 miles with sprint speeds between 20 and 30 mph, after training.

AUSTRALIAN CATTLE DOG
Pennsylvania breeder Monica Shifflet says the ACD is a "Velcro dog" whose athletic build, stamina and smarts mean yours will follow you everywhere. But remember that the ACD was bred to herd cattle—and might occasionally be tempted to run off and return with cows.

BRITTANY
The Brittany's legendary energy and endurance can boost your workout. As with all bird dogs, the hunting instinct can override caution, so keep your Brittany on a leash near roads.

POINTER
Pointers were bred to go all day long in the field, looking for game. That translates into a high-powered cycling companion. Watch that your dog's birding instincts don't take him near cars.

SIBERIAN HUSKY
The Siberian husky is the quintessential long-distance dog. Its love of running needs to be tempered in hot weather. Though their double coat won't grow as thick in warmer climates, it makes it harder for huskies to cool down.

WEIMARANER
The swiftest in the group, the weimaraner won't stop—even if it runs its pads off. "They are a nightmare without exercise," says dog handler and cyclist Mara Wildfeuer of California. Short, light coats prevent overheating, and what Wildfeur calls a "co-dependency gene" ensures they'll return to their human when they inevitably take off after birds or squirrels.

a slick film." To turn, exaggerate the normal cornering technique of driving weight into the lowered, outside pedal. This helps your tires grip the road as much as possible.

PAINT STRIPES. The slickest parts of any wet road are the lane markings, says Brinton. To stay safe, cross them as close to a right angle as you can. If you get forced onto a slick road line, avoid an abrupt reaction. "Clear the line gradually," he advises.

POTHOLES. Swerving around potholes makes sense—unless there's traffic or you're surprised by one while riding in the middle of a group. Learn to lightly roll or hop over holes. "Master popping the front wheel over small cracks," says Brinton. "Once you can do that, practice popping the rear wheel over the same crack." When you can clear both wheels separately, combine the two maneuvers. With your pedals parallel to the road, pull up on the handlebar while lifting your feet. "For most potholes you don't even need a full bunnyhop," says Brinton. "At 25 miles per hour, all you really need to do is take a little bit of your bike weight off the road and your wheels will float right over." And, as with all hazards, a pack should flow smoothly around a pothole rather than degenerating into a frenzy of bunnyhops. It's up to the lead riders to steer the pack from the front, gently weaving around hazards while pointing them out with a finger.

PARALLEL CRACKS. If your wheel gets caught in a crack running the length of the street, chances are you'll shred either rubber or skin. To cross a parallel crack, lean your bike slightly toward the damaged pavement, then pop your front wheel sideways so it clears the crack. If your wheels get caught in the crack, pull directly up on the front wheel, and it will automatically pop out and to the side.

ROADKILL. As with resolving the grief you feel for the poor critters, the key to avoiding them is to look ahead. It's a well-known adage that your bike goes where your eyes focus. Look about 20 yards up the road, not 5.

COBBLED AND BRICK ROADS. "Avoid death-gripping the bar," says Brinton, "and use your arms as a suspension system for the rest of your body." Push a bigger gear than normal, which floats your butt just above the saddle. Just like in mountain biking, let the bike find its own, natural line through cobbles. On brick roads, slot into the path smoothed out by car tires.

RIDER **RESOURCES**

Learn how to ride safely in traffic at one of the League of American Bicyclists' Smart Cycling classes (bikeleague.org).

Carmichael Training Systems (trainright.com) offers a variety of camps; topics include road skills, climbing and women's cycling.

If you're a police officer, firefighter, EMT or other public safety official, you may be eligible to take skills courses offered by the International Police Mountain Bike Association (ipmba.org).

IV

Bike Maintenance

IT'S TIME TO GET UP CLOSE AND PERSONAL WITH your bike. While the prospect of taking things apart can be daunting ("hmm, I'm pretty sure I had two of these little springs before . . . "), learning to perform simple repairs will make you more self-sufficient on the road, and can potentially save you money. Of course, if you screw something up, wrenching at home can end up costing you money— which is why we're here to help.

CHAPTER 11

Your Home Workshop

A well-equipped workbench can make the difference between a stellar ride and downtime at the bike shop. Here you'll find the tools and supplies every cyclist should own, instructions for building your own workstand, and a list of household items you can use to work on your bike in a pinch.

WORKSHOP ESSENTIALS

SPOKE WRENCH. No common household tool can replace a spoke wrench, used to true wheels and replace broken spokes. Spoke nipples come in a variety of sizes, so make sure to get the correct size wrench, or you'll round off the nipple. Steer clear of multi-size spoke wrenches, which tend to have a sloppy fit.

CHAINWHIP/CASSETTE LOCKRING. Removing and installing a rear cog is a two-minute job with these tools, and nearly impossible without them. The chainwhip holds the cassette in place while the lockring is loosened. Shimano lockrings are the same for road and mountain bikes, so its tool works on both (and on Shimano's Centerlock disc rotors, too). Campagnolo uses a different size lockring and tool.

CHAIN BREAKER. This allows the removal and installation of a chain. It precisely drives out the chain's pin, then drives in a replacement connecting pin. It's a tool you won't use often, but if you damage a chain or wear one out and want to replace it yourself, you'll be glad you have it.

TORQUE WRENCH. Almost every nut and bolt on your bicycle has a recommended torque setting—undertightening can cause slipping; overtightening can cause parts to fail. You want everything just right. Standard torque wrenches can be very expensive, but Park's bike-specific TW-1 ($\frac{1}{4}$-inch drive, 0-60 in./lb. range) and TW-2 ($\frac{3}{8}$-inch drive, 0-600 in./lb. range) are more economical beam-style wrenches that are very easy to use (parktool.com).

LUBE AND GREASE. Chain lube is essential to keep your drivetrain running smoothly. Some lubes, such as Tri-Flow (triflowlubricants.com), also work well on cables. Use quality grease, such as Finish Line with Teflon (finishlineusa.com), on bearings and bolt threads to prevent water contamination and corrosion.

TIRE LEVERS. Don't even think of going near your wheel with a screwdriver; you'll get the tire on or off but you're likely to damage the tire, tube and rim in the process. Plastic tire levers gently lift the tire's bead into place without marring the rim. They usually come in sets of three and cost less than five bucks, so throw a second set into your seatbag while you're at it.

HEX TOOLS. Once you own a Y hex wrench, you'll never want to be without one. It's made up of 4-, 5-, and 6-mm hex wrenches (the sizes needed for most bike repairs), and the convenient shape provides ample leverage on most bicycle fasteners. In addition, be sure you have a basic set of hex tools, from 2mm to 8mm, to cover what the Y tool doesn't. Full-size wrenches give you better torque and easier access to tight spots than folding or mini versions, and installing bottle cages and adjusting front derailleurs usually requires an individual hex wrench, due to space constraints. We like Park Tool's HSX-2, which has a few nice additions: a holder to keep wrenches organized and easy to grab, ball ends (which allow for angled usage in tight spots) and a short sleeve that allows you to spin the wrench to speed up installation of longer screws.

FLOOR PUMP. Tire pressure affects your bike's comfort, speed, handling—and even safety. And although your road tires may have a maximum pressure of 125 psi, that might not be the pressure you should use; most riders of average height and weight will experience optimal performance with less than the maximum stated pressure. Despite its inelegant name, Bike Hard's PumpHard 4.0 (bikehard.com) is one of the most fully featured pumps around. The large, heavy steel base makes it stable, the rubber-coated handle is comfortably contoured, and the action is smooth and precise. The generous stroke length fills tires quickly (700x23 to 100 psi in 20 strokes), the top-mounted gauge is clear and easy to read, the chuck automatically adapts to presta or Schrader, and there's a bleed-off button in case you overfill.

HEAVY-DUTY CITRUS DEGREASER. When it's time to overhaul a drivetrain, a dose of this stuff and a bit of scrubbing will have your chain, cassette and chainrings sparkling and ready for your favorite lube. You can also use it for overhauling bearings, removing adhesives and, diluted, it can be used to clean other materials. (Test it first, especially on plastics and rubbers, to be sure it doesn't cause damage.)

EZ ONE #5 BOX OF RAGS. Yup, it's five pounds of rags (nationruskin.com), all different sizes. Use them for a host of jobs: cleaning bikes, tools and hands; wiping excess grease or lube; mopping spills; as protective padding when packing your bike. The list is endless.

TORPEDO LEVEL, TAPE MEASURE, AND A BIKE FIT SYSTEMS PLUMB BOB. If you know your preferred saddle height, saddle offset and reach dimensions, these tools will help you set up a new bike quickly and accurately. Or use them to experiment with your positioning to find more performance or comfort. Start by writing down your original position (so you can return to neutral), then make small changes, one at a time, to your saddle offset or height. For info go to empirelevel.com and bikefit.com.

BUILD YOUR OWN REPAIR STAND

If you want to learn how to do your own bicycle wrenching, you'll need to start with one basic tool: a workstand. (After all, turning the cranks to make adjustments won't work if your wheels are touching the ground.) Commercial stands are nice, but they can be pricey. Besides, with 30 bucks, a trip to The Home Depot, and a couple of hours, you can build your own customized work station. Here, Jim Langley, author of the e-book Your Home Bicycle Workshop (roadbikerider.com/hbw_page.htm), shows you how it's done.

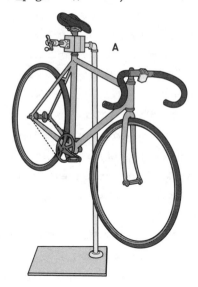

1. BRUSH BASE. Paint the plywood—the semi-gloss finish makes removing lube and dirt easier. When it's dry, position the pipe flange about 4 inches in from one corner and mark where the four flange holes are. Remove the flange and drill through the wood on the marks, making sure to countersink the holes on the underside of the plywood so the nuts are flush. Then bolt the flange into place with the 1x $\frac{1}{4}$-inch bolts.

2. POSITION PIPES. Screw the 5-foot section of pipe into the flange until it's tight. Then screw the reducer elbow onto the top until it's tight and facing in—toward the corner of the base opposite the flange. Then screw the 2-foot pipe to the elbow (A).

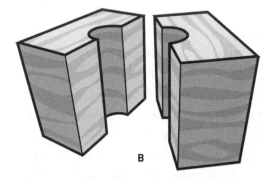

3. MAKE JAWS. Drill a hole a little larger than the diameter of your largest seatpost lengthwise down the middle of the 4x4 wood block. (For example, for a 27.2-mm-diameter seatpost, drill a $1\frac{1}{8}$-inch hole.) Then saw the block—and hole—in half lengthwise (B).

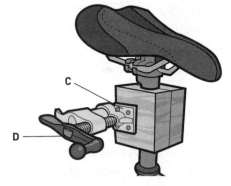

4. PREP PONY. Drill four holes into each Pony clamp jaw—one in each corner (C). Then slide the Pony clamp parts onto the horizontal arm and screw on the handle end, locking it in so the horizontal edge of the clamp is 10 degrees below parallel with the ground (D). This angle ensures that in

The Ingredients

→ One 3x3-foot piece of 1-inch plywood or particleboard (this is the base of the stand)

→ Semigloss paint (to paint the base)

→ One 1-inch threaded pipe flange (for joining the upright to the base)

→ Four each: 1 x ¼-inch bolts, washers and nuts (for attaching the flange to the base)

→ One 5-foot section (or whatever length best fits your height) of 1-inch diameter pipe, threaded on both ends (this is the upright)

→ One 1 x ¾-inch, 90-degree reducer pipe elbow (for joining the arm to the upright)

→ One 2-foot section of ¾-inch diameter pipe, threaded on both ends (this is the arm)

→ One 5-inch section of 4 x 4 (to make the clamp jaws)

→ One Pony clamp fixture (style no. 50; go here to see what it looks like: adjustableclamp.com/cf50)

→ Eight 1-inch screws (for attaching the jaws to the clamp)

the stand your bike's front wheel will be lower than the rear and not swing when you're working.

5. CLAMP IT. Holding the wood block together as it was before you cut it in half, place it between the Pony clamps so the seatpost hole is running vertically. Then tighten the Pony clamp to hold the block in place, and drill and screw it to the wood jaws using the 1-inch screws.

6. USE STAND. With the Pony clamp open, carefully lift your bike and place the seatpost between the jaws. Turn the handle to tighten the clamp and hold your bike in the perfect position. TIP: Line the wooden jaws with recycled innertubes to prevent scratching.

TOOLS ON HAND

If you feel a sudden urge to put the shine on your bike, but don't have the bike-specific tools for the job, look no further than home sweet home.

TOOTHBRUSH. When your Oral-B starts to look like you've been scrubbing the toilet with it, throw it into your bike-cleaning bucket. Use it to clean hard-to-reach spots and tiny bolts.

CARDBOARD. One corrugated box can floss a lot of grimy cassettes. The cardboard is just the right thickness to fit between and hit both sides of the cogs.

SCOTCH-BRITE. These fuzzy green pads not only remove baked-on lasagna, they can also clean brake pads and rim sidewalls for better braking. Another use: After a ride, lightly hold one against each tire while you spin the wheels in both directions; it'll snag debris from the rubber.

DISH DETERGENT. A mild, grease-cutting dish soap such as Dawn can gently clean your frame, but also has the goods to remove light gunk from your drivetrain. And dish sponges? Use old ones to clean chains, cassettes and pedals; use new ones on your saddle, bar tape and frame.

CHAPTER 12

Do It Yourself

Even if you plan on leaving the bigger repairs, such as truing wheels or overhauling your suspension fork, to the professionals, a little at-home maintenance can give you more hours to ride (especially during peak season, when shops won't be able to look at your bike right away). And giving your bike a little love between tune-ups will help it last longer.

In this chapter, you'll find a guide to your bike's parts—and instructions on when to replace them, advice on preserving the longevity of your components, and step-by-step solutions to some common problems and repairs. If any of the fixes described here take you out of your comfort zone, don't be afraid to take your bike to the shop—if you ask nicely, the mechanics might even pass on some of their knowledge. And when you're ready for a new maintenance challenge, check out the *Bicycling Guide to Complete Bicycle Maintenance & Repair* (rodalestore.com).

EASY SOLUTIONS TO COMMON PROBLEMS

Shut Up Your Bike

Here are three sounds every bike inevitably makes, and how to make them go away.

SQUEAKY SEAT. Your peaceful ride is interrupted by a distracting sound coming from your saddle—like a broken spring in a roll-out cot.

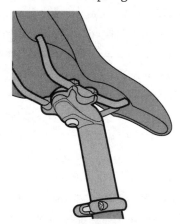

The problem: Your seat- and seatpost-clamp bolts may not be properly lubricated.

What to do: Remove your saddle from your post and treat the saddle bolt or bolts, depending on your type of seatpost, and seat rails with a small amount of grease such as Park Tool Poly Lube. Then remove the seat-clamp bolt and

Which Lube Goes Where?

Grease and oil—they're not the same thing. Before you slop any old lube onto your bike's moving parts, think logically (bike-specific grease: good; leftover French fry oil: bad)—and follow the instructions on the lubricant's label or in your part's manufacturer's manual. As a general rule, bike grease, because it's thicker and won't drip, is best used for ball bearings, threaded parts, axles and bottom brackets—places that not only need lubrication, but also have a tendency to get stuck over time with use and corrosion. Use oil-based bike lubricants on brake and derailleur pivot points, chain links, cassette bearings and cables—hard-to-reach areas and those prone to attracting crud.

grease not only the bolt, but also where the clamp contacts the frame. Before you put it back together, apply a light layer of grease inside the seat tube. If you have a carbon-fiber frame, use a carbon-prep paste such as Syntace's Friction Paste (syntace.com). Grease may damage clear coats or cause the composite laminate to swell.

CREAKING BOTTOM BRACKET. Every time you turn the cranks, it sounds like you're walking on loose floorboards.

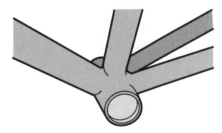

The problem: Your crank bolts, chainring bolts, or bottom bracket aren't properly torqued, or your BB shell is dirty.

What to do: First, snug the crank bolts (using the tool required for your crankset), the bottom bracket (using a BB tool) and the chainring bolts. If the creak remains, remove the cranks and bottom bracket, then clean the BB shell with a clean rag and Finish Line Speed Degreaser. Apply a

generous amount of grease inside the shell, reinstall the BB and cranks, and tighten everything.

SCREECHING BRAKES. You hear a sound like fingernails on a chalkboard when you squeeze a brake lever.

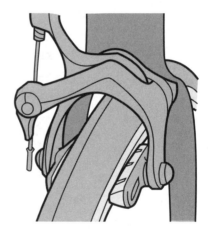

The problem: Your brake pad and rim surfaces have a buildup of crud on them.

What to do: Remove your wheel. Using a clean rag and Finish Line Speed Degreaser or plain rubbing alcohol, clean both sides of the rim. Then, with a flat file or a piece of medium-grit sandpaper, lightly scuff both brake-pad surfaces.

Before reinstalling the wheel, make sure your pads are properly toed in; the front of the pad should touch the rim right before the rear hits.

Anatomy of a Bike

Saddle

Stem

Shift/Brake levers

Head tube

Headset

Top tube

Seatpost

Seat collar

Rear brake

Seat tube

Cogs/Cassettes

Seatstay

Chainrings

Drop handlebar

Front brakes

Fork

Down tube

Crankarm

Rim

Rear derailleur

Chainstay

Front derailleur

Pedal

Hub

Chain

Stanchion

Brake lever

Trigger shifter

Compression strut

Pivots

Rear hydraulic brake caliper

Linkage

Cables

Fork

Spokes

Bottle boss

Tire

Lowers

Shock

Front disc brake rotor

Rear disc brake rotor

Chainstay

Front hydraulic brake caliper

DON'T TRASH IT

"Archimedes said he could move the world with a lever and a place to stand," says Jerry Kraynick, owner of Kraynick's bike shop in Pittsburgh. "Well, with the right tool and enough leverage, you can make any repair." Here's his best advice for getting through three of the most difficult repairs without damaging your bike.

Mount a Tire with Your Hands

It's better to put on a tire without levers if you can. Because the levers can pinch a tube against the rim and puncture it before you ever get a chance to ride it, hands are the best tools for this job. But many people say the tire is too tight to slip on by hand, says Jerry. "I threaten to get my wife in the shop to show them how it's done," he says, and the tire is usually on the rim before he can dial the phone. If you don't want to use the power of embarrassment, try Jerry's other method: While sitting, place the bottom of the wheel on your feet and brace the top of the rim on your knees. Wrap your hands around the top of the tire with your fingers on the bead. Pull the bead over the rim slowly, one finger at a time.

Remove a Rusted Seatpost

For a steel post, spray the seat tube-seatpost juncture with a penetrating oil, like PB Blaster; for aluminum, use ammonia. (Carbon posts are rare at Kraynick's, so you're on your own there.) Clamp the frame vertically, so it's pointing up and down, into a stand by the top tube. (Don't do this with thin-wall aluminum tubes or carbon tubes.) Grab the nose of your seat while a friend holds the down tube, then pull in opposite directions.

Unstick a Pedal

Clamp your bike upside down in a stand or set it on the floor on its handlebar and saddle. Stand in front of the bar. Turn the cranks so the stubborn pedal is farther away from you. Hold the opposite chainstay with your arm over the forward pedal to keep it stable. Position the pedal wrench slightly above horizontal and press down. For more power, slip a pipe over the wrench handle to extend your leverage.

MAINTAIN YOUR BRAKES

Bad weather can spell disaster for brakes. Mud, road grit and water accelerate wear, cause corrosion and may leave you stopping Fred Flintstone–style. Here are signs of wear to watch for and tips to keep your brakes working year-round.

Pro Tip

"IF YOU TOTALLY CLOG YOUR MOUNTAIN BIKE WITH MUD, WATER IS ALREADY IN THERE, SO GO AHEAD AND USE YOUR GARDEN HOSE TO SPRAY IT DOWN. JUST FOLLOW IT UP WITH A COMPLETE PROFESSIONAL OVERHAUL—ONCE A YEAR OR MORE FREQUENTLY IF YOU RIDE IN MUD A LOT—TO REPLACE HYDRAULIC OIL OR LUBE OIL. THE INNARDS GET DIRTY, NO MATTER HOW WELL YOU CLEAN THE OUTSIDE."—*"BICYCLE BOB" GREGORIO, MOUNTAIN BIKE HALL OF FAMER AND MECHANIC AT DURANGO CYCLERY IN COLORADO*

RIM BRAKES. Signs of wear: The grooves in your pads are thin or unevenly worn. You hear a grinding noise or braking feels less precise than normal.

Know this: Those grooves are there to channel debris away from your rims, and that noise may be coming from objects lodged in the grooves. Pads that lasted all summer and are half-worn can wear down to the metal in one wet, nasty ride. Even brand-new pads can wear out in one ride.

Do this: Check for embedded objects in the pads. Even if everything seems fine, check pads often and always put a fresh set on your rim brakes for the winter months.

DISC BRAKES. Signs of wear: Most disc brake manufacturers recommend pad replacement when there's 0.5 to 1mm of pad material left.

Know this: Disc brakes offer the most stopping power and wear the best in adverse conditions, but they can still succumb to the effects of winter—even wearing out in one muddy or wet, sandy ride.

Do this: Although hydraulic brakes are well sealed and rarely become contaminated, change the brake fluid at least once during the winter, because moisture inside the system can cause corrosion and heat-related brake fade. Mechanical discs work well as long as the cables are in good condition (see Cables, below).

CABLES. Signs of wear: Your brakes feel rough and are hard to pull when you squeeze them.

Know this: Water can contaminate cables and create friction caused by corrosion and dirt. Friction reduces overall braking power and your ability to modulate it. In really cold climates, water in the cables can freeze.

Do this: Pull the housing out of the frame stops, slide it back, and wipe the cable dry and clean. Apply a lightweight lubricant such as Rock N Roll's Cable Magic (rocklube.com) to reduce friction and help displace water. Also consider using sealed ferrules or shielded housing, such as Avid's Flak Jacket (avidbike.com), or running full-length housing to the rear brake to avoid contamination. Also, replace cables often during the winter and avoid blasting them with a strong hose when washing.

RIMS. Signs of wear: Your rim is worn so thin that it fails, causing the tire to blow off, the tube to explode and the sidewall of the rim to fold outward. If you're lucky, this will happen while you're pumping up the tire, not midride.

Know this: Rim brakes, when exposed to gritty road grime and off-road mud, can grind down the rim's surface.

Pro **Tip**

"CHECK THE TORQUE ON DISC BRAKE ROTOR BOLTS EVERY SIX MONTHS—THEY BECOME LOOSE OVER TIME FROM VIBRATION. ALSO CHECK PADS FOR WEAR—IF THERE'S LESS THAN 1MM OF PAD MATERIAL LEFT, THEY MUST BE REPLACED. PAY ATTENTION TO HYDRAULIC DISC BRAKE PADS. THEY SELF-ADJUST TO COMPENSATE FOR WEAR, SO EVEN IF THEY FEEL FINE THEY COULD BE JUST ABOUT SHOT. AND THE LAST THING YOU WANT TO EXPERIENCE ON AN EPIC RIDE IS METAL ON METAL."—*FRANK TROTTER, MECHANIC AND MANAGER FOR TEAM GIANT*

Do this: There's no easy fix for worn rims; replacement is the only answer. Some manufacturers machine depressions into the sidewall to serve as wear indicators. Place a straightedge against the rim; if it's concave, it should be inspected by an experienced mechanic and will likely need to be replaced.

Repair a Broken Chain

Neglect the string of links that keeps your drivetrain working, and your epic day of riding could turn into an even more epic day of walking. Follow these tips to care for, replace and repair your chain.

1. Lube your chain at least once a month, or more often if necessary. Use a dry lube, such as Rock "N" Roll Extreme ($6/4 oz.), if you ride in arid conditions, because it won't attract dust. If you ride in muddy, wet conditions, you need a more viscous grease that'll stay put, such as Finish Line's WET Lube ($5/2 oz.; finishlineusa.com). Drip lubricant onto each link of your chain as you backpedal. After a few rotations, wipe off the excess lube with a clean, dry rag. To make your chain positively spotless, use a clamp-on chain scrubber or remove the chain and clean it in degreaser.

2. Before installing a new chain, it's important to cut it to t he correct length. If you're replacing a chain that worked fine before, cut the new one to the same length. If you're starting from scratch or replacing a damaged chain, shift into the big ring/big cog combo and thread the chain through the derailleurs and around the big chainring. Pull the chain so the cage of the rear derailleur falls at about the 4 or 5 o'clock position (6 o'clock is too

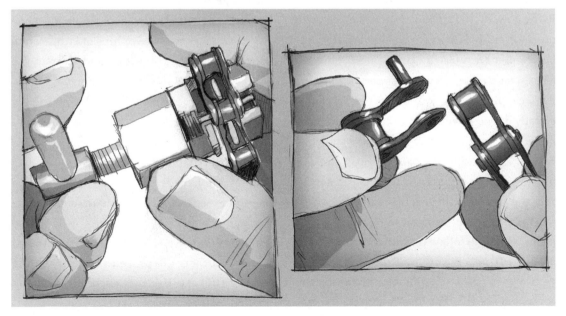

slack, 3 is too tight), then mark the pin you need to remove. If your bike has rear suspension, let the air out of the shock (or remove the spring if it's a coil-over shock) and bottom out the suspension before you measure—chainstay growth could snap the derailleur if you happen to be in the big ring/big cog combo and bottom out the suspension. The goal is to get the chain as short as possible without setting it up for potential failure.

Treat Your Carbon Right

Right now, there's a good chance that the bolts on the stem holding your carbon bar and carbon steerer are too tight. Let us guess: You used a hex wrench to tighten your stem bolts like you were capping a bottle of Coke. You may have already damaged your handlebar and just don't know it. Don't take a tiny crack in your bar lightly. It will eventually and without warning break, and the outcome could be disastrous. Whether you're riding what you think is a perfectly tight setup or installing a new bar and stem, be sure to follow these instructions.

BUY A TORQUE WRENCH. Then find out—in your owner's manual, online or by calling the company—your stem manufacturer's recommendations regarding torque. Once you have that information, use the torque wrench to tighten each bolt on your stem (where it connects to your handlebar as well as where it connects to your steerer tube). You don't have to be a genius; the wrench will let you know when to stop tightening. (In simple terms, a torque wrench is a tool that measures resistance to rotation.)

You'll have to apply very little pressure to reach the recommended torque, and it won't feel as tight as you think it should. Don't worry, you did it right.

MOVE AROUND. You've probably heard all about grease and carbon seatposts and never mixing the two. That's sort of true. While grease has been found to deteriorate the external layer of laminate and eventually weaken the post, a total absence of grease can downright fuse a post into the frame. Head to your local shop and pick up a carbon-prep paste—carbon's answer to grease. Use it to prevent sticking and slipping. Go one step further: Every two to three months, rotate your seatpost and move it up and down in the seat tube to make sure it's not stuck. Over time, your own sweat can actually cause corrosion at the contact points. Too late? See page 90.

Change Your Bar Tape

Wrapping a bar takes practice, and there are plenty of step-by-steps out there to guide you through the process (watch ours at bicycling. com/videotape). Still, there are functional wraps and there are those that approach the level of fine art. Use this expert advice, and your bar will be riding in style.

FLIP IT TO STICK IT. "When working with bar tape that has no sticky back, first wrap electrical tape around the bar end once, then flip the roll—don't cut it—so the sticky side is up, and wrap it around so it covers a couple inches. Turn the tape over again so the sticky side is down, and wrap it once more. This creates a very tacky start to a good tape job."—Mike Spilker, High Gear Cyclery; highgearcyclery.com

WHIP IT GOOD. "Rather than finish off the wrap with electrical tape, I spend a little extra time to cord-whip it. I make a loop with the cord—I like to use thin, round leather cord that you'd find at a craft store—and hold it with one hand under the bar while I start winding the cord around it. After a couple turns over the loop, it will hold itself in place. Start the cord neatly against the ferrule so you start winding nice and square, and wind back over the tape, which I like to stop about ¼-inch short of the ferrule to avoid bulkiness under the cord. When the cord covers about an inch of the tape, put one end through the loop and pull the other end, stopping when it's tucked neatly under the wound cord. Trim the ends of the cord with a sharp knife and apply several coats of clear urethane to waterproof and seal it so it doesn't unravel."—Dave Moulton, ex-framebuilder for Paris Sport, Masi Bicycles and under his own name; davesbikeblog. squarespace.com

MAKE IT SHINE. "I'd heard about shellacking handlebars and kind of laughed. I thought it might make the bar slippery or that it would ruin in the rain. Well, I finally caught the bug and shellacked my cork tape (it's usually done on cloth tape). A few coats made my cork glow—it almost matched my honey-colored Brooks leather saddle. Downside? I put the bike in a hot car and took it to my bike shop to show off. When I removed it, the finish had peeled. Disaster! So much for impressing the shop guys. Then I learned from iBOB, an online bike-lore group (see bikelist.org), that a light rubdown with denatured alcohol revives rumpled shellac. I tried it and it worked great."—Jeff Potter, publisher of *Out Your Back Door*; outyourbackdoor.com

HEAT TREAT IT. "End the tape at the bar top and finish it with electrical tape to hold it in place. Use scissors on the finish tape—don't tear it off. Begin and end the finish wrap on the underside, then use a soldering gun or hex wrench end heated by a cigarette lighter to spot weld the finish tape so it doesn't come loose."—Calvin Jones, director of education, Park Tool; parktool.com

Pro **Tip**

"THE ADVICE 'TIGHTEN ALL BOLTS' IS A BIT OVERSIMPLIFIED. MOST OF THEM, LIKE FOR CRANKS AND DERAILLEURS, YOU WANT TIGHT. BUT ON MORE-FRAGILE AREAS SUCH AS THE FACEPLATE BOLT OF YOUR STEM, STEM CLAMP BOLTS AND SOME SEAT BINDER BOLTS, YOU JUST WANT BOLTS HAND TIGHT TO THE POINT THAT YOUR HANDLEBAR AND SEATPOST DON'T SLIP. THESE ARE THE AREAS WHERE WE SEE THE MOST CRACKS AND FAILURES."—*EVA BARABAS, THE FIRST WOMAN TO WRENCH FOR A UCI-CERTIFIED MEN'S PRO TEAM*

Prevent a Stuck Seatpost

Your seatpost is the unsung hero of your bike's components. Its job is to hold you in the proper position for a pain-free ride. Your job is to pay attention to its wants and needs. If you experience a seatpost setback, one of these tips is sure to get you back in the saddle—safely—in no time.

1. Proper frame prep can have a dramatic impact on the life span of your seatpost. If the seat tube has a sharp edge at the seat clamp, it will dig into the seatpost, causing a stress riser and over time a broken post. Use a round file to smooth the edge to a bevel. If filing your frame makes you feel uneasy, take it to a shop. Seat-clamp torque values are fairly low, so use a torque wrench when tightening, especially on carbon-fiber posts.

2. Use grease or antiseize if your frame is steel, titanium or aluminum and your post is alloy or titanium. If either is carbon fiber, use carbon-prep paste to prevent slippage. If your post creeps down, don't overtighten the seat clamp. Instead, measure the seat tube and post diameters to see if they're compatible. If a slipping post strikes midride, sprinkle the seatpost with fine trail dirt to create friction and bite—a temporary fix.

3. If you didn't follow the previous advice, your seatpost might not budge when you try to move it. Corrosion may be the culprit. Start by applying penetrating oil to the top of the seat tube and through either the water bottle bosses (remove the screws) or by removing the bottom bracket. Let it sit for a day or two and

Pro **Tip**

"NOISE FROM YOUR HEADSET IS TYPICALLY JUST FROM THE DUST SEALS AT THE BOTTOM. A CLEANING AND A LIGHT COATING OF OIL SHOULD TAKE CARE OF IT. IF IT DOESN'T, BEFORE DOING AN OVERHAUL, CHECK THE CAPS ON YOUR CABLE HOUSINGS. IF THEY'RE METAL THEY SOMETIMES CREAK; A LITTLE LUBE OR REPLACING THEM WITH PLASTIC CAPS ARE QUICK FIXES."—*MIKE SPILKER, MANAGER AT HIGH GEAR CYCLERY, STIRLING, NJ*

try again. If this doesn't work, a good mechanic will be able to extract it without destroying your frame—the post may not be so lucky.

4. To quiet a creaking seatpost head, grease the bolts and any mating surfaces and apply a thin film of grease to the seat rails. Tighten the clamp to the recommended torque spec. If you bend a rail in a crash, replace the saddle—even if you straighten it, it'll likely break eventually. If you upgrade to a saddle with oversized rails, make sure your post can accommodate it. If proper fit requires that you set your saddle extremely fore or aft, the increased leverage on the seat rails may cause your post to bend or break. Replace your post with one that has more or less offset.

5. Mark your post (use a permanent marker; etching it can create a stress riser) with your preferred saddle height so you can return it to the proper position if you move it. Follow the maximum and minimum insertion recommendations for your post. If you don't, you could end up with a bent or broken post or frame.

6. Seatposts come in different diameters in increments of 0.2mm. Smaller diameter posts can fit larger seat tubes with the proper shim. Never tighten the seat clamp to make it fit— you'll risk breaking the frame. If you have doubts, your shop will most likely have gauges that accurately indicate the correct size.

Tune Your Suspension to Match Your Riding Style

As the technical training coordinator at SRAM Technical University, Hercules Castro has trained employees from hundreds of dealer locations in the finer points of SRAM's products, including extensive work on RockShox suspension repair, maintenance and tuning. Here are his tips for making your mountain bike ride the way you want it to.

Common knowledge: "The manual that comes with your fork includes everything you need to know, from the basics, like what damping means and what spring rates are, to the more detailed, such as how to set sag and damping. For example, to set rebound damping, stand next to your bike and compress the fork, then pull the handlebar up as fast as you can. The fork should rebound slightly slower than you can pull up. For compression damping, if your fork has little or no travel when it hits a bump, you have to increase low-speed compression damping. If it compresses too much, you have to increase high-speed compression."

Uncommon wisdom: "When changing travel, take into account speed, bumps, drops and all of that fun stuff, but don't forget about your bike's geometry. Having more travel means the fork is longer. This is great for downhilling because a longer fork creates a more relaxed head angle, which in turn creates more handling stability. At speed, you want that. Also, a longer fork keeps your weight farther back, which is important in steep sections. Dial your travel down for the climbs and the steering gets more responsive, which is great for maneuvering around obstacles and navigating more-efficient lines."

FIX IT, OR REPLACE IT?

Swap out your bike's smaller parts when they're worn, and you won't have to replace pricey components as often. Here's the damage to look for.

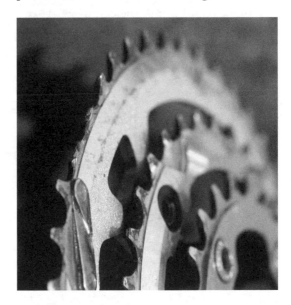

CHAINRING TEETH. We've seen teeth bent from rough handling, crashes and sloppy shifts (almost always on the outer ring). You'll know you've bent them: The chain will snag or derail as you pedal. Sometimes you can bend the teeth back into place (especially if you have a small adjustable wrench) long enough to get home, but aluminum teeth frequently snap. Missing teeth—torn off in a crash, usually—are more insidious because you can ride a long time without being able to pinpoint the cause of your lousy shifting. (The chain usually deserves most of the blame.) For either malady, replace the ring. If the teeth look fatally worn but intact, double-check the diagnosis with your bike shop; the teeth of modern chainrings and cassettes are so sculpted to enhance shifting that to an unpracticed eye they can appear misshapen even when new.

CHAIN. As the chain engages and pulls against the teeth of the cogs and rings, the bushings between the plates become worn. Play develops between the links until the distance between them is so great they no longer mesh evenly with the teeth. The drivetrain becomes clattery and shifting is balky or unpredictable. You can lengthen the life of your chain with regular cleaning and lubing; rather than recommend a time interval, we like the basic rule that your chain should never be dry or be wet enough to have anything stick to it. But even a well-cared-for chain will wear out, usually between 1,000 and 2,500 miles. Check your chain monthly with a Park Tool Chain Checker or by having your shop take a look. Ridden too long, a worn chain can in turn disfigure the teeth of the cassette and chainrings; if this happens, you have to replace those as well as the chain.

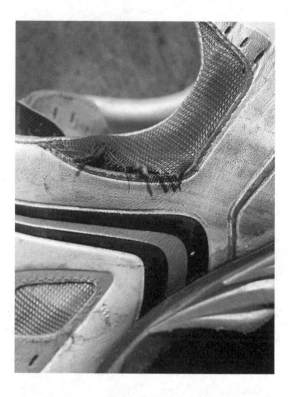

SHOES. There's a certain style that comes with running broken-in shoes, but once the wabi-sabi advances from blemishes and scratches to frayed uppers and failed stitching, you're robbing yourself of pedal power. The shoe won't cup your foot as snugly as it used to, and if you tighten the fasteners to get a better fit you're likely to create hot spots. We recommend overlooking (or even enjoying) cosmetic flaws but replacing a shoe when there's any structural damage.

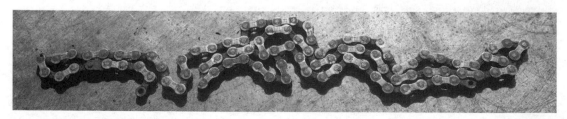

HANDLEBAR. Rigorous testing by major manufacturers has resulted in incredible durability and strength from carbon bars. But overtightened bolts, the impact of crashes or even a deep scratch can concentrate stresses in one area until the affected fiber fails catastrophically. Telling the difference between potentially dangerous damage and harmless wear to the outer clear coat can be difficult. Generally, if you can fit your fingernail into the scratch or clearly see a difference in layers between the clear coat and the fiber (as in the photo), there's no question that the bar needs to be replaced. We recommend asking a shop to check out marks. If you have an aluminum bar, any gouge deeper than the anodizing or paint (exposing bright silver) should trigger immediate replacement.

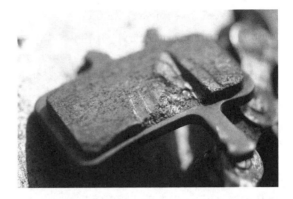

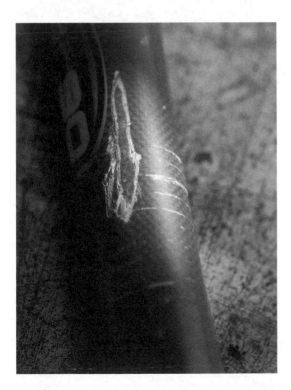

DISC-BRAKE PADS. Fair-weather riders might go a year without wearing out their pads, while others might ruin theirs in a single month of sloppy winter riding. Grit and grime that gather on the disc eat away the pad. Check weekly for large nicks or deep gouges, instead of even wear across a more-or-less uniform surface, and if you find any, replace the pads.

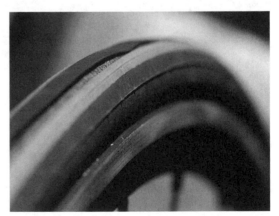

TIRES. There's no such thing as an average life expectancy for tires. Used for racing, some last less than 1,000 miles, while training or commuting tires can reach 5,000 miles or more. The commonality is that, while all types of tires can sustain some level of nicks, cuts and loss from normal wear, once you can see threads, belts or the innertube through an opening you have to replace the tire. If you don't, you risk splitting the tire (as in the picture on page 93) or violently popping a sidewall. Examine the tire at least weekly, ideally before every ride. One effective trick for prolonging the life span of road tires: When the rear is worn, swap your old front tire to the back and install the new one up front. The rear is the drive wheel and carries most of your weight, so it wears quicker.

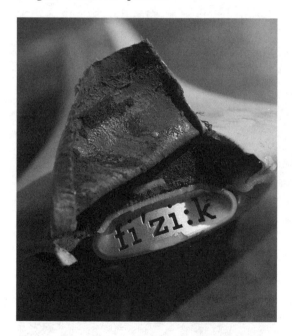

SADDLE. As with shoes, there is a certain romance to a tarnished saddle, but anything that harms its structural integrity should be your signal to get a new one. Such flaws include a peeled cover, bent or broken rails, chips or gouges that reach to the inner shell, or lumpy spots caused by shifted or hardened gel or padding. Any of these can concentrate friction and cause saddle sores, or force you to alter (and unbalance) your riding position in an effort to alleviate discomfort. Worse, a saddle that snaps at the rails can cause you to lose control and crash. In our experience, the average life span of a saddle that's ridden about 5,000 miles a year and doesn't experience undue damage is two to three seasons.

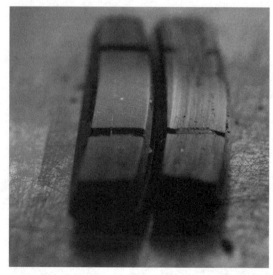

ROAD-BRAKE PADS. You compromise your ability to slow down (and could also harm the rim, an expensive replacement compared with $20 pads) if you use pads worn beyond the limit indicator. As shown with the pad in the above photo, when the bottom of the vertical gap is flush with the surface, the pad needs to be replaced. (As the pad wears toward this point, you can dial out the barrel adjuster to bring it closer to the rim so your braking power doesn't diminish.) Replace all four pads at once so you have an even application of force. To prevent damage to the rim, at least once a week use a small screwdriver or awl to remove embedded grit from the pads. To ensure your brakes grab predictably and smoothly, every two weeks roughen the surface of the pad with sandpaper or a file.

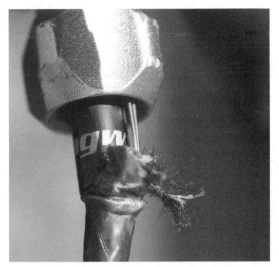

HOUSING. At the change of each season of the year, inspect the cable housings and replace those that are broken, bent, or cracked. Damaged housing causes undue stress and wear on the cables (necessitating more frequent replacement), detracts from shifting and braking, and, when undetected, can cause you to fruitlessly service all the other components on your bike in an effort to fix the clumsy shifting or braking.

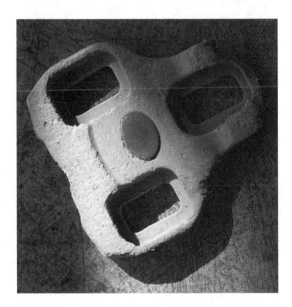

CLEATS. Replace them at the start of every year or when the wear indicator says you should. (For many plastic cleats, the signal for replacement is when a color indicator or line either disappears as it's worn away, or shows through a worn surface.) Cleats used beyond their effective life span often release unexpectedly or stick in the pedal; either can cause a crash. Walking on cleats causes the worst premature wear.

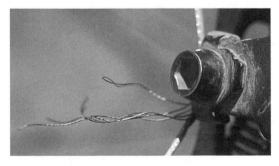

CABLES. Although many cyclists think that frayed ends are merely unsightly, the weakened cable is actually more likely to break. In addition, when you're fidgeting with a barrel adjuster or cleaning your bike, you can stab your thumb on one of the tiny, rusty wires that stick out. Don't twine the strands back together and put on a new end cap; ensure structural integrity by buying and installing a new cable. To maintain smooth operation, we recommend replacing cables once a year or whenever you spot rust.

CHAPTER 13

Never Walk Home: Flat Tire Fixes and Other Roadside Repairs

Mechanical mishaps such as flat tires and broken chains are unquestionably aggravating—depending on your levels of fitness and expertise, fighting with a stubborn component can raise your heart rate almost as much as a challenging climb. But these issues don't have to ruin your ride. The tips in this chapter will help you get out of almost any trailside jam, while keeping your swearing to a minimum. To start, here's a pre-ride checklist that can help prevent problems in the first place.

YOUR PRE-RIDE INSPECTION

Keith Schmidt, owner of K-Man Cycle & Run in Atascadero, California, has been performing bike-safety checks for 15 years as lead mechanic at the Wildflower Triathlon. Here's what he looks for, and what you should do, before your next ride.

Check: Stem for loose bolts; handlebar for side-to-side and up-and-down play. By: Bracing the front wheel between your knees and giving the bar a side-to-side tug, then applying downward pressure on the hoods. Fix: Tighten loose stem bolts with a torque wrench. Or Else: Your handlebar could unexpectedly turn sideways or slip downward midride, causing you to lose control.

Check: Wheels for trueness and broken spokes. By: Putting your bike in a workstand and spinning each wheel, using the brake pads as reference points to find wobbles. Fix: Replace broken spokes and tighten loose ones, then re-true your wheel. Or Else: A wobbly wheel can become unstable while riding, and may cause the tire to rub on the brake pad, which could lead to a dangerous blowout.

Check: Brakes for proper function. By: Giving the levers a firm squeeze; if the cable slips, the cable anchor bolt is loose. Also, take a look at the brake pads for alignment and excessive wear, and to make sure they're contacting the rim properly. Fix: Tighten any loose fasteners, adjust pads if needed and replace any worn parts. Or Else: You could lose your brakes without warning.

Check: Tires for proper inflation. By: Using a tire gauge or a pump with a gauge. Fix: Adjust air pressure according to the tire manufacturer's specifications. Never inflate your tires beyond the maximum pressure listed on the sidewall. Or Else: Underinflated tires are susceptible to pinch flats and can cause you to lose control. Overinflated tires can blow off the rim.

Check: Helmet for cracks and age. By: Inspecting it for visual damage. All organized rides and races require that you wear a helmet, and some have a helmet check. Some events have age limits on helmets—usually three or five years. Fix: Replace your helmet if it's damaged or more than three years old. Or Else: Your skid lid won't protect you in a crash, and you might not be allowed to participate in the event.

FLAT TIRES: THE CYCLIST'S NEMESIS

They come in catastrophic bangs, or with the sickening crunch of rim hitting rock, or a sibilant hiss that rises in volume until it inspires panic, or the flappy drumroll of tire unpeeling itself from rim. Or they come as sensation before sound—a vague squishiness, as if your wheel is squirming around on melty pavement, or an unsettling feeling, as if your bike has impossibly started to fold in on itself, or the rim grinding against asphalt so hard it makes your teeth hurt. Or, most rarely, a friend rides up beside you, puts a hand on your shoulder and says, simply, "I think you're going flat." No

matter: The outcome is the same. You are deflated.

But don't despair: A flat tire is not a disaster but rather an opportunity to learn, to test your character against the fates, to demonstrate your bicycle acumen (or just plain show off), to save the environment, maybe even to change your life. Really: Just ask Dan Ciammaichella. In 2005, the cyclist was a twice-divorced 45-year-old who had just moved back to Ohio, where he'd grown up. While riding the Ohio & Erie Canal towpath one day, he encountered a 14-year-old boy walking his mountain bike. The kid had a flat. Ciammaichella stopped, and as he changed the tube, they chatted. The boy, Brian, complained that he was going to miss the local MS 150 charity ride because his stepfather wouldn't ride with him. Ciammaichella, who'd already planned on doing the event, volunteered to ride with the kid if his parents said it was okay. With the flat fixed, they rode together to the parking lot where Brian's mother was waiting to pick him up. When they arrived, Ciammaichella froze in shock: The woman, Cheri, had been his high school sweetheart nearly 30 years earlier. After Ciammaichella and Brian rode the MS 150 together, Cheri started coming out for rides with them. The two adults rekindled their relationship—this time as friends, a situation that continued even after Cheri's marriage ended. Eventually the two former sweethearts became so close they wound up exchanging wedding vows. You should be so lucky to flat.

Six Simple Steps to Change a Flat

Here's an idiot-proof guide for you or a beginner friend.

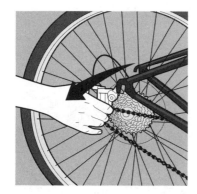

1. DETACH THE WHEEL FROM THE BIKE. The front is easy: Release the brake, open the quick-release lever, loosen the skewer and pull the wheel from the fork dropouts. The back is harder. Shift to the smallest cog to make reinstallation relatively easier. If you're on your bike when you notice the flat, shift as you slow down. Loosen the brakes and skewer, pull down on the derailleur and slide the wheel out. Lay your bike, chain side up, by the side of the road.

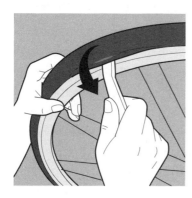

2. GET THE TIRE OFF THE WHEEL. You may or may not need tire levers. If you do, jam the flat end of the lever between the rim and the tire,

and scoop it under the bead. Then push down on the lever and hook the other end of it to the spoke. Insert another lever less than 2 inches away from the anchored one, and repeat, which should loosen the bead enough that you can unseat the bead all the way around. Remove the blown tube.

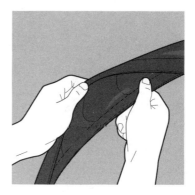

3. INSPECT THE TIRE. Using your fingers and your eyes, check the tire inside and out for whatever caused the flat. Take your time and remove all suspicious matter. Back-to-back flats are sure to kill the will to ride.

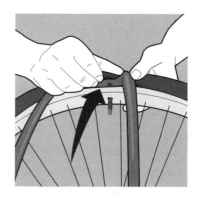

4. INSTALL THE NEW TUBE. Twist open the valve of the new tube and use your minipump to add a tiny bit of air, which makes it easier to stuff into the tire. Thread the valve into the hole in the rim; this will serve as an anchor as you push the rest of the tube into the tire.

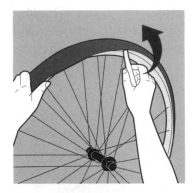

5. KNEAD THE TIRE BACK ONTO THE RIM. The key to not losing your mind by having the part of the tire slip off where you just put it on: Hold one hand at the top, and work around the wheel with the other. Once you have half the tire secure, you can let go with your anchor hand. Use a lever for the last little bit if you need to, but be very careful not to pinch any protruding bits of tube. Then give it a check: Squeeze both sides of the tire as you work around the wheel, making sure none of the tube is poking out under the bead. Pump it up. A CO_2 cartridge, a submarine-shaped vessel of air that attaches to the tube's valve via a special chuck, is easy to use if you follow the instructions on the packaging. Minipumps take a lot of elbow grease, but are good for an infinite number of tires.

6. REATTACH THE WHEEL. On the front: Fit the fork onto the skewer (the QR lever goes on the left side of the bike) and tighten; don't forget to flip the brake QR down. For the rear: Hold up the bike's back half, then focus on one thing: getting the wheel positioned so that the cogs are any-

where in between the chain. Then set the bike down and tweak until the frame and wheel are properly mated—this could take at least a minute. Tighten the skewer and brake, then roll.

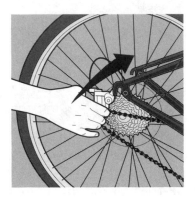

Three Ways to Prevent Another One

Changing flats fast makes you a rock star on a group ride. But don't hustle so much you make a mistake that flats your spare. Here are three smart steps:

DIAGNOSE THE CAUSE. Look at the tire and failed tube before crumpling it into your jersey pocket. See if you can spot one of these telltale signs:

→ A jagged puncture or pinhole on the top or side of the tube usually is made by an object—glass or thorns, for instance—that has become embedded in the tire. To find and remove the intruder (if it hasn't already fallen out), rotate the tire with one finger lightly brushing the interior. If you don't feel anything, rotate the tire again, examining the outer tread for slits; when you spot one, pinch it open to see if anything is buried in it.

→ If you find two short, parallel rips on the bottom of the tube—a "snakebite"—your underinflated tube got squashed between the rim and a hard object (like a rock), or you simply rode too heavily into an obstacle such as a curb or pothole. When you reinflate the tire, make sure you pump it to the recommended pressure.

→ A round hole on the bottom of the tube often occurs when the rim strip moves or tears over a spoke hole, exposing a rough edge. Wriggle the strip back into place; if it's damaged beyond usefulness, lay a dollar bill, energy bar wrapper or similar material over the exposed spoke hole.

→ A huge, jagged hole in the side of the tube or the tire's sidewall comes from a blowout—the easiest type of flat to identify because of its gunshot sound. A few potential causes: The tube failed due to advanced age or a manufacturing defect; it got squeezed between the tire bead and rim (when you hit a rock hard enough to unseat the tire's bead, for example); or something, like a stick or curb, ripped the sidewall. If the tire is damaged, line the hole with a tire boot such as a folded dollar bill or energy bar wrapper, which should get you home.

INSTALL IT RIGHT. Double-check that the tube is completely tucked inside the tire bead before inflating. If even the tiniest fold emerges, you'll cause another blowout when you inflate the tube to 60 psi or so. To properly seat it: After rolling the tire beads onto the rim, work your hands around the circumference, pinching it inward and looking into the gap between tire and rim to make sure no tube is visible.

→ Before inflating, push up on the valve to seat that portion of the tube (which is thicker) fully into the tire, then pull the valve back into proper position.

→ Don't tear off the valve stem when inflating the new tube. This happens more often with pumps than CO_2 cartridges, but if you're hasty and fatigued, anything's possible. Be careful not to jiggle the adapter too much when you screw in the CO_2. With a pump, grip the valve, rim and tire in the palm of one hand, or pump with the valve propped against your thigh.

JUST SAY NO. Don't try to save the last bit of CO_2 for a miniature whippet. It's a much better high to roll on a fully inflated tire.

Tubular and Tubeless Tires

A tubular is a one-piece tire sewn around a tube. It is glued onto a rim in a multistage process that often spans days. The rim-and-tire combination almost always weighs less than the lightest clincher combo, usually has lower rolling

Fun **Fact**

In 1926, newly invented Mavic aluminum rims were banned from the Tour de France over concerns the metal would heat during braking and pop tubes. Some racers snuck them in by using wood-colored paint.

resistance and often feels more responsive in corners. This is why pros use them almost exclusively. But tubs—that's the correct nickname, not "tubies"—are problematic when you flat on the road.

Your best bet is to carry a can of aerosol tire sealant such as Vittoria Pit Stop (vittoria.com; more on that later) or Hutchinson Fast'Air (hutchinson.fr). After checking your tire to remove glass or thorns, open the valve and thread on the pump. Empty the sealant into the tire until it's fully inflated, then finish your ride. Unfortunately, your lightweight tubular has now gained weight.

You can also fold up and carry a spare tubular (about the size of a water bottle) strapped under your seat. (You need one anyway if the puncture is too large for sealant to patch.) To change: Remove the wheel and let out the remaining air. Unseat the tire by digging under the tubular with a tire lever on the opposite side of the rim from the valve. Once you have enough loose tire to grab, pull the rim away with your other hand. Roll the new tub onto your rim and inflate. Air pressure and the remaining glue will hold the tire on if you take care in the corners.

Pro **Tip**

"MY FAVORITE GLUE BRUSHES ARE ACID BRUSHES FOUND AT ACE HARDWARE FOR 25 CENTS EACH. THEY'RE CHEAP, SO I USUALLY GET A BIG HANDFUL OF THEM EACH YEAR TO GLUE TIRES AND WHEELS."—*VINCENT GEE, MECHANIC FOR TEAM RADIOSHACK*

A tubeless tire is like a car tire—there's no innertube. Air pressure (and sealant) secure the tire bead against the rim. Popular in mountain biking, and gaining acceptance for road bikes, tubeless tires can run at lower pressure for greater traction and comfort without risking a pinch flat. They're almost impervious to flats, in fact, thanks to their puncture-plugging sealant, unless the sidewall tears. To get rolling again after gouging your sidewall, carry a spare tube, pump and tire boot. Unscrew and remove the valve (or remove the rim strip if the valve is attached). With your tire on the rim, one bead off, place the tube in the tire and add a little air. With the tube gently pressing against the tire, slide in the tire boot, which will prevent the tube from pushing through the tear. Reseat the tire bead and inflate your tire to the minimum pressure necessary to ride home. Too much pressure will blow out the boot.

Recycle Your Rubber

Bikes are green. No secret there. Ride just 20 miles a week instead of driving and you single-handedly cut half a ton of CO_2 emissions in a year. But the inconvenient truth is that spent tubes help trash the environment. In 2007, 130 million new bikes were sold worldwide. That's 260 million tubes. If just half of those flatted and got tossed, that's nearly 100,000 tons of cast-off rubber.

There are few effective options for reusing the rubber, but if there's a receptive recycling center nearby, bundle the used tubes (maybe work with a shop) and deliver them in bulk.

More Uses for Old Tubes

FRAME PROTECTOR
Wrap an old tube around your chainstay and affix with electrical tape to reduce chain slap—it'll cushion your frame and cut down on noise.

BAND AID
Use pieces of a damaged tube to patch a reparable tube. Apply it the same way you would a repair-kit patch.

CUSTOM RUBBER BANDS
Slice and dice your tube into skinny and wide bands. You'll never again have to rely on that infamous junk drawer where you toss gratuitous bands from the morning paper or the fresh-cut flowers your gal bought for her, um, self.

BE CREATIVE
Cut into various lengths, sizes, shapes, strips and pieces, old tubes become bungees to hold things down, clamps to keep things in place, garden ties to attach plants to stakes, supporters to keep saplings upright, sleeves to protect seatposts, and waterproof pockets to store iPods and IDs.

The best solution: Patch your tubes. Don't do it midride; carry a spare and repair the punctured one at home later. Kits with a tube of glue, square of sandpaper and multiple patches sell for around $5. Buy one, then follow these steps:

1. Locate the hole. If it's not visible, inflate the tube and hold it near your cheek, rotating it until you feel an airflow. If that fails, submerge the tube bit by bit in water and watch for air bubbles.

2. Dry the tube if necessary, then rough up the area around the hole with sandpaper.

3. Spread a light layer of glue on the tube in an area slightly larger than the patch. Be careful not to rush here; let the glue dry until the adhesive turns tacky.

4. Apply the patch and press it evenly onto the tube with the heel of your hand.

MORE MID-RIDE FIXES

Fixing a bike in a garage full of tools and spare parts is admirable. But solving a mechanical failure on the road or trail can be downright heroic. Here are some impromptu fixes that have let our readers and contributors ride it out.

Difficulty Gauge

1 = Baby Wrench
2 = Boy Scout
3 = Handyman
4 = MacGyver

Let Nature Mend a Broken Frame
Difficulty: 3

We wouldn't have believed it without the step-by-step photos he sent us. Mike Shannon was out with more than a dozen buddies, riding the Chilliwack trails near Vancouver, British Columbia. "We were all taking turns going off this drop," says Shannon, a typical North Shore freerider who can handle higher drops than most riders— or frames, it seems. "It wasn't anything big— maybe between shoulder and head high. But when I landed, the frame snapped." Shannon faceplanted into the dirt, unhurt thanks to his full-face helmet and body padding.

His Santa Cruz Super 8, on the other hand, snapped in two, with the down tube and top tube shearing off at the same spot a few inches behind the head tube. The bike wasn't only unrideable; at 55 pounds and in two pieces limply strung together by brake and shift cables, it was also a chore to carry. So the computer-security-expert-by-day took quick inventory of his group's potentially useful supplies: a Leatherman tool, a few large zip-ties and an abundance of sticks in the woods around him. With a shrug, he set about making the bike one again.

"I just picked up a few pieces of wood and whittled them down with the Leatherman so they'd fit inside the frame tubes," he says. "We had to hammer them in a bit." He first fit the wood pieces into the main-triangle side of the bike, then cut the branches off with the Leatherman's saw blade to leave just the right length stub hanging out. As a friend squeezed the frame, Shannon wiggled and pounded the head-tube section onto the sticks. He then ran a zip-tie around the head tube and back through the frame's shock bracket, to cinch everything down tight. "The whole thing took maybe 10 minutes," says Shannon.

He rode off down the trail with a hoot and grin. But freeriders just can't contain themselves. "After pedaling along for 20 minutes I saw another, smaller drop I just had to do," says Shannon. "But the zip-tie broke. And it deformed the wood so the bike was unrideable." In the end, he faced an hour-long march out of the woods with the beast. "I definitely wanted to save the bike," he says. "I think the head tube could be made into one of the best bongs ever." Ah, freeriders.

Poach a Bolt

Difficulty: 2 (Catch: If the threads don't match up, you're out of luck.)

When something on your bike breaks, you might not have the right spare part—but you do have a bike full of options. A creative switcharoo could save the day, or at least make your predicament less dire.

Consider the case of Dave Kingsbury, a market research executive who frequents mountain trails near his home just west of Boulder, Colorado. "We did a huge climb a couple of years ago, and stopped at the top for a minute," he says. There, poised on the sweet end of one of his favorite descents, Kingsbury noticed the arm of his front Shimano XTR V-brake hanging off the side of his Santa Cruz Superlight. "There was no way I could do the descent without a front brake," he says. "So I spread out the contents of my seatbag and started looking for what I could poach."

Kingsbury thought his spare tube looked promising. Or at least the threaded presta valve did. So he cut the valve out of the tube and broke off the pointy screw nub. Then he screwed the makeshift bolt into the brake boss—bingo! It was the right thread and diameter. The ragged rubber at the valve's bottom even gave him something to twist with. Kingsbury's valve was just the right length, but if yours is too long, you can cinch it down with the jam nut (you know, the one you always throw away).

Other switcheroos: One reader accidentally stripped the nut on his front quick-release skewer due to some overly enthusiastic tightening. The on-the-spot replacement came from the plate in his shoe that the cleat screws into—better to have one foot unattached to the pedal than a loose front wheel. Other eligible donor bolts include those holding on your water-bottle cages and the cap bolt on top of threadless stems (not the clamp bolts on the side, or the single bolt on quill-style stems—double-check by making sure the stem doesn't loosen), which can often sub for a seatpost bolt.

Pro **Tip**

"DROPPED THE CHAIN? DON'T TOUCH IT WITH YOUR BARE FINGERS. INSTEAD, SHIFT THE FRONT DERAILLEUR TO THE INNER CHAINRING. FIND A SHORT STICK OR PIECE OF DEBRIS ALONG THE ROAD. USE THE STICK TO HOOK THE CHAIN ONTO THE FIRST FEW TEETH ON THE UNDERSIDE OF THE INNER CHAINRING. SPIN THE CRANKS BACKWARD UNTIL THE CHAIN IS COMPLETELY ENGAGED AROUND THE RING."—*ALEX STIEDA*

The Multitalented Quick-Release

Change a Flat

Difficulty: 1 (It's a hassle to undo that second skewer.)

Chain Fix

Difficulty: 4 (Requires wrenching chops.)

Whip that quick-release skewer out of your wheel and you've got a multi-tool, of sorts. An easy fix: If you break your only tire lever fixing a flat, simply flip open your front quick-release lever, remove the nut from the opposite side, and slide the skewer out of the hub (make sure not to lose the springs—one goes on each side of the hub, small end facing inward). Now use the rounded, flat end of the lever to pry the tire bead over the sidewall of the rim. You may need a second lever, conveniently located on the bike's other wheel.

For a much more advanced maneuver, turn your quick-release into a chain tool. The trick lies with the quick-release's cam action: When you close a QR, it squeezes like a miniature press—plus it's conveniently located next to your chain. To mend a broken chain, start by properly threading one end through the rear derailleur (remember the chain wraps around the back of the lower derailleur pulley wheel) and up around the smallest rear cog. Then pull the same end through the front derailleur, but don't wrap it around a chainring—you want as much slack as possible. Instead pull the chain through until you can make both ends meet at the bike's rear dropout. Open the rear quick-release, unscrew it a few turns (removing the skewer springs helps), and place a link in the space between the drop-out and skewer nut. By positioning a link just right and flipping the QR closed, you can drive a pin through the chain sideplates. The tricky part is first getting a pin pressed out—try using the orphaned pin from the link that broke—but if you made it this far you don't need us anymore.

The All-Time Best Roadside Fix

If Lance Armstrong or any current Tour de France rider has a mechanical problem, he just waits by the side of the road until a team car speeds up with a new part or whole new bike. It takes seconds. But during the 1913 Tour, when there were strict rules about riders being self-sufficient, Frenchman Eugene Christophe pulled off the most incredible mid-ride fix of all time.

Christophe ground his way over the top of the Tourmalet—still one of the Tour's most feared climbs—in second place, only to have the fork on his one-speed bike snap on the descent of the Pyreneean mountain. Undaunted, he schlepped his bike nine miles to the town of Sainte Marie-de-Campan, where he found a blacksmith shop and proceeded to braze his own fork back together. The piece de resistance? He still received a time penalty for accepting outside assistance—a helper worked the bellows for him. Christophe crossed the line nearly four hours behind the winner, but continued on to Paris, finishing a plucky seventh place overall. Christophe's name later adorned millions of steel toeclips—almost every 1970s' 10-speed had 'em.

MYTH BUSTERS

Some famous claims for mid-ride fixes aren't what they seem.

MYTH: Patch a punctured tube by melting latex from a glove or condom.

REALITY: The melted rubber turns to a thin, sticky mess that can't seal a hole, plus the latex easily catches fire.

MYTH: If you don't have a pump, inflate your presta tube by blowing.

REALITY: Try it—you won't even get to 2 psi.

MYTH: You can't fix a Campy chain with a standard chain tool, or fix a Shimano without the special pin.

How a Chain Tool Works

If your chain snaps mid-ride, this quick fix will get you home.

Carefully line up the pin you want to remove in the chain tool. (If it's slightly off, you risk damaging the chain and bending the tool.) Slowly turn the tool clockwise until it pushes the pin through the rollers, but not past the outer plate. Remove the damaged link. If you don't have a spare link, you can reconnect the ends of the chain. It will be a little shorter, so take it easy for the remainder of your ride, and stay in the smaller chainrings/cogs. Set the reconnected link into the tool and push the pin back to its original position, leaving equal amounts of the pin on either side of the plates.

REALITY: We've done both. Using a standard chain tool, one staffer has rejoined busted chains of both makes, with sufficient strength to finish the rides. Both times, he had someone standing behind him telling him it wouldn't work.

IMPROMPTU FIXES ANYONE CAN DO

Limp home with the help of these old standbys.

→Boot a gashed tire with an energy bar wrapper, dollar bill, or a segment from an old tire. Be sure the piece is large enough to overlap an inch of tire on either side of the cut, to prevent slippage and tube blowouts.

→Use a chain tool to turn your bike into a one-speed if the derailleur gets trashed. How? Bypass the derailleur by wrapping the chain directly from front chainring to rear cog and removing enough links (with the chain tool) to make the chain taut.

→Straighten a tacoed wheel by wedging it into a tree or slamming it on the ground. Do this last-hope maneuver by eyeballing the section that's out of plane with the rest of the rim and brute-forcing it back into approximate position.

→Stuff a flat mountain bike tire full of leaves. It takes a lot of leaves. Seriously, a lot. And the tire will still be semi-flaccid at best, just enough to protect your rim.

→No spare tube? Cut and knot a flat one at the puncture. The knots make the tube lumpy and short, so expect a tire that thunks with each revolution.

Pro **Tip**

"IF YOU THINK YOUR BRAKE PAD IS RUBBING, GIVE THE BRAKE LEVERS A PUMP, THEN LIFT EACH WHEEL AND SPIN IT. LOOK BETWEEN THE SPINNING RIM AND THE BRAKE PADS. IF ONE BRAKE PAD IS CLOSER TO THE RIM OR ONE IS RUBBING, YOU NEED TO CENTER THE BRAKE. OFTEN, YOU CAN SIMPLY PULL OUTWARD ON THE OFFENDING PAD TO REALIGN IT. IF THAT DOESN'T WORK, USE A 5-MM HEX WRENCH TO LOOSEN THE BOLT THAT ATTACHES THE CALIPER TO THE FRAME, CENTER THE PADS AND RETIGHTEN THE BOLT."—*ALEX STIEDA*

→Secure a slipping handlebar grip with a dab of energy gel.

→Quiet a squeaky cleat or pedal with lip balm or sunscreen.

→Guzzle what's left in your water bottle, then turn it upside down and slip it over a broken seatpost. A small seat is better than no seat.

THE KLUDGE THAT WON THE TOUR DE FRANCE

Going into the final stage of the 1989 Tour, a 24-kilometer time trial into Paris, American Greg LeMond trailed Frenchman Laurent Fignon by a seemingly insurmountable 50 seconds. At the 11th hour—the waiting in part to keep his new-fangled equipment secret—LeMond had his bike fitted with a then-radical (at least to Euro pros) aero handlebar. But the aero bar's mounting clamps were too large and could not be cinched down tightly enough on the handlebar. So his team of mechanics whipped up shims by cutting strips of aluminum from a Coke can, then wrapped them (going with the curve of the can) around the handlebar to fill in the extra space between the handlebar and the clamps. LeMond went on to win the stage and take the Tour by just eight seconds—the smallest margin of victory ever in the Tour. It was calculated that, without the aero bar, LeMond would have ridden about 30 seconds slower. Of course, for years enterprising cyclists have used aluminum-can shims to stop wiggles on aero bar attachments, stems and, most often, seatposts—but never were the stakes so high.

AVOIDING OUR ADVICE

Every jam seems to have its own peculiar set of circumstances, so there's no perfect list of what to carry. But pack the following, and most push-it-out, hitchhike-home disasters can be avoided:

Pump

Spare tube

Patch kit with tire-booting material

Multi-tool that includes a chain breaker, tire levers, and spoke wrench

Mini pocket knife

Money

Cell phone

CHAPTER 14

30 Days to a Beautiful Bike

We know how it is—work, family, happy hour and those endless airings of Dog the Bounty Hunter *all conspire to make it impossible to set aside even a measly hour to concentrate on bike maintenance. But if you devote a little time to bike care every day for a month, you can accomplish much more than you would by squeezing in a spare hour here and there on weekends. Our simple, 30-day plan assumes you want to keep riding your bike. Aside from a scheduled three-day stint at the bike shop to take care of the major stuff, there's no forced downtime. Happy wrenching.*

DAY 1. Start off the month by giving your bike a light cleanup. This isn't the full-on Silkwood shower—we'll get to that. For now, use a damp cloth to remove the first layer of grime from the frame, rims, derailleurs, crankarms, brakes, stem and handlebar. Wipe with a dry rag. Now you can touch your bike without getting filthy.

DAY 2. Check the frame for cracks. This is satisfying to do for two reasons: First, you probably won't find any. Second: If you do, you just saved your life, or at least one of your collarbones. Cracks usually occur near welded areas, or where the frame is butted. Probably the most common spot is the underside of the down tube, just below the head tube. On carbon frames, it can be difficult to tell if you're looking at a

scratch in the clear coat or a crack in the frame. General rule: If your fingernail can catch on the blemish, it might be a crack. If you have your suspicions, go to the bike shop tomorrow for a learned opinion.

DAY 3. Even if your frame checked out, head over to the bike shop today and get everything you might need for the month: two tires, three tubes, two sets of brake pads, a set of cables and housings for shifters and brakes, handlebar tape, degreaser and frame wax. You might not use all this, but at least you'll have spares.

DAY 4. All seatposts can bond to the frame—take five minutes and avoid this disaster. Mark the height of your seatpost with tape or a pencil, then remove it, wipe it clean and, if it's steel or aluminum, smear a light layer of grease over the section that goes inside the frame. For carbon, apply a layer of carbon-prep paste, which, like regular grease, prevents the post from bonding to the frame but is gritty enough to stop the common problem of slippage.

DAY 5. Inspect each tire. Deflate the tube to about half its pressure, so the tire is still shaped but pliable. Rotating the wheel in the frame, manipulate the tire with your hands to expose cuts in the sidewalls or tread. If you find any that go either entirely through the tire, or are deep enough to make you anxious, replace the tire. Rule of thumb for mountain bike tires: If five or more treads are ripped away, the tire is ready to fail systemically and should be replaced if you want to avoid lots of flats.

DAY 6. Look at the underside of your down tube: All those disgusting black warts are road tar that was thrown up onto your bike at some point and dried there. At first pass of the rag, removing them will seem impossible. Keep soaking them with diluted degreaser or a solution of equal parts dish soap and water, and scrub hard. That's a noble 20 minutes you just spent doing something no one but you will ever appreciate.

DAY 7. It's Obvious Day: Spin the wheels and see if they're running crooked. Hold your bike 4 inches off the ground and drop it onto its tires, listening for rattles and clinks, then pinpoint them. Think back to all those clunks you've heard on your recent rides and catalog them. Think about how your bike has felt: Sticky steering? Loose feeling from the rear on descents? Write everything down, then call the bike shop and make an appointment to bring your bike in midweek to check on those things. (Weekends are rush time.)

DAY 8. Remove each wheel from the frame. Hold the wheel between your hands and slowly turn the axle. If the motion feels rough or the axle seems to catch, try slightly loosening the cones inside the hub to reduce pressure on the bearings. (There are various methods, ranging from two cone wrenches to one hex; all are simple but can seem intimidating. You might want to just add this to your list of concerns for the bike shop.) If the axle spins smoothly, check it for looseness: Using your index finger and thumb, wiggle the axle around; if it moves enough to cause a knocking feeling, tighten the hub or add it to your shop list.

DAY 9. Scuff up your shoes today. Glazed brake shoes cause weak braking and impolite squeals. Use sandpaper, a file or an emery board to buff off the glaze and roughen up the pads. Also pick out dirt, grit or pieces of metal that have become embedded in the pad. If the pad has hardened so much that you can't scratch it with your fingernail, or if it's worn past the indicator line, replace it.

DAY 10. Take your bike to the shop for its appointment. While you're there, buy two new matching water bottles. Never buy just one.

DAY 11. When the shop calls, tell the respectful young man with the pleasant phone manners that you know your cables and housings need to be replaced but you're going to do it yourself later because you're spending a whole month pampering your bike. Pretend the sound you hear is coughing, not laughing.

DAY 12. Organize and clean your tool bench or tool chest; if you don't have either, go buy something, even if it's just a generic tool box. Get two buckets while you're at it, plus two sponges, a bag of rags and a car-washing brush. Store the sponges, rags and brush in the nested buckets.

DAY 13. Buy a case of Dale's Pale Ale—the world's best canned beer—for your mechanic. Its artisanal blue-collar vibe will make him swoon.

DAY 14. Pick up your bike today and drop off the case. Have one with the shop personnel—yes, they'll ask, and it's your duty. If you're a guy, set yourself apart from the pack by refraining from flirtation with the foxy female mechanic while still acknowledging her. Women: Drop one double entendre about bottom-bracket stiffness and make a clean, classy exit.

DAY 15. Detail-clean your derailleurs with degreaser. Saw the rag back and forth through open areas in the derailleur's structure, or use cotton swabs. Dry with a clean rag, then apply one drop of light oil to each spring or pivot.

DAY 16. Clean the rims with a slightly abrasive pad, or just scrub hard with a rag soaked in dish soap—then rinse and dry. Over time, road spray and gunk from the brake pads coat the rim, which interferes with stopping power.

DAY 17. It's Chain Day: First, check chain wear. Place the edge of a 12-inch ruler over the pin of one link. (It's easiest on top of the chain, above the chainstay.) The 12-inch hash mark should sit over another pin. If it doesn't, the chain is worn, which reduces shifting efficiency and causes excess wear on the rings and cassette; replace it. If the chain is fine, clean it: With your bike in a workstand, grasp the chain with a clean rag soaked in degreaser as you backpedal. Then apply a drop of lube to each link as you slowly backpedal. Wipe off excess lube so you don't attract more dirt to your chain.

DAY 18. De-grime the crankset. Use a toothbrush and degreaser to clean the rings, then wipe with a dry rag. Clean between each tooth; if there's dirt in there, it wears the chain.

DAY 19. Clean the cassette. Remove the rear wheel and hold it vertically but slightly slanted so the cassette angles toward the ground; this will prevent degreaser from dripping into the freehub. Spray the cassette with degreaser and use a shoe brush or an old toothbrush to scrub grit from between the teeth. It's messy. Then use a screwdriver or awl to pick out weeds, string or anything else entwined around the cassette body. (Check the hollowed-out back of the body, too.) Hold or set the wheel horizontally and swipe a rag soaked with degreaser between the cogs, then over the face of the cogs, for a sparkly finish.

DAY 20. Cable and housing replacement appears labyrinthian, but can be goof-proof simplified if you're willing to work slow and deliberate (think of a sloth). Loosen the pinch bolt on one brake, clip the cap off the cable, then push it through the housing until the other end pops out of the lever. Pull the cable out. Note the position of the housings (which will still be in place), then remove one piece at a time and, measuring against the new housing, cut a fresh section. When the housings are done, push the new cable through the lever, then through the housings. Run the end through the pinch bolt and hex it tight. For brakes, hold the arms so the pads are against the rims as you tighten the pinch bolt. There's usually enough residual slack along the cable to create clearance between the pads and rims when you let go.

DAY 21. Remove the pedals. (Remember to turn the wrench clockwise on the left pedal—the opposite of usual.) Clean them—and if your pedal has a visible spring, lube it. Apply a coat of grease to the pedal threads before reinstall-ing so they'll budge the next time you remove them.

DAY 22. Tune up your bike computer: Remove it from the mount and clean the contacts on the mount and computer head with a pencil eraser. Cut the zip-ties holding the sensor on the fork, strip off the electrical tape or pad, then clean off the grit lines. Replace the batteries to avoid a blackout halfway through next season. Put it all back together again. Use fingernail clippers to trim the zip-ties for a smooth edge.

DAY 23. Measure the distance from the nose of your saddle to the center of your stem. Then loosen the seat clamp, pull the saddle off the post and clean the rails with degreaser. Add a light layer of lube to the rails, then wipe them dry. Clean the clamp parts as well, then apply a dry lube to the grip surfaces and wipe clean. Reassemble everything, matching the saddle-to-stem dimension. You've just ensured yourself a season free of saddle squeaks.

DAY 24. Your new cables should have stretched by now. To fix clattering shifting: If the chain is having trouble jumping from big cogs to small, turn the barrel adjuster on the rear derailleur half a turn clockwise. If the chain hesitates from small to big, go half a turn counterclockwise. Shift again and repeat. For the front derailleur: With the derailleur in its lowest position over the small ring, loosen the pinch bolt and pull the cable to remove slack, then retighten the bolt—don't make the cable so taut it twangs. For mushy brakes: Pinch the arms in with your fingers until the pads just contact the rims, loosen the pinch bolt and pull through the slack. Or you can dial out the cable adjuster, which is easier now but limits the amount of adjustment you'll have later.

DAY 25. Flip open your quick-release levers, unscrew them and pull them out of the axle (yes, you can do this with the wheel still in the frame, if you're careful). Screw the cap all the way off, remove the two springs, then clean the rod with degreaser, wipe it dry with a rag, apply a light layer of grease, then rebuild and reinstall the whole thing. (Remember to orient the springs with the tiny side facing inward.) When was the last time you took care of your bike down to that level of detail?

DAY 26. Today you will get cranky: Slip the chain off the little ring and loop it over the bottom bracket. Spray degreaser on the rings. Then prepare to drive yourself mental. With a rag, clean the space between each tooth on the big and little rings. Spray on more degreaser. Then, using a fresh rag, floss all those hard-to-reach spots between the rings (like where they meet at the arms of the crank). Spray on more degreaser, then clean the faces, and the inside, of both rings. Painstaking—and satisfying, because you have just completed a task only about two percent of all cyclists ever do.

DAY 27. If you don't own a torque wrench, borrow or buy one and check crank bolts, chainring bolts, stem clamp bolts, stem faceplate bolts and the seatpost binder bolt for proper tightness. You can find torque recommendations for every component on the manufacturers' websites.

DAY 28. Washing Day: Fill one bucket with clean water, and one bucket with water plus dish soap or degreaser. With one of your new sponges, soak your bike with plain water. Then soap up the second sponge and scrub the frame first, then wheels (don't forget the spokes), then drivetrain. Soap the brush, then scrub the cassette, chainrings and rims. Soak the clean sponge and use it to sluice the soap off the bike. Soak it again, wring it dry, and go over the whole bike again, drying it. Finish drying with clean rags, using the last two or three to swipe the nooks and crannies dry. The entire wash takes 15 to 20 minutes.

DAY 29. Break out the bar tape. Methods for taping are numerous and sometimes ridiculously complex, but don't be intimidated. All you need to know are the basics: Roll back the brake/shift hoods and stick the two tiny pieces of tape across the shifter clamp. Now take one of the big rolls and start at the bar end. Wrap toward the frame (counterclockwise for the right half; clockwise for left). On the first wrap, let half the width of the tape hang over the end of the bar, so you can stuff it in at the end to hold the plug tight. Wrap in spirals, overlapping half the width or less, and slightly stretch the tape as you pull it around. Make a figure 8 around the lever—it's more intuitive than it sounds, but you'll probably have to make two or three passes to get the tape right. Stop wrapping a little less than a hand's width from the stem. Cut off excess tape. Then cut a lengthwise slant in the tape so that the final wrap aligns directly against the edge of the previous wrap—don't worry, that'll make sense when you see it. Secure the last wrap with one or two layers of black electrical tape, half on the tape and half on the bar. Shove in the plug; you're done. For a visual, go to bicycling.com/videotape.

DAY 30. Top off the month by polishing your gem to a sheen with the frame wax. Pretty, isn't it?

RIDER **RESOURCES**

For more repair help and tricks from Langley, go to jimlangley.net and jimlangley.blogspot.com. Watch how-to videos on a variety of fixes at bicycling.com.

PART

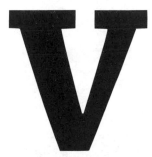

V

Riding for Transportation

IT'S SOMETIMES EASY TO FORGET—AS WE OGLE 13-pound, carbon-fiber race machines at the bike shop, or watch 130-pound men suffer their way through the French Alps on TV— that cycling is more than a sport. It's also a wonderful means of transportation. Consider this: The average American drives 29 miles per day. That means that if you used a bike instead of a car just one day per week, in one year you could save more than $1,000 in gas and auto maintenance costs, and burn 15 pounds' worth of calories, according to the Colorado advocacy group SmartTrips. And every mile you ride instead of drive prevents about a pound of carbon dioxide from entering the atmosphere.

CHAPTER 15

Getting There Is (At Least) Half the Fun

Consider yourself warned: By the time you finish this chapter, you won't have any excuses for not riding to work, or at least on the occasional errand. If you're not sure where to begin, check out our simple, five-step guide to getting started. If you're already a dedicated commuter, you'll find tips for making the journey easier and smoother. We'll also introduce you to four utility riders of varying degrees of commitment—a biking newbie, two commuter evangelists and one intrepid cyclist who gave up his car for an entire year.

HOW TO DUMP THE PUMP

You can find the safest route to work—and go from gas guzzler to bike commuter—with these five simple steps. Follow them, and you'll be a seasoned commuter faster than you can say, "You want how much for a gallon?"

THINK ON TWO WHEELS. The next time you drive to work, think like a cyclist. Pay attention to the entire route. Make mental notes of the roads that have shoulders wide enough to accommodate a bike as well as narrow stretches that are too dangerous. Use this as a starting point when mapping out your bike route.

MAP IT OUT. Pick up a detailed road map of the area your route will traverse—or download a bicycle-specific one from Google Maps (maps.google.com/biking). Highlight only the parts of your driving route that you know are safe. Find alternate routes that run parallel to the sections you want to avoid—choose side streets, parks and neighborhoods rather than high-traffic, high-speed roads. Also be sure to plan your route through well-lit streets—remember, you'll most likely be riding alone and, often, in the dark. The most direct route may not be the best cycling route.

TROUBLESHOOT YOUR ROUTE. Take the map of the route you've roughed out and go for a test drive. Troubleshoot as you go. Be on the lookout for busy intersections and shopping strips (where cars will be pulling out of parking lots). A section of road that initially looked rideable may turn out to be more dangerous than you thought. Find a way around it and mark it on your map. Do this until you've reached your destination. Test-drive it on the way back.

MAKE A DRY RUN. On a day off, test-ride your planned route to make sure it's safe and to see how long it will take you. You may find that your trip has too many small turns and not enough long stretches, or that you can save time by taking shortcuts on paths, or through parks or alleys where cars can't go. Experiment until you get it right.

EXPAND YOUR HORIZONS. Once you've nailed down your route and the time it takes to complete it, you'll be riding to and from work without even a second thought. Now's the time to change it up. Turn down a different road on your way home, check out a new neighborhood or incorporate a greenway. Keep the ride exciting and the scenery entertaining, and soon you'll be sad on the days you drive your car.

COMMUTER SPOTLIGHT: SEAN CRYAN AND KEN BOYD

Sean Cryan of Seattle, who received a Bicycling *BikeTown bike in 2005, says bike commuting helped him recover from open heart surgery:*

In February of 2005, I was diagnosed with mitral-valve regurgitation—the cords that operate the valve had snapped. I wanted to be in prime condition when I had surgery in June. When I went in for pre-op testing, my resting heart rate was in the low- to mid-50s. All these people kept saying, "Wow, you're a real athlete." I said, "Athlete? All I do is ride my bike to work."

For the first three weeks I wasn't allowed to lift more than five pounds per hand, so I couldn't put any weight on a handlebar. I had to wait three months for my sternum to set before riding outside. They cut the sternum down the center and closed it with stainless-steel wire. I have a titanium ring and some Gore-Tex in my heart, too. I was able to ride my BikeTown bike on the trainer five weeks after surgery. I was pretty tentative the first week, but the next week I rode the equivalent of 65 miles. I had a good incentive. My coworkers started the Cryan Bicycle Challenge: Our architectural firm would contribute a dollar for every mile employees biked or walked to work during Bike to Work Week. We raised $1,600 for two new office bikes, Wilbur and Orville. We have a lot of local projects, and it's easier to bike to the sites than to try to park downtown.

Why I Ride

"When you're not in a cab or bus, you make your own decisions about which way you want to go, or what you want to look at or how long you want to stay somewhere. On a bike you have a sense of freedom. If you want to stop and check something out, you just stop."—DAVID BYRNE, LEAD SINGER FOR THE TALKING HEADS

After his recovery, Sean lent his BikeTown bike to a coworker, Ken Boyd, who was recovering from knee surgery. Here is his story:

I tore my ACL playing soccer last winter. After surgery, the physical therapists suggested I get on a bike. I had an old Trek 800, but I'd taken it apart and couldn't get it back together again.

I set Sean's bike up in a trainer, and I would start by rocking back and forth on the pedals for about five minutes to loosen my knee. At first I could go only 15 or 20 minutes, tops. I felt lopsided—the muscles on that side had atrophied, so I had to make a conscious effort to use both legs. By summer, I started commuting. At first, I took the bus part of the way because I couldn't stand up on the pedals or use clips because of my knee. By the end of the summer I'd worked up to riding the whole route, 16 miles. I'm not a die-hard cyclist, so when the weather turns I switch back to running. But yeah, I'll ride again this spring. I may have to get my own bike—or get my brother to fix mine.

Fun **Fact**

Replacing your car or second car with a combination of bicycling, transit, and an occasional cab or rented car could help you save as much as 25 percent of your income.
—*SMARTTRIPS.ORG*

WHAT EVERY CYCLIST SHOULD KNOW ABOUT COMMUTING

➔Riding for transportation is real cycling. Add the miles to your training log and watch your fitness improve as you put in extra saddle time. And if your commute is long enough to serve as your training ride, you've just added more free hours to your day.

➔If your trip is less than five miles, there's not much excuse for driving instead of riding. It could take you just as long to drive to your destination and find a parking spot as it does to ride.

➔Quit using "there's no shower at work" as an excuse. In a survey of hundreds of bike commuters in North America, Dave Glowacz, author of *Urban Bikers' Tips and Tricks*, found that 85 percent don't bother to shower after reaching their destination. Change your clothes, and keep a stash of baby wipes in your desk drawer for quick cleanups.

➔A rural bike commute isn't much different than your regular road ride, but riding in urban traffic requires you to ride more like you would drive. Traffic will be heavier, but also slower than you're used to, so you may be able to take the whole lane. Also, signal where you're going and ride predictably.

➔It's not always fastest to ride fast. The need for sudden stops can hijack momentum. Commuting becomes almost a zen art, and a hell of a lot of fun, if you go with the flow of timed lights and traffic.

➔The best bike for your commute depends on the distance and terrain you cover, and whether or not you'll have to lock up. It could be the rusty hardtail or cruiser in your garage, your regular road bike or a dedicated

Why I Ride

"Car commercials portray driving as fun: Buy this car, and you can go this fast. But a more accurate commercial would be sitting on a freeway in rush-hour traffic—that's not a fun activity. Riding a bike is a fun activity."—DAVE ZABRISKIE, PROFESSIONAL CYCLIST AND FOUNDER OF THE ADVOCACY ORGANIZATION YIELD TO LIFE (YIELDTOLIFE.ORG).

commuter bike. The one bike that will work for every commute: a cyclocross bike.

→Commuting doesn't have to be an all-or-nothing endeavor. Bring a few changes of clothes to the office when you drive there on Monday morning. Commute back and forth by bike Monday evening through Friday morning. Drive home Friday after work. Or, drive partway (preferably beyond that dangerous stretch of highway), park your car and ride the remaining distance to work. You can also drive in and ride home one day, then ride in and drive home the next. Even commuting by bike just once a week helps keep the air—and you—healthier.

Reader Tip

"IF YOUR COWORKERS SEEM UNCOMFORTABLE WITH THE SPANDEX PARADE, CONSIDER WEARING BAGGY SHORTS OVER YOUR BIKE SHORTS, AT LEAST WHILE INDOORS. IT MAY KEEP YOUR BIKE COMMUTING FROM BECOMING AN ISSUE WITH MANAGEMENT."—*KEVIN UTSEY, BIKETOWN CHARLOTTE, 2005*

COMMUTER SPOTLIGHT: KEITH GATES (AKA THE COMMUTER DUDE)

Keith Gates took up cycling because of a guitar. "I threw the strap over my shoulder, looked down and couldn't see the strings," says the 38-year-old systems support analyst from Olathe, Kansas, who weighed 245 pounds at the time. "I started Weight Watchers the next week." He also started riding on weekends—once around the block at first, then on a local rec trail. Before long, "weekends just weren't enough," Gates says, so he began riding to work a couple times a week. "Eventually I realized I hadn't filled my car with gas in three months." The Commuter Dude was born.

Today Gates, who has lost nearly 100 pounds, commutes 25 miles round-trip and is on a mission to help others do the same—by dishing out advice and shooting down excuses at his website, commuterdude.com. Here are some of his best tips for getting started.

TAPE YOUR FRAME. The first year Gates commuted, he noticed that "more cars were cutting in front of me as the days got shorter. At first I thought 'What jerks,' but then I realized that they probably couldn't see me." In addition to using front and rear lights, Gates recommends applying easy-to-remove electrical tape to your frame, then sticking reflective tape to the electrical tape.

USE YOUR EARS. "You can often tell by the pitch of the tires and engine whether or not a driver sees you," Gates says.

AVOID BURNOUT. Commuting can leave you overtrained, especially if you also ride on weekends, says Gates. "I used to feel guilty about taking a day off, but we all need a break every once in a while."

JOIN THE CLUBS. "I try to support as many of the local bike clubs as I can," says Gates, who rides with several Kansas City–area groups and uses his website to publicize their advocacy efforts. "You never know what they might be doing that will benefit your riding, even if you don't commute."

Fun **Fact**

In one British study, car commuters stuck in traffic had anxiety levels comparable to those of fighter pilots or riot policemen. To keep your cool, ride your bike instead.

THE IN-A-PINCH MESSENGER BAG

The problem with cell phones is that wherever you are, you can be reached. And when your significant other rings you during your spin through town to ask you to pick up a few things at the market, this excuse won't fly: "Anything for you, my love, but I have no way of carrying the groceries home." Because all you need to get one bag of goods from point A to point B (without even bruising the produce) are three plastic grocery bags. Just make sure to booby-trap your bike (see p. 127) while you're inside feeling the melons.

1. At checkout, fit all of your items into one grocery bag.

2. Tie an empty grocery bag to one handle of the filled bag.

3. Tie another to the other handle.

4. Tie the second and third together at the top to create a plastic messenger bag.

5. Sling it over your shoulder and ride. And for the love of Mother Earth, find a creative way to reuse the bags.

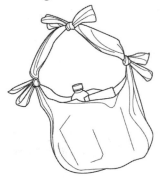

COMMUTER SPOTLIGHT: MICAH DEFFRIES

As part of New Belgium Brewing's Tour de Fat bike-trade program, Micah Deffries received a custom-built Black Sheep bike. In exchange, he signed over the titles of his two cars to the brewery, and lived car-free in Boise, Idaho, for 1 year. Here's what he learned:

CRUSH THAT DEBT. "About 2 years ago, I bought a bike and I gradually started using it," says Deffries. He credits riding with helping him emerge from debt. Now that he's completely carless, he saves about $400 a month.

PLAN EARLY AND OFTEN. Riding forces Deffries to plan his activities in advance, which has made him more organized. "If I need to go to the grocery store I need to have panniers with me. And if I take it to the shop for repairs I have to walk home."

PILFER-PROOF YOUR RIDE. Deffries secures his bike with a U-lock and a cable lock around the wheels. He's had lights and a cyclecomputer stolen, so he keeps them in his bag when he's not riding. "At least they didn't take my bike," he says.

SOMETIMES, ASK FOR HELP. When Deffries's roommate told him they needed to move,

Fun **Fact**

More and more government officials are recognizing the benefits of utility cycling, so much so that in March 2010, Transportation Secretary Ray LaHood instructed states and agencies nationwide to "consider walking and bicycling as equals with other transportation modes." That's good advice for all of us—and it's easier than you think.

he pulled most of his belongings across town in a BOB trailer, and loaded his bed and recliner into his roommate's truck. "That was the only time I've asked someone for a ride," he says.

AVOID CARS. Deffries tries to choose low-traffic routes. "I'm out there to make a statement, so I ride wherever I think I can," he says. "But in places where there's no shoulder and the sidewalks are horrendous, I think I can make a statement somewhere else."

CHAPTER 16

Be Careful Out There

While all cyclists need to learn to handle their bikes on the road (see Part III, Road Skills), it's an especially important skill for bike commuters, who are often riding when traffic is heaviest and tempers are shortest. And unlike most recreational riders, cyclists running errands on two wheels must lock their bikes securely—or risk being stranded. With the advice on the following pages, you'll learn how to navigate traffic and obstacles with ease, and prevent the most common cycling accidents.

BE STREETWISE

Former *Bicycling* Editor-in-Chief Loren Mooney, a New York City bike commuter, shares her best strategies for riding safely in traffic:

The light was green, so I pedaled toward the intersection, looking right just in time to see the black Lincoln Town Car gun into the crosswalk. I slammed on my brakes as the driver slammed on his, and we came to rest just a few feet apart. His window was open, and in the awkward moment of stillness, I glanced at his traffic light and said, "That looks red to me." He ignored me, then the light changed and he gunned it again. I waited for the intersection to clear, then pedaled through.

In 6 years of commuting by bike in New York City, I've also had near-run-ins with taxis, pedestrians, hot dog carts and police cars—and every one of them was breaking a traffic law.

My point is that the age-old cycling advice, "Ride like you're a car, and obey all traffic laws," is correct, but it won't necessarily keep you safe on a busy street. But these strategies have served me well.

ANTICIPATE. Being a self-involved urbanite gives me an advantage as a cyclist. Constantly considering how every little incident affects me helps me avoid accidents every day. I try to notice everything up to half a block ahead: There's an intersection; a car could speed through. That parked car's wheels are turned out; it could pull into my path. There's a woman hailing a cab; one could dart in front of me and stop. This works in suburban or rural environments, too: That dog isn't wearing an invisible-fence collar; he could chase me.

BE HUMAN. I may be one of the only cyclists in New York City who signals. I do it not only to let

Three Key Handling Skills for Riding in Traffic

STOP FAST
With your body weight over the rear of the saddle to prevent skidding, squeeze both brake levers, using strong force for the left (front brake) lever and moderate for the right (rear). If the rear wheel skids, let up slightly on both levers before squeezing again.

PEDAL SLOWLY
As you approach a red light or slow-moving obstacle, gently squeeze both brake levers and pedal lightly. The pressure on the cranks keeps your center of gravity low, making balancing at slow speeds easier. To go ultraslow: With constant pressure on the brakes, stand with your weight over the bottom bracket and ratchet one pedal (whichever feels more comfortable) between 2 and 3 o'clock. As you barely inch forward, swing the handlebar left and right for balance.

ROLL POTHOLES
On a crowded street, sometimes the safest path is over the asphalt divot, not around it. Unweight the front of your bike so it glides over the pothole instead of nose-diving into it. With a loose and light grip on the handlebar, squat so that most of your weight is on your pedals, and your butt is resting lightly on the back of your saddle.

drivers know I'm turning, but also because it's humanizing. When cyclists don't interact with drivers, it's too easy for drivers to see us as just another road hazard. When I signal, "I'm turning left," the subtext is, "Hi, I have arms just like you and am using this road, too." Likewise, making eye contact with drivers at intersections is a good way to ensure that you're seen.

DON'T ALWAYS DO THE RIGHT THING. Hugging the right side of the road generally keeps you out of harm's way, but riding three or so feet into the lane is safer if parked cars line the street (a car door could open). Likewise, riding a few feet into the lane can be a good idea if you're approaching an intersection—if a car passes you, then cuts you off to turn right, you can escape by riding around on the left. Or if the color-blind driver of a Town Car suddenly surges in from the right, you are deep enough into the intersection to avoid being hit.

HERD THE PEDESTRIANS. When you happen upon unsuspecting jaywalkers, aim to pass behind them rather than cut in front of them as they cross the street. Like a deer in headlights, a walker's natural reaction to an oncoming vehicle is to freeze, then hurry forward. Cutting behind them gives you both a better chance for safe passage.

THE GOOD FIGHT. We've found this general script effective (though not perfect) for defusing heated confrontations with drivers.

First, introduce yourself and put your hand out to shake. If you rolled through a stop sign

Pro **Tip**

ALWAYS WRAP YOUR THUMBS AROUND THE HANDLEBAR, INSTEAD OF LAYING THEM ACROSS THE TOP. I CAN'T TELL YOU HOW MANY TIMES I'VE SEEN A RIDER GO DOWN AFTER HIS HANDS WERE JARRED OFF THE BAR WHEN HE HIT A BUMP.

—*ALEX STIEDA*

Turning Points

Under the Uniform Vehicle code, cyclists must signal their intention to turn right or left continuously for the last 100 feet before the turn. (If your hand "is needed in the control or operation" of your bike, you are not legally required to signal.) If the cyclist is stopped and waiting to turn, the cyclist must signal when stopped, although that signal need not be continuous. Some states also require cyclists to signal stops.—Bob Mionske

STOPPING

RIGHT-HAND TURN (OPTION 2)

RIGHT-HAND TURN (OPTION 1)

LEFT-HAND TURN

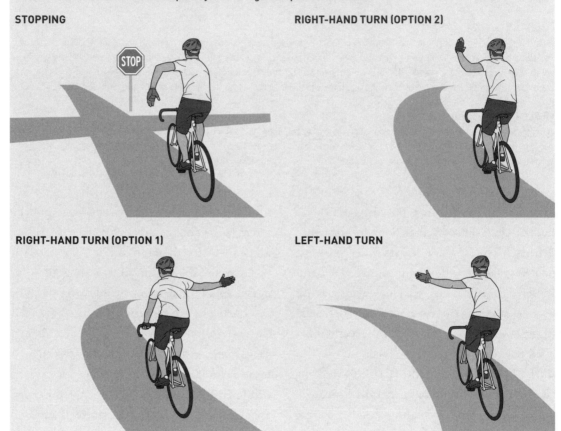

or did something even remotely wrong, apologize.

If the driver cites an incorrect belief about road rules, point it out, with empathy: "Actually, it is legal to ride two abreast in this state. But I know it can be frustrating to wait to pass."

Cite the bottom line: "It's extremely danger-ous for cyclists out here when people lose their tempers. Two cars can have a minor fender bender but if you and I collide, I could die. It's not worth it for either of us."

Cut off the interaction to avoid further escalation: "I have to take off now. I hope that next time we see each other it can be on better terms."

THE MOST COMMON CAR-BIKE COLLISIONS—AND HOW TO AVOID THEM

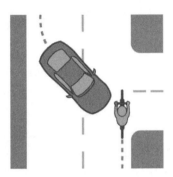

LEFT CROSS: A motorist fails to see a cyclist and makes a left turn—it accounts for almost half of all car-bike crashes, according to the Pedestrian and Bicycle Information Center (PBIC).

AVOID IT: If you see a car turning into your path, turn right into the lane with the vehicle. "Don't creep into the intersection at red lights to get a head start," says Laura Sandt, program specialist for the PBIC.

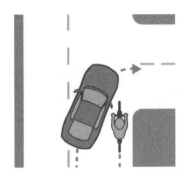

RIGHT HOOK: A motorist passes a cyclist on the left and turns right into the bike's path.

AVOID IT: Passing stopped or slow-moving cars on the right places you in a driver's blind spot. Take the lane—it's your right in all 50 states. "If

you're in the lane, the driver will slow down and stay behind you and wait to make the turn," says Preston Tyree, who runs the Community Mobility Institute in Austin, Texas.

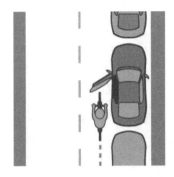

DOORED: A cyclist traveling next to parked cars lined up on the street strikes a car door opened by the driver.

AVOID IT: "Always be looking several cars ahead," Sandt says. Ride at least three feet from parked cars, taking the lane if necessary. Be prepared to stop suddenly. Keep your weight over your rear wheel and apply strong force to the front brake lever, with moderate force to the back.

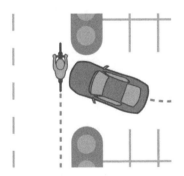

PARKING LOTTED: A motorist exits a driveway or parking lot into the path of a bicyclist.

AVOID IT: No bike-handling tricks can overcome the danger of riding on a road with numerous parking-lot exits. Just take a less-direct route. If you don't change routes, follow the law and ride fully in the road. Most of all: Stay off the sidewalk—motorists aren't looking for you there, Sandt says.

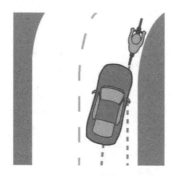

THE OVERTAKING: A motorist hits a cyclist from behind.

AVOID IT: "Make yourself as visible as possible and ride predictably," Sandt says. Use reflectors and lights on your bike at night; when moving to the left, signal with your arm; and hold a straight line while checking traffic over your shoulder, because even the most diligent driver could hit a swerving bike.

LOCK YOUR BIKE

Bike thefts account for 3.7 percent of all larceny and theft crimes in the United States. To keep your bike from contributing to this statistic, don't just chain it up and cross your fingers. Know where to lock it, how to lock it and what to lock it with. Then cross your fingers.

PICK THE RIGHT LOCK. U-locks are the most secure, followed by the chain-and-padlock style. Cable locks place third—but even a thick cable can be cut. High-security locks use pick-resis-

tant flat keys with disc tumblers. Standard house-type keyways are the easiest to pick. Look for good ratings from independent testing agencies like Sold Secure (silver or higher) and ART (three or more stars). Don't forget to register for your lock's antitheft guarantee. Smart tip: Use two types of locks. Because thieves use different techniques or tools for each style of lock, using both a U-lock and a cable lock, for example, will make a theft more difficult.

USE PROPER TECHNIQUE. Look for a sturdy object that's secured to the ground. A bike rack is best, but street-sign poles and parking meters are good options. Never lock your bike to something that can be cut or broken, such as a flimsy sapling, or to an object that the bike can be lifted up and off of.

To secure your bike with a single lock, slide a U-lock's shackle around the wheel where it passes closest to the seat tube. If your front wheel has a quick-release, unfasten the wheel and lean it against the rear wheel so the U-lock shackle secures it, too. If you're using two locks,

Pro **Tip**

TO LOOK LEFT, MOVE YOUR RIGHT HAND TOWARD THE CENTER OF THE HANDLEBAR NEAR THE STEM, THEN DROP YOUR LEFT HAND OFF THE BAR AS YOU TURN YOUR HEAD TO LOOK BACK. TRACK RACERS USE THIS TECHNIQUE WHEN DOING A MADISON RELAY CHANGE—LOOK IT UP ON YOUTUBE TO SEE SOME MAGIC BIKE HANDLING. KEEP YOUR UPPER BODY RELAXED, AND PRACTICE, IDEALLY IN AN EMPTY PARKING LOT WITH LINES YOU CAN FOLLOW.—*ALEX STIEDA* secure the down tube and the bike's front wheel to the object, then use a secondary cable lock to secure the rear wheel to the frame, front wheel and object. With expensive bikes, don't overlook the seat and post. A carbon post and top-quality saddle can cost $300 to replace, and even a standard seat binder can be unfastened in seconds. If you can't take the seat with you, simply unfasten it and run the cable lock through the seat rails. You can also lock your helmet by passing the U-lock or secondary cable lock through the straps.

BREAK THE PATTERN. The same $2,500 mountain bike parked in the same rack at the same time every day is an easy target. Shake it up: Park in different locations, ride different bikes and use different combinations of high-security locks. Take the front wheel with you one day, lock it with the bike the next. Unpredictability makes you less of a target.

PLEAD YOUR COMMUTER CASE. The best place to put your bike if you ride it to work is inside your office, but that's not always feasible. Ask HR about a secure storage room or a rack in the building's garage—many are equipped with surveillance cameras or other security. Point out that riding a bike to work saves parking spaces for other employees.

NO LOCK? NO PROBLEM

Three ways to booby-trap your bike. Say you're out for a ride when you remember that your faithful feline ran out of 9Lives that morning. The problem: You don't have a lock with you. You could go home and break the

Pro Tip

"IF YOU ARE IN AN ACCIDENT DURING DARKNESS AND YOU HAVE REMOVED YOUR BIKE'S REFLECTORS, YOU MAY BE EXPOSING YOURSELF TO CLAIMS THAT YOUR OWN NEGLIGENCE PREVENTED A MOTORIST FROM SEEING YOU."
—BOB MIONSKE

news to Salem that there's no dinner, or you could rig your rig to make it harder to swipe while you make a quick stop. These tips won't prevent your bike from being stolen, but they will slow down a potential thief and buy you some time. Just remember, whatever you do or undo, you have to undo or redo. Or something like that.

YOU: Rig the chain. As you're coasting near your stopping point, shift into the big-ring/big-cog combo. When you stop to park your bike, shift just your shifters (don't pedal) into the small-ring/small-cog combo.

THE THIEF: Jumps on, tries to pedal—only to have the gears go crazy and the chain drop off—then freaks out and splits.

YOU: Open the rear quick-release skewer.

THE THIEF: Pedals for a bit—until the wheel starts to wobble and the bike eventually becomes unrideable—then drops the bike and runs.

YOU: Use your minitool to loosen the side pinch bolts on your stem and turn your bar 90 degrees; loosen your seat clamp bolt and turn your seat backward.

THE THIEF: Looks at bike, thinks he's losing his mind, wants nothing to do with it, and moves on.

CHAPTER 17

Taking Action

Make your community safer, more friendly—and more accountable—to cyclists.

Commuting by bike can expose you to things you'd never noticed from your car: uniquely designed houses or gardens; smiles from crossing guards; the smell of your neighbor's backyard barbecue. But once you start riding around town, you'll probably also start seeing areas that could stand to be improved: an open grate or pothole that forces you to swerve into traffic, or a street that could really use a bike lane. Here's how to change laws, create an effective campaign or advocacy group, and improve the cycling infrastructure where you live.

FIND LOCAL FRIENDS. Don't go it alone—like-minded enthusiasts make everything from organizing to politicking easier. "Most cities have some kind of bike-advisory committee or group that has a seat at the table when you're dealing with cities and local agencies," says Andy Clarke, executive director of the League of American Bicyclists. "It's a good idea to be involved with people who are already involved."

LEARN FROM THE LEADERS. If no formal organizations exist in your area, or the groups seem weak and disorganized, educate yourself by associating with bigger nationwide or regional groups. Avery Stonich, former marketing and communications manager for the Bikes Belong Coalition, suggests taking cues from other successful bike-advocacy groups. "Our organization provides support so people don't have to reinvent the wheel every time they want to get involved," she says.

SET GOALS. "Do your homework before you do anything," Clarke says. Find out what the bike laws are in your area and compare them with laws nationwide. Determine your community's needs and use them to focus your goals. "Is it changing the law, or is it changing the community's culture?" Clarke says. Stonich urges aspiring bike advocates to avoid frustration. "One of the challenges is that it's a slow process," she says. "You can start work today and you might not see results for several years." If you want to create a relatively quick change with measurable results, target one law that stands out as the weakest in comparison with nationwide norms. A good longer-term goal: the creation of a bicycle master plan for a city.

NETWORK. Find out who pulls strings in your community: Who knows the mayor or your congressional representative? Ask around—you might be surprised to find out who has influence. Use any venue available for getting face time with legislators. "Often all it takes is saying the word 'bicycle,'" Clarke says. "You'd be amazed how all of a sudden people want to be on your side." Even sending a handwritten letter to a town VIP can make a difference. Attend public meetings about bike or public transportation plans, or parks and recreation, Stonich says, so you'll stay on the minds of powerful people.

BE SPECIFIC. When speaking face-to-face with a legislator, avoid being overbroad. "The more open you are, the more room there is for interpretation," Stonich says. Instead of saying, for example, that your city needs to be friendly to cyclists, request that bike lanes be placed in a certain part of town, or that a city bike coordinator be instated. "If you're making a presentation and you just talk about how bad everything is, it's easy for your listener to cluck and say, 'Well I wish you all the best,'" Clarke says. "Ask for something specific, and you'll be hard to ignore."

DON'T GIVE UP. Earl Jones, president of the Louisville Bicycle Club, in Kentucky, pushed cycling for years with no results. Louisville had no bike lanes and two shared-use paths. "Then our mayor, Jerry Abramson, realized that bicycling can add a certain kind of spice, buzz, whatever to a city," Jones says. Abramson called a citywide bike summit in 2005, and the city made progress. In 2006, Louisville earned the Bike Friendly Community distinction from the League of American Bicyclists, and in 2008, *Bicycling* named it one of America's most-improved cities for cycling.

RIDER **RESOURCES**

The Bikes Belong Coalition (bikesbelong.org), League of American Bicyclists (bikeleague.org), Alliance for Biking and Walking (peoplepoweredmovement.org) and Pedestrian and Bicycle Information Center (pedbikeinfo.org) are armed with statistics and resources that can help you improve cycling conditions in your town.

Calculate the amount of money you could save by leaving your car at home at smarttrips.org.

Find car-style taillight signals and other bike lights from the American Bike Safety Company at safetybikesignals.com.

Know someone who could use a bike to get around? Check out Bicycling.com/biketown to see if we're giving away bikes in your city this year.

VI

Fitness, Training, and Racing

FOR SOME PEOPLE, RIDING IS SIMPLY A WAY TO GET from point A to Point B, and that's great. But sooner or later, most of us are tempted to try to pedal faster—or farther. Whether your goal is to win a race, lose 20 pounds, or just to reach the top of your local hill without stopping, we can help you get there.

CHAPTER 18

Training Tips and Workouts Galore

You'll find five of our favorite plans on the following pages, along with plenty of advice on tackling everything from hills to hot days. (Note: If you're aiming for a century ride, also see Chapter 22.)

FIRST, FIND YOUR THRESHOLD

Your lactate threshold (LT) pace is, in riding terms, the fastest speed you can maintain for 30 minutes without feeling like your legs are on fire. You'll know you've hit it when your breathing becomes short, quick and rhythmic (but not gasping). Raise your LT, and "you can produce more power at a comfortable heart rate, which makes you a better rider and racer in every situation," says USA Cycling expert coach Margaret Kadlick.

Pros test their LT in a lab, where they pedal against ever-increasing resistance while technicians take blood samples to measure the increasing lactate levels. But you can find your LT with a do-it-yourself time trial:

Map a three-mile route that you can ride without stopping. Strap on a heart rate monitor, warm up for 20 minutes, then ride the route at the fastest pace you can sustain. Recover for 10 to 20 minutes by riding back to the start of your route at an easy pace. Repeat the test. Your LT is

approximately the average heart rate of the two efforts. (More accurately, it's 103 percent of that figure.) Jot down your times and average paces.

Like most things body-related, LT is partially genetic. But it's also quite trainable—which is where some of the workouts in this chapter come in. Repeat the test in eight weeks to see your progress.

PLAN #1: BUILD YOUR BASE IN FOUR WEEKS

Purists preach that to properly prepare for the cycling season, you need to roll out six weeks ahead and do nothing but low-heart-rate, low-intensity rides before you throw the hammer down and go out and play, especially if your idea of fun is a frisky group ride. It's no problem if you're a professional rider with nothing but time and a salary to ride, but for the rest of us, it's precious pedal time we simply don't have. Thankfully, it's also unnecessary.

"For pros who can ride 20 to 30 hours a week, a long base period is appropriate," says expert coach Jeb Stewart, CSCS, owner of the online coaching company Endurofit. "But if you struggle to squeeze in half that amount, it's almost counterproductive because you aren't clocking enough saddle time to elicit a training stress." Stress is key. If you don't have hours to slowly tax your system, you need to do shorter rides with focused efforts to stimulate fitness adaptations, says Stewart. "You can get the same amount of training stress in a 90-minute tempo interval workout as you can in a three-hour endurance ride."

You'll still need to build in saddle time to condition your body to sit on a bike for longer rides, but Stewart's focused four-week plan will lay down a solid fitness foundation for the season ahead. To stave off early-season aches and pains, warm up and cool down before and after each workout, and recover for five minutes between intervals.

Heart Rate Zones and Threshold Power

Threshold heart rate (T HR): Average HR or power for a 20-minute time trial or 1-hour hard group ride

Threshold power (T power): Average power for a 20-minute time trial minus 5% of this number

Threshold (T) pace: 95–105% of T HR/91–105% of T power

Active Recovery pace: <68% of T HR/<55% of T power

Endurance pace: 69–83% of T HR/56–75% of T power

Tempo pace: 84–94% of T HR/76–90% of T power

WEEK 1

Monday: Off

Tuesday: 1 hour w/5 sets of 5x15-second Fast Pedaling intervals

Wednesday: 1 hr. in the Active Recovery zone

Thursday: 1 hr. w/3x10-min. Big Gear Tempo intervals at 50–70 rpm

Friday: 1 hr. in the Active Recovery zone

Saturday: 2–3 hrs. in the Endurance zone

Sunday: 1 hr. in the Active Recovery zone

WEEK 2

Monday: Off

Tuesday: 1.5 hrs. w/4 sets of 5x30-sec. Fast Pedaling intervals

Wednesday: 1 hr. in the Active Recovery zone

Thursday: 1.5 hrs. w/3x15-min. Big Gear Tempo intervals at 60–80 rpm

Friday: 1 hr. in the Active Recovery zone

Saturday: 3–4 hrs. Hills

Sunday: 1.5–2 hrs. in the Active Recovery zone

WEEK 3

Monday: Off

Tuesday: 2 hrs. w/3 sets of 5x1-min. Fast Pedaling intervals

The Midday Stress-Buster

You can do this workout on a loop as short as half a mile. With warm-up and cool-down, it takes around 45 minutes. Pick starting points, such as mailboxes, for one-minute intervals. Accelerate to maximum effort over 20 seconds, then hold that intensity for the rest of the minute. Space the starting points so you can do the interval, then cruise for less than three minutes before the next one. Complete four intervals, then ride easy for six minutes before starting a second set. Do two sets; experienced riders can add a third.

Wednesday: 1 hr. in the Active Recovery zone

Thursday: 2 hrs. w/2x20-min. Tempo intervals

Friday: 1 hr. in the Active Recovery zone

Saturday: 4.5 hrs Hills

Sunday: 1.5–2 hrs. in the Active Recovery zone

WEEK 4

Monday: Off

Tuesday: 1 hr. of easy pedaling

Wednesday: 1.5 hrs. w/5x30-sec. Fast Pedaling intervals and 1x10-min. Tempo interval

Thursday: 1 hr. in the Active Recovery zone

Friday: Off

Saturday: Group ride, century or hammerfest

Sunday: 1 hr. in the Active Recovery zone

The Workouts

FAST PEDALING. Spin quickly with proper form. Active and recovery periods are the same duration. Improves pedaling efficiency and increases workout intensity.

BIG GEAR TEMPO. Ride a bigger gear at a specified cadence in the Tempo zone. (If your knees begin to hurt, decrease the gear and increase the cadence to do regular tempo work instead.)

Improves muscular endurance and increases training stress.

TEMPO. Ride intervals at 90+ rpm in the Tempo zone. Increases aerobic fitness, muscular endurance and training stress.

ENDURANCE. Ride for two to five hours in the Endurance zone at a comfortably high cadence. Boosts muscular endurance, aerobic fitness and fat-burning capacity.

HILLS. Ride in the Endurance and Tempo zones on hilly terrain using gearing and cadence to control effort. Improves muscular endurance and overall strength.

WORKOUTS FOR WEIGHT LOSS

For most of us, shedding those last ten pounds doesn't mean riding more. It means riding smarter. The secret is EPOC. Though it sounds like something the U.S. Anti-Doping Agency might ban, EPOC is a biological process known as excess post-exercise oxygen consumption or, more plainly, the number of calories your body burns after you've racked the bike. The higher your afterburn, the more fat you fry.

"A variety of workouts infused with high intensity is the key to enhancing EPOC," says exercise physiologist Len Kravitz, PhD, of the University of New Mexico. The harder your body needs to work to replenish oxygen stores, repair muscles and remove metabolic waste, the more post-ride calories you burn. During a recent research review, Kravitz's lab identified the top workouts for maximizing exercise afterburn, which lasts about two hours before fading. The following five cardio workouts (the two other top workouts were circuit training and high-intensity strength training) led the pack.

Workout Type: Tempo

EPOC Boost: Warm up for 10 minutes. Crank the intensity until your heart rate is between 80–85% of your max. Stay there for 30 minutes. Cool down.

How It Works: Tempo pace hugs the redline between aerobic and anaerobic efforts, pushing your lactate threshold higher, so you can ride longer—and burn more fat—at higher intensities.

Do It: Once a week. Each week, add 3–5 minutes to the tempo interval until you hit 45- to 50-minute efforts.

Workout Type: LSD (long slow distance)

EPOC Boost: Saddle up and keep the pace easy. Intensity should be very light to somewhat hard (65–70% of your max HR) for 1–2 hours or longer.

How It Works: LSD beefs up your mitochondria—the little furnaces in your cells that blast stored fat and carbs with O_2 to make aerobic energy. The bigger your furnaces, the more fat you can burn and the higher your capacity for intense interval work.

Do It: Once a week. These can be extended to as long as you like. Best done solo or with a small, like-minded group to quell the urge to hammer.

Workout Type: Splits

EPOC Boost: Warm up for 10 minutes. Turn up the intensity to 80–85% max HR. Hold it there for 15–20 minutes. Recover for 5 minutes at a very low intensity (50% max HR). Repeat three more times. Cool down.

How It Works: Repeating bouts of high-end tempo-intensity efforts forces your body to dig deep into its reserves, boosts fitness and trains the body to recover quickly.

Do It: Perform Splits OR 3-Minute On-Off Intervals OR Supramaximal Intervals once a week.

Workout Type: 3-Minute On-Off Intervals

EPOC Boost: Warm up for 10 minutes. Ramp up to 85–90% of max HR for 3 minutes. Recover for 3 minutes at 50% max HR. Repeat intervals for a total duration of 30 minutes. Cool down.

How It Works: These anaerobic efforts improve your body's ability to use oxygen, and thereby burn more fat at higher intensities.

Do It: Perform 3-Minute On-Off Intervals OR Supramaximal Intervals OR Splits once a week. Work up to doing 45–50 minutes' worth of 3-Minute On-Off Intervals.

Workout Type: Supramaximal Intervals

EPOC Boost: Warm up for 15 minutes. Blast up to >90% of max HR. Hang on, maintaining good form, for 60 seconds. Recover for 2–5 minutes at 50% max HR. Repeat 15–20 times. Cool down.

How It Works: Supramaximal intervals elicit metabolic changes that increase your lactate buffering capacity. They also push the upper limits of your exercise capacity, which ultimately improves endurance.

Do It: Perform Supramaximal Intervals OR Splits OR 3-Minute On-Off Intervals once a week.

PLAN #2: RACE THE CLOCK

Want to crush your buddies in the group ride? Or blister the competition in a local crit, road race, or even triathlon? Train like a time-trialist. (For a triathlon-specific plan, see p. 146.) To master the discipline, you need to spend most of your interval time at an intensity near your lactate threshold, that burn point at which your muscles accumulate lactic acid faster than your body can flush it. The benefit of pedaling at this uncomfortable pace is that you edge your threshold higher, which enables you to ride harder and longer while feeling great—any day, any time. During the rest period between intervals, keep a high cadence (80–100), with little or no resistance.

Beginner (>9:00 in a flat, windless 3-mi. time trial) = workouts in black; advanced (<9:00 in a flat, windless 3-mi. TT) = variations in white where they appear

All rides at conversational pace (easy to moderate) on flat to rolling terrain, unless otherwise noted Recovery Ride = Easy ride in a light gear at moderate cadence

LT Intervals = Pace just below lactate threshold (LT), or the point at which your breathing goes from deep and rhythmic to fast, almost gasping, with a perceived exertion of about 7 on a scale of 1–10, or 85–89% of your max heart rate

VO_2 Intervals = As hard as possible, paying no attention to heart rate, to boost maximum oxygen consumption (VO_2 max) levels

Power Intervals = Pace above lactate threshold, with a perceived exertion of 8–9, or 90–95% of your max heart rate

THIS 40K TIME TRIAL PLAN CAN MAKE ANYONE FASTER.

Want to crush your buddies in the group ride? Or blister the competition in a local crit, road race, or even triathlon? Train like a time-trialist. To master the discipline, you need to spend most of your interval time at an intensity near your lactate threshold, that burn point at which your muscles accumulate lactic acid faster than your body can flush it. The benefit of pedaling at this uncomfortable pace is that you edge your threshold higher, which enables you to ride harder and longer while feeling great—any day, any time. Plan Tip: During the rest period between intervals, keep a high cadence (80–100), with little or no resistance.

Beginner (>9:00 in a flat, windless 3-mi. time trial)=workouts in BLACK; advanced (<9:00 in a flat, windless 3-mi. TT)=variations in WHITE where they appear ▪ All rides at conversational pace (easy to moderate) on flat to rolling terrain, unless otherwise noted ▪ RECOVERY RIDE=Easy ride in a light gear at moderate cadence LT INTERVALS=Pace just below lactate threshold (LT), or the point at which your breathing goes from deep and rhythmic to fast, almost gasping, with a perceived exertion of about 7 on a scale of 1–10, or 85–89% of your max heart rate VO₂ INTERVALS=As hard as possible, paying no attention to heart rate, to boost maximum oxygen consumption (VO₂ max) levels POWER INTERVALS=Pace above lactate threshold, with a perceived exertion of 8–9, or 90–95% of your max heart rate

WEEK	MONDAY	TUESDAY	WEDNESDAY	THURSDAY	FRIDAY	SATURDAY	SUNDAY
1	REST DAY	1 hr. 30 min. w/ 3x4-min. LT Intervals; 10 min. rest w/ 3x8-min. LT Intervals; 8 min. rest	1 hr. 30 min. w/ 4x4-min. LT Intervals; 8 min. rest w/ 4x7-min. LT Intervals; 8 min. rest	REST DAY	30 min.	2 hrs. w/ 3x6-min. LT Intervals; 8 min. rest w/ 3x10-min. LT Intervals; 8 min. rest	1 hr. 30 min.
2	REST DAY	1 hr. 30 min. w/ 3x6-min. LT Intervals; 8 min. rest w/ 3x10-min. LT Intervals; 8 min. rest	1 hr. 30 min. w/ 3x4-min. LT Intervals; 8 min. rest w/ 3x8-min. LT Intervals; 8 min. rest	REST DAY	30 min.	2 hrs. 30 min. w/ 4x6-min. LT Intervals; 10 min. rest w/ 4x10-min. LT Intervals; 10 min. rest	2 hrs.
3	REST DAY	1 hr. 30 min. w/ 3x2-min. Power Intervals; 4 min. rest w/ 3x4-min. Power Intervals; 4 min. rest	1 hr. 30 min. w/ 4x20-sec. VO₂ Intervals; 45 sec. rest w/ 4x30-sec. VO₂ Intervals; 30 sec. rest	REST DAY	1 hr. w/ 3x4-min. LT Intervals; 8 min. rest w/ 3x8-min. LT Intervals; 8 min. rest	3 hrs. w/ 4x8-min. LT Intervals; 10 min. rest w/ 4x12-min. LT Intervals; 10 min. rest	2 hrs. 30 min.
4	REST DAY	1 hr.	1 hr. 30 min. w/ 3x6-min. LT Intervals; 8 min. rest w/ 3x10-min. LT Intervals; 8 min. rest	REST DAY	30 min.	2 hrs. w/ 3x2-min. Power Intervals; 4 min. rest w/ 3x4-min. Power Intervals; 4 min. rest	1 hr.
5	REST DAY	1 hr. 30 min. w/ 3x2-min. Power Intervals; 4 min. rest w/ 3x4-min. Power Intervals; 4 min. rest	1 hr. 30 min. w/ 4x6-min. LT Intervals; 10 min. rest w/ 4x10-min. LT Intervals; 10 min. rest	REST DAY	1 hr. w/ 4x6-min. LT Intervals; 10 min. rest w/ 4x10-min. LT Intervals; 10 min. rest	2 hrs. w/ 4x8-min. LT Intervals; 10 min. rest w/ 4x12-min. LT Intervals; 10 min. rest	1 hr. 30 min.
6	REST DAY	1 hr. 30 min. w/ 4x3-min. Power Intervals; 4 min. rest w/ 4x4-min. Power Intervals; 4 min. rest	1 hr. 30 min. w/ 4x8-min. LT Intervals; 10 min. rest w/ 4x12-min. LT Intervals; 10 min. rest	REST DAY	1 hr. w/ 2 sets of 4x20-sec. VO₂ Intervals; 45 sec. rest; 2 min. b/t sets w/ 2 sets of 4x30-sec. VO₂ Intervals; 30 sec. rest; 2 min. b/t sets	2 hrs. 30 min. w/ 4x10-min. LT Intervals; 10 min. rest w/ 4x15-min. LT Intervals; 10 min. rest	1 hr. 30 min.
7	REST DAY	1 hr. 30 min. w/ 3x2-min. Power Intervals; 4 min. rest w/ 3x4-min. Power Intervals; 4 min. rest	1 hr. 30 min. w/ 3x4-min. LT Intervals; 5 min. rest w/ 3x8-min. LT Intervals; 5 min. rest	REST DAY	1 hr. w/ 4x20-sec. VO₂ Intervals; 45 sec. rest w/ 5x30-sec. VO₂ Intervals; 45 sec. rest	3 hrs. w/ 4x8-min. LT Intervals; 10 min. rest w/ 4x12-min. LT Intervals; 10 min. rest	1 hr. 30 min.
8	REST DAY	1 hr. w/ 3x2-min. Power Intervals; 4 min. rest w/ 3x4-min. Power Intervals; 4 min. rest	1 hr. 30 min. w/ 3x4-min. LT Intervals; 8 min. rest w/ 3x8-min. LT Intervals; 8 min. rest	REST DAY	30 min.	1 hr. w/ 2x1-min. VO₂ Intervals; 6 min. rest w/ 3x1-min. VO₂ Intervals; 6 min. rest	1 hr. 30 min.
9	REST DAY	1 hr. 30 min. w/ 3x2-min. Power Intervals; 4 min. rest w/ 3x3-min. Power Intervals; 4 min. rest	1 hr. 30 min. w/ 4x8-min. LT Intervals; 10 min. rest w/ 4x12-min. LT Intervals; 10 min. rest	REST DAY	1 hr. w/ 4x20-sec. VO₂ Intervals; 45 sec. rest w/ 5x30-sec. VO₂ Intervals; 45 sec. rest	2 hrs. w/ 4x8-min. LT Intervals; 8 min. rest w/ 4x12-min. LT Intervals; 8 min. rest	1 hr. 30 min.
10	REST DAY	1 hr. 30 min. w/ 4x3-min. Power Intervals; 3 min. rest w/ 4x4-min. Power Intervals; 3 min. rest	1 hr. 30 min. w/ 4x8-min. LT Intervals; 8 min. rest w/ 4x12-min. LT Intervals; 8 min. rest	REST DAY	1 hr. w/ 2 sets of 4x30-sec. VO₂ Intervals; 45 sec. rest; 2 min. b/t sets w/ 2 sets of 4x45-sec. VO₂ Intervals; 45 sec. rest; 2 min. b/t sets	2 hrs. 30 min. w/ 3x15-min. LT Intervals; 10 min. rest w/ 3x20-min. LT Intervals; 8 min. rest	1 hr. 30 min.
11	REST DAY	1 hr. 30 min. w/ 3x3-min. Power Intervals; 4 min. rest w/ 3x4-min. Power Intervals; 4 min. rest	1 hr. 30 min. w/ 4x8-min. LT Intervals; 5 min. rest w/ 4x10-min. LT Intervals; 5 min. rest	REST DAY	1 hr. w/ 4x30-sec. VO₂ Intervals; 30 sec. rest w/ 4x45-sec. VO₂ Intervals; 30 sec. rest	3 hrs. w/ 4x12-min. LT Intervals; 10 min. rest w/ 4x15-min. LT Intervals; 8 min. rest	1 hr. 30 min.
12	REST DAY	1 hr. w/ 3x2-min. Power Intervals; 4 min. rest w/ 3x3-min. Power Intervals; 4 min. rest	1 hr. 30 min. w/ 3x4-min. LT Intervals; 8 min. rest w/ 3x6-min. LT Intervals; 8 min. rest	REST DAY	30 min.	1 hr. w/ 3x30-sec. VO₂ Intervals; 6 min. rest w/ 3x45-sec. VO₂ Intervals; 6 min. rest	EVENT OR RACE DAY

Chris Carmichael's Weight-Loss Workout

This one-hour workout delivers the double whammy of torching calories and building high-end aerobic power you can put to good use the rest of the season. It's strenuous, so do it a maximum of three times a week to allow for adequate recovery and best results.

- → 6 min.: warmup
- → 1 min.: fast pedal, spinning a light gear as fast as you can
- → 1 min.: recovery spinning
- → 1 min.: fast pedal
- → 1 min.: recovery spinning
- → 5x2 min. at maximum intensity, with 2 min. recovery spinning between each
- → 6 min.: recovery spinning
- → 5x2 min. at maximum intensity, with 2 min. recovery spinning between each
- → 8 min.: cooldown
- → Total time: 60 min.

HOW TO . . . CRUSH CLIMBS

Often, a climb will loom in the distance for miles, giving us time to ponder its difficulty and worry about our fitness. "People get very intimidated by hills," says Jim Rutberg, a Carmichael Training Systems pro-level coach who helps run the company's climbing camps. With practice and some improvements in technique, says Rutberg, that same climb will become easier every time you do it.

For Instant Gratification

Try these techniques on your next ride.

SIT AND SPIN—MOST OF THE TIME. Sitting and spinning an easy gear is the most efficient way to climb. Standing puts more weight on your leg muscles—they work harder, and you use 10 percent more energy and increase your heart rate by 5 to 10 percent. On gradual grades, sit back on the saddle; for steeps, move toward the nose of the saddle and gently pull the bar to assist you up the hill. But there are times when standing is in order, like when your body needs a break on a climb or if you want to accelerate.

SHIFT BEFORE YOU STAND. Shift up a gear, move your hands to the brake hoods and stand as your power foot comes to the top of the pedal stroke. This will push you forward and boost your momentum. Gently push on the bar and rock the bike beneath you as you climb.

STAY ABOVE 75. You may feel mighty mashing uphill in a monster gear at 50 rpm, but you won't make as much progress as you would if you dropped into a lower gear and ramped up to 75, even 85 rpm. An easier spin is more sustainable and won't leave your legs as fatigued.

HERE IS THE FASTEST WAY TO THE TOP OF THE MOUNTAIN.

To climb fast, start by climbing slowly, with controlled intervals, then even slower with muscle-tension work—it's like strength training on the bike. Plan Tips: Beginners, take Mondays and Fridays as rest days ■ Find a breathing rhythm on climbs, and your body will follow.

 Beginners (7–10 hrs./week)=workouts in BLACK, advanced (11–15 hrs./week)=variations in WHITE where they appear ■ All rides at a conversational pace (easy to moderate) on flat to rolling terrain, unless otherwise noted ■ RECOVERY RIDE=Easy pace in a light gear, at a cadence of 75–85 rpm CLIMB REPEATS=Steady climb at 78–83% of MHR, cadence 70–85 rpm TEMPO=Pace at 80% of max heart rate (MHR) in a moderately hard gear, cadence 70–75 rpm MT INTERVALS=Gradual hill in a big gear at low cadence (50–60 rpm) with low heart rate, to achieve muscle tension (MT), to increase strength STEADY STATE=Long effort at your lactate threshold (85% + 3 beats per minute of your MHR), cadence 85–95 rpm

WEEK	MONDAY	TUESDAY	WEDNESDAY	THURSDAY	FRIDAY	SATURDAY	SUNDAY
1	REST DAY: 1 hr. RECOVERY RIDE	1 hr. 15 min. w/ 2x8-min. Climb Repeats; 8 min. rest / 1 hr. 45 min. w/ 3x8-min. Climb Repeats; 6 min. rest	1 hr. 2 hrs. 15 min. w/ 2x20-min. Tempo; 10 min. rest	1 hr. 15 min. / 1 hr. 30 min. w/ 2x10-min. Tempo; 10 min. rest and 3x5-min. MT Intervals; 3 min. rest	REST DAY: 1 hr. TO 1 hr. 30 min. RECOVERY RIDE	1 hr. 45 min. / 2 hrs. 30 min. w/ 3x8-min. Steady State on a climb; 8 min. rest	1 hr. 45 min. 2–3 hrs.
2		1 hr. 30 min. w/ 3x8-min. Climb Repeats; 8 min. rest / 1 hr. 45 min. w/ 3x10-min. Climb Repeats; 8 min. rest	1 hr. 2 hrs. 15 min. w/ 2x27-min. Tempo; 8 min. rest	1 hr. 30 min. w/ 2x10-min. Tempo; 5 min. rest and 4x4-min. MT Intervals; 2 min. rest		2 hrs. / 2 hrs. 45 min. w/ 3x10-min. Steady State on a climb; 8 min. rest	2 hrs. 2 hrs. 30 min. to 3 hrs. 30 min.
3		1 hr. 45 min. w/ 3x10-min. Steady State; 10 min. rest / 2 hrs. w/ 3x12-min. Steady State; 8 min. rest	45 min. 2 hrs. 30 min. w/ 2x30-min. Tempo; 10 min. rest	1 hr. 45 min. w/ 2x15-min. Tempo; 8 min. rest and 3x5-min. MT Intervals; 3 min. rest		2 hrs. 15 min. / 2 hrs. 45 min. w/ 3x12-min. Steady State on a climb; 8 min. rest	2 hrs. 15 min. 3 hrs. w/ 2x25-min. Tempo; 8 min. rest
4		45 min. 1 hr.	1 hr. 1 hr. 30 min.	1 hr. 15 min. 1 hr. 30 min.		2 hrs. 30 min.	2 hrs. 2 to 3 hrs.
5		1 hr. 15 min. w/ 2x10-min. Climb Repeats; 8 min. rest / 1 hr. 45 min. w/ 3x10-min. Climb Repeats; 6 min. rest	1 hr. 2 hrs. 30 min. w/ 2x30-min. Tempo; 10 min. rest	1 hr. 15 min. / 1 hr. 30 min. w/ 2x15-min. Tempo; 10 min. rest and 4x4-min. MT Intervals; 3 min. rest		2 hrs. 15 min. / 2 hrs. 45 min. w/ 3x12-min. Steady State on a climb; 10 min. rest	2 hrs. 3 hrs. w/ 30-min. Tempo
6		1 hr. 30 min. w/ 3x10-min. Climb Repeats; 10 min. rest / 1 hr. 45 min. w/ 3x12-min. Climb Repeats; 8 min. rest	1 hr. 2 hrs. 30 min. w/ 2x35-min. Tempo; 10 min. rest	1 hr. 45 min. w/ 3x10-min. Tempo; 5 min. rest and 4x5-min. MT Intervals; 3 min. rest		2 hrs. 30 min. w/ 3x14-min. Steady State; 8 min. rest / 2 hrs. 45 min. w/ 3x16-min. Steady State on a climb; 6 min. rest	2 hrs. 15 min. 3 hrs. 30 min. w/ 2x20-min. Tempo; 5 min. rest
7		1 hr. 45 min. 2 hrs. w/ 2x20-min. Steady State on a climb; 5 min. rest	45 min. 2 hrs. 30 min. w/ 2x40-min. Tempo; 10 min. rest	1 hr. 45 min. 1 hr. 30 min. w/ 2x15-min. Tempo; 5 min. rest and 5x4-min. MT Intervals; 4 min. rest		2 hrs. 45 min. 3 hrs. w/ 2x20-min. Steady State on a climb; 8 min. rest	2 hrs. 45 min. 3 hrs. 30 min. w/ 2x30-min. Tempo; 5 min. rest
8		1 hr.	Rest 1 hr. 30 min.	1 hr. 30 min. w/ 2x15-min. Tempo; 5 min. rest and 4x3-min. MT Intervals; 3 min. rest		2 hrs.	2 hrs. 30 min.
9		1 hr. 15 min. w/ 3x8-min. Climb Repeats; 6 min. rest / 2 hrs. w/ 3x12-min. Climb Repeats; 6 min. rest	1 hr. 2 hrs. 30 min. w/ 2x35-min. Tempo; 8 min. rest	1 hr. 15 min. / 1 hr. 45 min. w/ 2x10-min. Tempo; 5 min. rest and 5x5-min. MT Intervals; 2 min. rest		2 hrs. 15 min. / 2 hrs. 45 min. w/ 3x12-min. Climb Repeats; 5 min. rest	2 hrs. 3 hrs. w/ 30-min. Tempo
10		1 hr. 30 min. w/ 3x10-min. Climb Repeats; 8 min. rest / 2 hrs. 15 min. w/ 3x12-min. Climb Repeats; 8 min. rest	1 hr. 2 hrs. 30 min. w/ 2x45-min. Tempo; 8 min. rest	1 hr. 30 min. / 1 hr. 45 min. w/ 2x10-min. Tempo; 5 min. rest and 5x5-min. MT Intervals; 5 min. rest		2 hrs. 30 min. / 2 hrs. 45 min. w/ 3x12-min. Climb Repeats; 8 min. rest	2 hrs. 15 min. w/ 40-min. Tempo / 3 hrs. w/ Tempo
11		1 hr. 45 min. w/ 2x15-min. Climb Repeats; 10 min. rest / 2 hrs. 30 min. w/ 4x10-min. Climb Repeats; 8 min. rest	45 min. 2 hrs. 30 min. w/ 2x45-min. Tempo; 10 min. rest	1 hr. 45 min. 2 hrs. w/ 2x10-min. Tempo; 5 min. rest and 4x7-min. MT Intervals; 5 min. rest		2 hrs. 45 min. 3 hrs. w/ 4x10-min. Climb Repeats; 6 min. rest	2 hrs. 45 min. w/ 50-min. Tempo / 3 hrs. 30 min. w/ 30-min. Tempo
12		1 hr.	Rest 1 hr.	1 hr. 30 min. w/ 20-min. Tempo		1 hr.	EVENT OR RACE DAY

BACK IT DOWN 10. The ideal climbing intensity is just below threshold (where your legs start to burn). To find it, ride a hill as hard as your legs will allow (you should be able to sustain it for more than 30 seconds), then back it down about 10 percent. This gives you a reserve to dig into so you can handle changes in pace and pitch without popping. If you're already at threshold, you have nowhere to go but down.

Should You Ride When Sick?

Sometimes a good ride is just what you need to blow out the pipes and breathe better, at least temporarily. Other times, well, not so much.

The American College of Sports Medicine recommends using the general "above the neck" rule: If your symptoms are above your shoulders, such as a drippy nose and stuffy head, go ahead with a low-intensity workout (it's not a good idea to push it when you're even a little sick). Just be sure to stay well hydrated. If your symptoms are below the neck—diarrhea, a cough based in your chest, fever or vomiting—you're better off riding your sofa.

Here is a more detailed guide to help you make the right call.

Symptom: Sniffles
Ride if: You generally feel okay otherwise.
Rest if: You're so blocked up you can barely breathe, even after 10 minutes of light spinning.

Symptom: Fever
Ride if: It's 100 degrees F or below.
Rest if: It's above 100.

Symptom: Headache
Ride if: It's mild enough to not be distracting.
Rest if: Your head is pounding like it did the morning of your 21st birthday.

Symptom: Muscle aches or chills
Ride if: Don't ride.
Rest if: Aches and chills indicate a more serious full-body infection. Your body needs all its reserves to fight it.

Symptom: Sore throat
Ride if: It's just a little scratchy.
Rest if: Your glands are swollen.

Symptom: Cough
Ride if: You're coughing just to clear your throat of excess mucous.
Rest if: You feel like you're hacking up a lung.

Why I Ride

"In cycling, even for pros, there's always something to improve on. If I ever felt like I had it all figured out, it would be because I didn't want to figure anything else out, and it would be time to quit."—LEVI LEIPHEIMER, PROFESSIONAL CYCLIST

For Long-Term Gains

The obvious way to climb better is to climb more often. But to improve your strength and stamina when the road turns up, add these drills to your hill days. For the best results, do them twice a week.

HILL ACCELERATIONS. Improve power on rolling hills, which last one to two minutes each but come at you one after another. **The Workout:** Ride the majority of the roller at a steady and sustainable pace until you're 200 to 300 meters from the top. Stay seated and accelerate until you're about 10 seconds past the summit. Focus on increasing your cadence to create the initial acceleration, then use your gears to keep increasing speed as you reach and pass the top of the hill. Recover with five minutes of easy spinning and repeat. Novice riders should complete four hill accelerations, intermediate riders (Cat 3 and masters) should complete two sets of four with 10 minutes of recovery between sets, and advanced riders can do two sets of six.

OVER-UNDERS. These intervals alternate between a sustainable pace and a higher intensity to help you develop better power at lactate threshold so you can handle changes on sustained climbs. **The Workout:** During a six-minute climb, ride "under" at a steady and sustainable climbing pace (86 to 90 percent of your maximum sustainable power output or 92 to 94 percent of your maximum sustainable heart rate) for the first two minutes; for the "over" portion of the drill, accelerate to your maximum sustainable pace (95 to 100 percent of your maximum sustainable power output or 95 to 97 percent of your maximum sustainable heart rate) for one minute. Return to your under intensity for another two minutes before accelerating again to your over for the final minute. Stronger riders can add another cycle to make a nine-minute interval. Do three six-minute intervals with six minutes of easy spinning recovery

Pro **Tip**

"PLUNKING YOUR BUTT DOWN IN THE SADDLE WHEN YOU SIT BACK DOWN IS A SIGN OF FATIGUE. DON'T DO IT, AND IF YOU SEE SOMEONE AHEAD DO IT, ATTACK."—*BRIAN WALTON, THREE-TIME OLYMPIC CYCLIST AND 1996 SILVER MEDALIST*

TRAIN FOR TERRAIN THAT MAKES YOU REDLINE, RECOVER, THEN REDLINE AGAIN.

When you blast beyond the bounds of your aerobic fitness, your technical skills take a dive. This plan builds base fitr while honing your top speed. Plan Tips: Beginners, take Mondays, Wednesdays and Fridays as rest days. ■ Try to d least half of the interval sessions on dirt.

Beginner (7.5–9.5 hrs./week)=workouts in BLACK, advanced (9–14 hrs./week)=variations in WHITE where they appear ■ All rides at a conversational pace (easy to moderate) on flat rolling terrain, unless otherwise noted ■ RECOVERY RIDE=Easy ride, light gear, moderate cadence CLIMB REPEATS=Steady climb at 78–83% of max heart rate (MHR), cadence 70–85 STEADY STATE=A longer effort at your lactate threshold (85% + 3 beats per minute of your MHR), cadence 85–95 rpm HILL ACCELERATIONS=Pedal normally until the final 500 yards of hill, then gradually accelerate to near MHR; start the interval the last few yards of the hill, out of the saddle at max effort POWER INTERVALS=Pace above lactate threshold, with a perc exertion of 8–9, or 90–95% of MHR TEMPO=80% of MHR in a larger gear, cadence 70–75 rpm VO₂ INTERVALS=As hard as possible, paying no attention to heart rate, to boost max oxyge consumption (VO₂ max) levels HILL SPRINTS=All-out sprint on a hill

WEEK	MONDAY	TUESDAY	WEDNESDAY	THURSDAY	FRIDAY	SATURDAY	SUNDAY
1	REST DAY	1 hr. 30 min. w/ 3x10-min. Climb Repeats; 10 min. rest / 2 hrs. w/ 3x15-min. Steady State; 10 min. rest	REST DAY; 2 hrS. TO 3 HRS. AT CONVERSATIONAL PACE; REST DAY—WEEKS 4, 8 AND 11	1 hr. 30 min. w/ 3x8-min. Climb Repeats; 8 min. rest / 2 hrs. 15 min. w/ 4x15-min. Steady State; 10 min. rest	REST DAY; 30 min. TO 1 hr. 30 min. RECOVERY RIDE	2 hrs. 30 min. / 3 hrs.	2 hrs. / 2 hrs. 45 min
2		1 hr. 45 min. w/ 3x12-min. Climb Repeats; 10 min. rest / 2 hrs. 15 min. w/ 4x15-min. Steady State; 10 min. rest		1 hr. 45 min. w/ 3x10-min. Climb Repeats; 8 min. rest / 2 hrs. 30 min. w/ 3x20-min. Steady State; 10 min. rest		2 hrs. 45 min. / 3 hrs. 15 min.	2 hrs. 30 min. / 3 hrs.
3		1 hr. 45 min. w/ 3x15-sec. Hill Accelerations; 3 min. rest / 2 hrs. 30 min. w/ 3x20-sec. Hill Accelerations; 2 min. rest		1 hr. 45 min. w/ 3x6-min. Climb Repeats; 6 min. rest / 2 hrs. 45 min. w/ 3x8-min. Climb Repeats; 6 min. rest		3 hrs. 30 min. w/ 2 sets of 2x3-min. Power Intervals; 3 min. rest; 6 min. b/t sets	2 hrs. 45 min. / 2 hrs. 15 min.
4		1 hr. / 1 hr. 30 min.		1 hr. 30 min.		2 hrs. 30 min.	2 hrs. 30 min. w/ 30 min. Tempo
5		1 hr. 30 min. w/ 2 sets of 3x3-min. Power Intervals; 3 min. rest; 8 min. b/t sets / 2 hrs. 15 min. w/ 3x20-min. Steady State; 10 min. rest		1 hr. 30 min. w/ 2 sets of 2x3-min. Power Intervals; 3 min. rest; 8 min. b/t sets / 2 hrs. 30 min. w/ 3x10-min. Climb Repeats; 8 min. rest		2 hrs. 30 min. / 3 hrs. 15 min. w/ 3x3-min. Power Intervals; 10 min. rest	2 hrs. 30 min. w/ 3x10-min. Steady St 10 min. rest
6		1 hr. 30 min. w/ 3 sets of 3x3-min. Power Intervals; 3 min. rest; 6 min. b/t sets / 2 hrs. 30 min. w/ 3x10-min. Climb Repeats; 8 min. rest		1 hr. 30 min. w/ 4x6-min. Climb Repeats; 6 min. rest / 2 hrs. 30 min. w/ 4x8-min. Climb Repeats; 6 min. rest		2 hrs. 30 min. / 3 hrs. 30 min. w/ 2 sets of 2x4-min. Power Intervals; 4 min. rest; 10 min. b/t sets	2 hrs. 45 min. / 3 hrs. 15 min. w/ 3x15-sec. Hill Acce tions; 3 min. rest
7		2 hrs. w/ 4x30-sec. VO₂ Intervals; 30 sec. rest / 2 hrs. 45 min. w/ 6x30-sec. VO₂ Intervals; 30 sec. rest		1 hr. 45 min. w/ 4x8-min. Climb Repeats; 8 min. rest / 3 hrs. w/ 4x10-min. Climb Repeats; 8 min. rest		2 hrs. 45 min. w/ 6x10-sec. Hill Sprints; 5 min. rest / 4 hrs. w/ 3x4-min. Power Intervals; 4 min. rest	3 hrs. / 2 hrs.
8		1 hr. / 1 hr. 30 min.		1 hr. 30 min. w/ 20-min. Tempo		2 hrs. / 2 hrs. 30 min.	3 hrs. w/ 30-min. Tempo
9		2 hrs. w/ 2 sets of 3x3-min. Power Intervals; 3 min. rest; 8 min. b/t sets		2 hrs. w/ 3x6-min. Climb Repeats; 6 min. rest / w/ 4x10-min. Climb Repeats; 8 min. rest		3 hrs. w/ 4x3-min. Power Intervals; 4 min. rest / w/ 4x4-min. Power Intervals; 3 min. rest	2 hrs. 30 min. / 3 hrs. 15 min.
10		1 hr. 30 min. / 2 hrs. 45 min. w/ 3 sets of 4x30-sec. VO₂ Intervals; 30 sec. rest; 8 min. b/t sets		1 hr. 45 min. / 2 hrs. 45 min. w/ 2 sets of 3x3-min. Power Intervals; 3 min. rest; 8 min. b/t sets		2 hrs. / 3 hrs. w/ 45-min. Tempo	2 hrs. 30 min.
11		1 hr. 45 min. / 2 hrs. w/ 5x10-sec. Hill Sprints; 5 min. rest		1 hr. 30 min. w/ 3x2-min. Power Intervals; 2 min. rest / w/ 6x10-sec. VO₂ Intervals; 2 min. rest		2 hrs. w/ 45-min. Tempo	2 hrs. 30 min. w/ 2 sets of 2x3-min. P Intervals; 3 min. rest; 8 b/t sets
12		1 hr. 30 min. w/ 2 sets of 5x30-sec. VO₂ Intervals; 30 sec. rest; 8 min. b/t sets		1 hr.		1 hr. / 1 hr. 15 min. w/ 3x2-min. Power Intervals; 5 min. rest	EVENT OR RACE DA

between them. If you do nine-minute intervals, keep recovery at five minutes.

HILL SPRINTS. These hard-charging intervals will give you the brute force you need to punch your way over short, steep walls. Just remember, after you hit the summit, use your gears to bring your cadence up so you don't get dropped after the climb. **The Workout:** Find a short, steep hill with a flat road leading up to it. Ride toward the base of the hill at a moderate speed (15 to 20 mph). With your hands in the drops, get out of the saddle and start sprinting about 25 to 50 meters before you start going uphill. Continue sprinting for 10 seconds. Recover with five minutes of easy spinning between sprints. Novices should complete four hill sprints, intermediate riders should complete two sets of three sprints with 10 minutes between sets, and advanced riders should complete two sets of five sprints with four minutes between sprints and eight minutes between sets.

Watts Your Climbing Power?

Forget heart rate, perceived exertion or the time it takes to drop your buddy: Power is the true measure of your performance on the bike. But even if you're not ready to shell out $1,000-plus for a power meter, you can approximate your power output on climbs with a couple of relatively simple formulas.

The pros talk about VAM, or vertical ascent in meters—the height you can climb in an hour. At the peak of his career, Lance Armstrong was capable of climbing more than

Fun **Fact**

Losing just 5 pounds could save you about 30 seconds on a 5-kilometer climb (averaging an 8 percent grade).

1,800 meters (about 6,000 feet) per hour during the Tour de France. Your results may differ. But regardless of your ability, it takes a known amount of energy to raise a known weight a given height, which means you can estimate power output if you know your VAM (or VAF for us nonmetric types). All you need is a climb of known length and height, or a cyclecomputer with a percent-grade function.

First, weigh your bicycle and yourself in full cycling kit. This is the total weight you will be dragging uphill. Next, calculate your VAF. For example, if it takes you 20 minutes to ascend a 1,000-foot climb, you are ascending at 3,000 feet per hour. Climbing a 6 percent grade at 10 mph is a VAF of 3,168 (10 mi/hr x 5,280 linear feet/mi x 0.06 vertical feet/linear foot). Your power output is equal to: gravitational power (the energy you use working against gravity) + rolling power (energy used to overcome rolling resistance) + aerodynamic power (energy used to overcome air resistance).

For climbing, especially at speeds below 12 mph and at grades above 6 percent, many experts, such as power guru Allen Lim, PhD, advisor to Team RadioShack, just use gravitational power as the total measurement:

Gravitational power = (rider weight + bike weight) x VAF x fudge factor

The fudge factor, 0.0004, includes the gravitational constant, a time conversion from hour to seconds and metric converters (use a fudge factor of 0.0028 if you're working with VAM). Based on this formula, a 180-pound rider-and-bike climbing at a VAF of 2,000 generates a power output of approximately 144 watts—almost enough juice to power two sewing machines. While figuring out your number is easy, you'll have to get sweaty to increase it: Visit bicycling.com/powerup for workouts that have been scientifically proven to boost power output.

PLAN #3: WIN A SPRINT

If you're not fit enough to be with the front pack at the end, you won't win the sprint. This plan helps you develop a good aerobic base, then builds leg speed with explosive efforts. Teaching muscles to fire more quickly is a neuromuscular adaptation, rather than an aerobic one. You'll see results fast, especially if you don't typically do sprint training.

Plan tips: Beginners, take Mondays and Fridays as rest days throughout. For sprints, form is vital; position your hands in the drops, and be sure that you are in a hard-enough gear to stand and get good leverage on your first two strokes.

Beginner (8–9.5 hrs./week) = workouts in black; advanced (9–12 hrs./week) = variations in white where they appear.

All rides at a conversational pace (easy to moderate) on flat to rolling terrain, unless otherwise noted.

Recovery Ride = Easy ride in a light gear at moderate cadence

Power Intervals = Pace at 90–95% of your max heart rate (MHR)

VO$_2$ Intervals = As hard as possible, paying no attention to heart rate, to boost max oxygen consumption (VO$_2$ max) levels

Tempo = Pace at 80% of max heart rate (MHR) in a moderately large gear at a cadence of 70–75 rpm

Flat Sprints = on a flat road, begin at moderate pace and gearing, and accelerate to max-effort sprint

High-Speed Sprints = on a flat road or slight downhill and in a moderate to high gear, jump out of the saddle for a max burst of speed

HOW TO . . . BLAST THE FLATS

"People see a flat ride and think, 'Oh, it'll be cake,' but if you're not conditioned for it, cycling on endless flat roads can be monotonous and demoralizing," says elite-level cycling coach Andy Applegate of Carmichael Training Systems. Here's how to keep your strength (and spirits) up when the road is long and level.

TRAIN ON THE EDGE. On long endurance training rides, aim for 50 percent of your effort being easy and 50 percent being at the upper end of your aerobic zone—just hard enough that you need to concentrate to keep from drifting back into easy, says Applegate. "This drill will help you stay fast on the flats."

BUILD BLAZING SPEED YOU CAN COUNT ON UNTIL THE END.

If you're not fit enough to be with the front pack at the end, you won't win the sprint. This plan helps you develop a good aerobic base, then builds leg speed with explosive efforts. Teaching muscles to fire more quickly is a neuromuscular adaptation, rather than an aerobic one. You'll see results fast, especially if you don't typically do sprint training. Plan Tips: Beginners, take Mondays and Fridays as rest days throughout. ■ For sprints, form is vital; position your hands in the drops, and be sure that you are in a hard-enough gear to stand and get good leverage on your first two strokes. Ⓑ

WEEK	MONDAY	TUESDAY	WEDNESDAY	THURSDAY	FRIDAY	SATURDAY	SUNDAY
1	REST DAY; 1 hr. RECOVERY RIDE; REST DAY—WEEKS 4, 8 AND 12	1 hr. 15 min. / 1 hr. 45 min. w/ 4x3-min. Power Intervals; 3 min. rest	1 hr. / 1 hr. 30 min.	1 hr. 30 min. / 1 hr. 45 min. w/ 4x30-sec. VO₂ Intervals; 30 sec. rest	REST DAY; 1 Hr. RECOVERY RIDE	2 hrs. 15 min. w/ 4x3-min. Power Intervals; 3 min. rest	2 hrs. 15 min. / 2 hrs. 30 min. to 3 hrs.
2		1 hr. 30 min. / 1 hr. 45 min. w/ 5x3-min. Power Intervals; 3 min. rest	1 hr. / 1 hr. 30 min	1 hr. 30 min. / 1 hr. 45 min. w/ 5x30-sec. VO₂ Intervals; 30 sec. rest		2 hrs. 15 min. w/ 5x3-min. Power Intervals; 3 min. rest	2 hrs. 30 min. / 3 hrs. to 3 hrs. 30 min.
3		1 hr. 45 min. / 2 hrs. w/ 2 sets of 3x3-min. Power Intervals; 3 min. rest; 6 min. b/t sets	1 hr. / 1 hr. 30 min.	1 hr. 30 min. / 1 hr. 45 min. w/ 2 sets of 3x30-sec. VO₂ intervals; 30 sec. rest; 3 min. b/t sets		2 hrs. 15 min. w/ 2 sets of 3x3-min. Power Intervals; 3 min. rest; 6 min. b/t sets	2 hrs. / 2 hrs. to 2 hrs. 30 min.
4		1 hr.	1 hr. 15 min. / 1 hr. 30 min.	1 hr. 30 min. w/ 3x3-min. Power Intervals; 3 min. rest / 1 hr. 45 min. w/ 4x3-min. Power Intervals; 3 min. rest		2 hrs. 30 min.	2 hrs. 15 min. / 3 hrs. w/ 30-min. Tempo
5		2 hrs. w/ 5x3-min. Power Intervals; 3 min. rest	1 hr. / 1 hr. 30 min.	1 hr. 30 min. / 1 hr. 45 min. w/ 2 sets of 3x30-sec. VO₂ Intervals; 30 sec. rest; 3 min. b/t sets		2 hrs. 15 min. w/ 5x3-min. Power Intervals; 3 min. rest	2 hrs. 30 min. / 3 hrs. w/ 2x20-min. Tempo; 10 min. rest
6		2 hrs. w/ 2 sets of 3x3-min. Power Intervals; 3 min. rest; 6 min. b/t sets	1 hr. / 1 hr. 30 min.	1 hr. 30 min. / 1 hr. 45 min. w/ 2 sets of 4x30-sec. VO₂ Intervals; 30 sec. rest; 3 min. b/t sets		2 hrs. 15 min. w/ 2 sets of 3x3-min. Power Intervals; 3 min. rest; 6 min. b/t sets	2 hrs. 45 min. / 3 hrs. w/ 2x25-min. Tempo; 10 min. rest
7		2 hrs. 15 min. w/ 2 sets of 4x3-min. Power Intervals; 3 min. rest; 6 min. b/t sets	1 hr. / 1 hr. 15 min.	1 hr. 45 min. / 2 hrs. w/ 3 sets of 3x30-sec. VO₂ Intervals; 30 sec. rest; 2 min. b/t sets		2 hrs. 30 min. w/ 2 sets of 4x3-min. Power Intervals; 3 min. rest; 6 min. b/t sets	2 hrs. 30 min.
8		45 min. / 1 hr.	1 hr. 30 min.	1 hr. 30 min. w/ 5x2-min. Power Intervals; 2 min. rest / 1 hr. 45 min. w/ 5x3-min. Power Intervals; 3 min. rest		2 hrs. 30 min.	2 hrs. 30 min.
9		1 hr. 30 min. w/ 2 sets of 3x2-min. Power Intervals; 2 min. rest; 6 min. rest b/t sets / 2 hrs. w/ 2 sets of 3x3-min. Power Intervals; 3 min. rest; 6 min. b/t sets	1 hr. / 1 hr. 15 min.	2 hrs. w/ 2 sets of 4x10-sec. Flat Sprints; 2 min. rest; 6 min. b/t sets		1 hr. 45 min. w/ 6x10-sec. High-Speed Sprints; 2 min. rest	2 hrs.
10		1 hr. 45 min. / 2 hrs. w/ 2 sets of 3x4-min. Power Intervals; 4 min. rest; 8 min. b/t sets	1 hr. / 1 hr. 15 min.	2 hrs. w/ 2 sets of 5x10-sec. Flat Sprints; 2 min. rest; 6 min. b/t sets		2 hrs. w/ 8x10-sec. High-Speed Sprints; 2 min. rest	2 hrs.
11		1 hr. 45 min. / 2 hrs. 15 min. w/ 2 sets of 4x4-min. Power Intervals; 4 min. rest; 8 min. b/t sets	45 min. / 1 hr. 15 min.	1 hr. 45 min. w/ 6x10-sec. High-Speed Sprints; 2 min. rest		2 hrs. 15 min. / 2 hrs. 30 min. w/ 10x10-sec. High-Speed Sprints; 2 min. rest	1 hr. 45 min.
12		45 min. / 1 hr.	1 hr. 30 min.	1 hr. 45 min. / 2 hrs. w/ 5x10-sec. Flat Sprints; 2 min. rest		30 min.	EVENT OR RACE DAY

PEDAL NONSTOP. When training on undulating terrain, avoid coasting on slight declines. "Keeping the pedals turning will train your legs to match the effort needed to cruise on flat roads," he says.

SWITCH GEARS. When on a long, flat stretch, periodically click up and then down a gear. The variation in cadence will keep your legs feeling fresher.

CHANGE POSITION. Keep your supporting muscles from getting sore by shifting your weight, riding the hoods and the drops, or by standing up and stretching.

WORK THE WIND. Head wind is your enemy. Resist the temptation to shift into a big gear to gain power and speed. "You'll wear yourself out," says Applegate. Instead, gear down, spin fast and enjoy the ride.

PLAN #4: TRAIN FOR A TRI

As a dedicated cyclist, you'll enjoy a decided performance advantage in a triathlon. The bike leg accounts for approximately 50 percent of the total time in an Olympic-distance race (1.5-K swim, 40-K bike, 10-K run), which effectively skews the playing field in favor of a cyclist. This simple program, from Matt Fitzgerald, senior editor at Competitor Group, will help you maximize this advantage, while also allowing you to develop your swimming and running fitness so that they don't undo your greatest strength.

Ride Even Stronger

To properly train for a 40-K bike leg, do these three key workouts each week for 6 weeks. If you ride more than three times a week, the additional rides should be low-intensity efforts.

THRESHOLD RIDE. Because the cycling portion of a triathlon is essentially a time trial, you should modify your bike training to boost your TT fitness. In other words, "you need to work on your lactate threshold," says Troy Jacobson, head coach of the Triathlon Academy, in White Hall, Maryland, and creator of the Spinervals cycling workout DVDs. Your lactate or anaerobic threshold, the cycling intensity at which lactic acid (not a direct cause of fatigue but an indicator of biochemical events that are) begins to accumulate rapidly in the muscles, roughly corresponds to the speed or power output level you'd sustain in a 40-K TT. **The Workout:** Warm up with 15 to 30 minutes of easy spinning interspersed with four to six jumps in speed (90 percent efforts) of 20 to 30 seconds. The threshold portion of the workout consists of 2x20 minutes at your lactate threshold speed/power (or the max speed or power level you can sustain for one hour) with 10 to 20 minutes of easy spinning between efforts. Cool down with another 10 to 20 minutes of easy spinning. In the final weeks before your triathlon, these workouts should be done on the bike you plan to race. "Getting comfortable in a time-trial position is important," says Jacobson. "Put in some miles in the aero bars instead of sitting up on the hoods."

LONG RIDE. Priority number two is endurance. "Keep your long ride on the weekend," says Gale Bernhardt, former head coach of the U.S. Olympic triathlon team and author of *Training Plans for Cyclists*. "If you can easily do a three-hour ride, you don't need to build endurance, just maintain it." After you've built a foundation with moderate-paced long rides, it's time to bump up the intensity. "A common problem with cyclists and triathletes is that they tend to ride at a conversational pace too often," says Dave Scott, six-time Hawaii Ironman winner and now a Boulder, Colorado–based tri coach. **The Workout:** Ride for two to three hours at moderate intensity (70 to 75 percent of your threshold speed/power). In the six weeks before your race, make your long ride a tempo ride: Shorten the duration and, after warming up, ride at 75 to 90 percent of threshold speed/power. "Bringing up the intensity teaches your body to burn fuel more efficiently," says Scott.

RECOVERY RIDE. The rest of your weekly rides should be easy. Follow one with a short run to get your body accustomed to running in a fatigued state. Resist the temptation to do more than two hard rides per week unless you're highly competitive. "There's more of a distinction between hard and easy days in triathlon than there is in cycling," explains Jacobson. **The Workout:** Ride for 45 to 90 minutes at a comfortable pace (50 to 60 percent of your lactate threshold speed/power). Maintain a cadence of 90 to 95 rpm. "This will prepare your legs for the run," says Scott, "which you should do at the same cadence."

Work Your Weaknesses

If simply finishing the swim leg leaves you exhausted by the time you reach your bike, you won't be able to take advantage of your cycling ability. And if you haven't worked hard enough on your running, your butt-kicking bike leg will go to waste. Fortunately, it doesn't take a huge commitment to develop basic swimming and running fitness. "You can get by on two swims and two runs per week," says Bernhardt.

IN THE DRINK. If you're new to swimming, your top priorities should be building the stamina to comfortably swim the full distance of your upcoming race and learning proper technique. "Gradually build your swimming distance until you can comfortably swim a mile," says Bernhardt. "That's something most beginners can do in eight to 12 weeks." Developing a good freestyle swim stroke is not something you can do on your own. "It's important to have a knowledgeable person watch your stroke," says Bernhardt. "I've been swimming a long time, and I still have people watch me and point out mistakes." To find a swim coach in your area, contact U.S. Masters Swimming (usms.org).

ON YOUR FEET. The top priority of your running should be avoiding injury while gradually adapting your fitness from two wheels to two feet. Build your running mileage slowly, by roughly 10 percent per week. "Don't hurry the early part of your run training just because your heart tells you that the effort is easy," says Scott. "It takes a while for the tissues of the lower leg to adapt to the trauma of impact." According to Bernhardt, combined bike-run, or brick, workouts are an excellent way to increase your running fitness. Start by tacking a five-minute run onto the end of a 30- to 60-minute bike ride. "Each time you repeat the workout, subtract a little time from the cycling portion and add time to the running segment," says Bernhardt. "Once you're running 30 minutes off the bike, make it a separate workout and continue building it up to about an hour." To keep your legs accustomed to running off the bike, continue to follow one of your weekly rides with a run of 10 to 30 minutes.

THE NEXT LEVEL. Once you have developed a decent swim stroke and built some running fitness, and perhaps completed one or more triathlons, "the next step is to add speed work to your second swim and run of each week," says Bernhardt. "Then add a third swim and run—those workouts should be easy to moderate."

HOW TO . . .
BEAT THE HEAT

Heat is the ultimate enemy of an endurance athlete, because after a point, the higher your body temperature rises, the slower you'll go. Read on for Chris Carmichael's advice on pedaling strong when the mercury rises.

Part of the problem with the heat is that your body generates its own heat when you exercise. Only a small portion of the energy liberated from food is used for mechanical work, such as walking or pedaling. The rest radiates from your body, which can be a big problem when it's already hot outside. Fortunately, with some planning and attention to detail, even hot days won't slow you down, and you'll be able to continue to maximize your training and racing.

EXPOSE YOURSELF. Consistency is a key to acclimating to hot, humid weather. Active exposure, such as moderate-intensity cycling, leads to faster and greater adaptations than passive exposure, such as sitting in a sauna or a house without air-conditioning. Chances are if you've been riding all summer, your body has already made the key adaptations of increasing blood plasma volume (to allow you to produce more sweat), and sweating earlier and over more of your body. Acclimating typically takes two weeks of consistent heat riding, not necessarily every day, but hot training sessions every two or three days.

Staying hydrated and well fed is also critical to temperature acclimation, and it's important to note that it's totally ineffective to restrict liquid intake purposely in an attempt to teach the body to perform well without it. Not only does it not work, but it's also dangerous.

PICK YOUR TIME. Riding in the morning or evening to avoid the heat of the day falls into the obvious-advice category, but there are other cooler times to ride, such as in the rain or soon after a thunderstorm. Training in the rain also offers the bonus of gaining the wet-riding skills and confidence you'll need when the sky opens up at your next race or century. If the mercury is scaring you away from hard intervals, which generate the most body heat, consider doing your intervals in an air-conditioned room with fans before going outside to complete the rest of your training volume at a steady, moderate intensity.

WARM UP TO COOL OFF. A thorough warm-up is vital in hot weather because it lets your evaporative cooling system get up to speed before you do. Jumping right into a hard effort spikes your body temperature before you've started sweating enough for your system to begin cooling you. One of the benefits of greater fitness and acclimation is that your body begins sweating earlier—it's much easier to keep a body cool than to use sweat to cool it once it's overheated. To stay on the safe side, start workouts off slowly.

GET WET. Tour de France riders grab bottles from fans on epic hot days, but not to drink. These bottles are for drenching their bodies. Cyclists have an edge over other athletes in this type of cooling because we move fast enough to have constant airflow over our wet clothing. On heat-alert days, carry extra bottles or stop and refill often to ensure you have enough liquid to keep your head and body wet. If you overheat to the point of heat illness, find a way to immerse yourself in cool or cold water, which is the best way to reduce core temperature, according to the American College of Sports Medicine. Jump into a creek or a pond, stand in a sprinkler, or use a hose—whatever you have to do to completely soak yourself. The wetter you get, the more quickly you'll dissipate heat.

PLAN #5: BREAK OUT OF THE DEAD ZONE

Dead Zone Syndrome, common among cyclists, is brought on by repeated training at a single, moderately hard intensity, known as Zone 3. It afflicts enthusiasts who push the pedals hard but don't follow a training program, as well as amateur racers who have the great Eddy Merckx's famous maxim, "Ride lots," indelibly burned into their brains.

Symptoms and Signs

Those suffering from the malady may not be aware of it, due to the syndrome's insidious nature. That's because, at a minimum, it maintains fitness, says Neal Henderson, a USA Cycling and USA Triathlon certified coach: "You're sweating, you burn calories and you get good endurance out of it." A former hard case

The Ideal Dog-Day Workout

It's hot and sticky outside, and your inner voice is telling you not to stray too far from the air-conditioning. But you know you'll feel better about yourself after you ride, and there's no reason to spend more time than absolutely necessary out there, so use this quick and effective workout, with short bouts of intensity and longer recovery periods to cool off. Start the ride with two bottles on the bike and two in your jersey pockets—half for drinking and half for dousing. Ride slowly for at least 20 minutes to warm up. Before the first interval, liberally squirt the front and back of your jersey with water. Then complete three all-out efforts of two minutes each, with three minutes of easy recovery, spinning between each. When you've finished the set, pour a full bottle of water over your body while spinning for eight minutes, and then repeat the interval set. Cool down on your ride home, and by the time you get there all four bottles should be empty.

himself, Henderson is now the sports science manager at Colorado's Boulder Center for Sports Medicine and is best known for coaching Taylor Phinney to a spot on the 2008 U.S. Olympic team. Many of his clients are former sufferers.

Dead Zone Syndrome often strikes in summer, after the body has reaped as much training benefit as possible from single-zone riding. It can manifest as a feeling of monotony, both physical and psychological. "Moderate-level intensity provides a constant stimulus to your sympathetic nervous system, your 'fight or flight' response," Henderson explains. "So if you're stressing that system to the same degree day-to-day, there'll be less recovery." In other words, you're wearing yourself down.

There's a plateau in Zone 3. "You're working kind of hard, but not doing a lot to change your physiology," Henderson says. In order for your body to adapt and improve, you need to follow a program that hits the extremes, he says, especially the high end.

Treatment

Try Henderson's "16+5" program for three weeks. Training is stacked in cycles of 16 "on" days with five days of recovery between cycles, which can be repeated as necessary. The time-crunched will experience better training benefit in less time than usual (it requires no more than 10 hours a week). Those with stale legs should note improvement in as little as one full cycle. Finally, this plan reduces the potential for overuse injury, because you're riding less overall and varying the intensity to give yourself time to recover.

The Rx: The 16+5 Plan

Because most cyclists have more time to ride on the weekends, this program begins on a Saturday and includes only shorter rides during the workweek.

WEEK 1: INTENSITY

Saturday: 2 hr. intense group ride, spending time in each Zone, 1 through 5

Sunday: 3 hr. Zone 2 w/optional 10x30 sec. high-cadence spin-ups

Monday: OFF or 30 min. Zone 1

Tuesday: 60 to 90 min. w/intervals; 4x5 min. in Zone 4 w/3 min. Zone 1 recovery

Wednesday: 90 min. Zone 2, optional 5x10 sec. max sprints w/full recovery

Thursday: 30 min. Zone 1

Friday: 90 min. w/intervals; 5x90 sec. in Zone 5 w/3 min. Zone 1 recovery

WEEK 2: VOLUME

Saturday: 3 to 3 hr. 30 min. Zone 2

Sunday: OFF or 30 min. Zone 1

Monday: 90 min. w/intervals; 6 to 10x3 min. Zone 3 (at 60 rpm) w/2 min. Zone 1 recovery (at 90 rpm)

Tuesday: Optional 30 min. a.m. Zone 1 ride; 60 min. p.m. Zone 2

Wednesday: OFF

Thursday: 60 to 90 min. w/a 15 to 30 min. steady effort in Zone 3 or 4

Friday: 30 to 45 min. Zone 1

WEEK 3: RECOVERY

Saturday: 3 hr. group ride, spending time in each Zone, 1 through 5

Sunday: 2 to 3 hr. Zone 2

Monday: OFF; get a massage

Tuesday: 30 min. Zone 1

Wednesday: OFF

Thursday: 30 min. Zone 1 w/optional 4x30 sec. high-cadence spin-ups

Friday: OFF; next cycle starts tomorrow

NOTES: This training plan assumes that you ride six to 10 hours per week and have an adequate training base. If you slacked off all summer, put in at least three weeks of Zone 2 or 3 riding before adding intensity. Before starting any interval workout, always do a 10- to 20-minute warm-up in Zone 1, and cool down 5 to 15 minutes in Zone 1 afterward. Spin-ups: In a low gear, begin at a comfortable cadence and end at the highest possible cadence without bouncing in the saddle. To build climbing strength, do Zone 3 intervals on an uphill.

The Zones

Power-based training, using watts, is the best, most cutting-edge way to maximize your potential. But the trusty Zone system, which has been around for years, offers a bare-bones approach that will take you far.

1. Recovery

   RPE (Rate of Perceived Exertion): 1 or 2 (out of 10)

   Feels Like: Taking your bike for a walk

   You're Thinking: I'm working out right now?

2. Endurance/Base

   RPE: 3 or 4

   Feels Like: An easy ride, conversational pace

   You're Thinking: Hey, I never noticed that cool old barn before.

3. Tempo

   RPE: 5 or 6

   Feels Like: Moderate pace; can talk, but not necessarily in full, flowing sentences

   You're Thinking: All right, now this is a workout.

4. Threshold/Steady State

   RPE: 7 or 8

   Feels Like: Hardest pace you can go for 20 to 30 minutes; can talk, but only in four-letter words

   You're Thinking: Man, I hope (ugh) the pace backs off (snort) soon.

5. Max Power

   RPE: 9 or 10

   Feels Like: An all-out effort you can sustain for only a couple of minutes, max

   You're Thinking: Not much, because you have tunnel vision, and self-preservation instincts have taken over.

HOW TO . . .
MAKE THE MOST OF
THE OFF-SEASON

To Spin, or not to Spin? Chris Carmichael can help you decide.

Every gym or health club has some form of indoor cycling class, and in the dead of winter it's tempting to jump in rather than face the elements or slave away on a trainer alone in your basement. There's nothing inherently wrong with these classes, but it's important to find one that will actually improve your performance on the bike. I encourage athletes to evaluate classes based on how well they address the core principles of training: overload and recovery, specificity, individuality and progression. I address each of these below.

OVERLOAD AND RECOVERY. Classes generally fall into two categories: sufferfests and structured workouts. Both have their merits, and I understand the psychology of the sufferfest fan's desire to reach the end of a class exhausted, but as a coach I prefer the latter approach. Though a sufferfest might feel excruciatingly difficult, your actual power output may be too low to improve your fitness due to inadequate recovery periods. Check in with the instructor: If the primary feature of the workout is that it's ridiculously intense, but he or she can't identify what you'll get out of it, find a different class.

SPECIFICITY. The fact that you're pedaling is a step in the right direction, but some classes have very little to do with actual cycling performance. And that's okay—I'm all for classes that burn calories and get people sweating. But if you're looking to improve your performance on the road or trail, you need workouts that target the energy systems and power demands of actual cycling. These classes can be harder to find because effective interval sets are often not the most entertaining, crowd-pleasing kind. The intensities are consistent and repetitive instead of all over the map, and while you may do some pedaling out of the saddle, no cycling-specific class will have you doing push-ups on the handlebar.

INDIVIDUALITY. This is where technology comes into play. The absolute best indoor cycling classes use power meters, whether that's in the form of CompuTrainers, power-equipped stationary bikes or personal bikes with power meters. And the best ones also set individual power-training ranges for each athlete. The next-best scenario is a class that uses heart-rate monitors and individual training intensities. The self-selected "turn the knob to the right" method is fine, but not optimal.

PROGRESSION. Progressive classes are pretty rare, and to find one you'll most likely need to go to a cycling performance center. To address the progression principle, a class needs to be designed with the idea that the same people will be coming back week after week, and that the workload will thus take into account the developing fitness of these participants. In the standard gym model, in which classes are accessible to anyone anytime, the programming tends to be static. (This is also partly why these classes often are sufferfests.) In a progressive class, some of the workouts may well be more moderate in intensity, and while that's good from a long-term training perspective, it's not as appealing to the intermittent class user.

Then again . . . Incorporating indoor classes into your winter training need not be an all-or-nothing proposition. There's nothing wrong with an occasional—even weekly—sufferfest. Even cyclists following well-structured, scientifically based, progression-driven indoor programs sometimes should forget the numbers and just open the throttle.

But if all you do all winter is pummel yourself, your progress will be blunted. The best option: Follow a scientifically based program, but incorporate some "hard for the sake of being hard" classes, just for fun.

Pimp Your Indoor Ride

Most sun-loving cyclists treat indoor training like a necessary trip through purgatory to reach the promised land come spring. But indoor training can become more productive and entertaining if you infuse it with speed drills and the elements that make real rides enjoyable—friends, variety and plenty of stimulation, says elite-level coach Andy Applegate. "Done right, indoor training can not only deliver benefits that reach beyond outdoor riding, but it can also be fun," he says. Here are six living-room workouts that will keep you fit, fast and sane. Note: Always warm up at least 15 minutes before interval work, and do these intervals no more than twice a week.

THE DRILL: High-cadence spin-ups

Spin at 70 rpm in a low gear, increasing by 5 rpm each minute until you bounce in the sad-dle. Then back off to being stable again and hold for a minute. Drop your cadence 5 rpm each minute until you're back to 70 rpm.

THE BENEFIT: Teaches you how to spin a small gear at a fast cadence, which spares your leg muscles so they stay fresher longer. Off-season is the perfect time to practice this, because you can convert the strength you build in the weight room to speed on the bike.

PIMP IT UP: Slide a copy of Fox Racing's *Chain-Smoke II* into the DVD player and spin like mad while off-road hotrods perform jaw-dropping stunts. The lightning-fast footage and raging soundtrack will amp up any speed session.

Fun **Fact**

If you're stuck riding indoors, bring your iPod—studies show that listening to music while exercising helps you work at greater intensity and for longer, and may even boost brainpower.

THE DRILL: Big-gear force drills

Click into the biggest gear that will allow you to maintain a 60-rpm cadence. Ride steady for five minutes, then shift down and spin easy for five. Repeat four times. Add three to five minutes to the intervals until you're up to two 20-minute repeats, recovering for 10 to 15 minutes between. (Avoid big-gear intervals if you have knee problems.)

THE BENEFIT: Builds leg strength and increases the force you can apply to the pedals with each pedal stroke.

PIMP IT UP: Create a "Use the Force" playlist. Studies prove driving music makes you work harder while feeling less pain. Here's a peek at our big-gear faves: "Seven Nation Army" (White Stripes), "Get Free" (The Vines), "Vertigo" (U2), "The Magnificent Seven" (The Clash), "Back in Black" (AC/DC), "Fire Woman" (The Cult), "Cochise" (Audioslave), "Nighttrain" (Guns N' Roses), "Ode to Joy" (Beethoven).

THE DRILL: Hill surges

Raise your front wheel 6 inches. Set the trainer's resistance to high. Pedal 80 rpm for 30 seconds. Click up one gear and maintain 30 seconds. Click up one more, stand and accelerate 15 seconds. Recover for one minute in an easier gear. Repeat eight times.

THE BENEFIT: Increases climbing power and improves your ability to crest and finish a climb stronger than you start it.

PIMP IT UP: Perform while watching one of your favorite mountain stages of the Grand Tours (worldcycling.com). Try to hang onto the wheel of your favorite rider throughout the drill.

THE DRILL: Speed play

Controlled-chaos training. Perform random intervals, ranging from 10 seconds to several minutes in length.

THE BENEFIT: Prepares your body for real-life cycling situations, like chasing breakaways and bridging gaps in races or hard rides.

PIMP IT UP: Do them when your favorite college or NFL team plays. Choose sprint cues, like first downs and time-outs, and sprint like crazy when they move the chains or take a break in the action.

THE DRILL: Single-leg pedaling

Rest one foot on a chair next to the trainer, and pedal with the other. Pedal smooth strokes, aiming for 90 rpm for 30 seconds, then switch legs. Increase the time up to four minutes as you improve.

THE BENEFIT: Trains your neuromuscular system to eliminate dead spots in your pedal stroke, which improves pedal efficiency and makes you a smoother, faster rider with less effort.

PIMP IT UP: Try these challenging drills while watching *A Sunday in Hell*, the classic DVD of 1976 Paris-Roubaix. Pretend you're riding buttery smooth over the cobbles as you work on perfecting your pedal stroke.

THE DRILL: Low-intensity endurance sessions

Spin for one to two hours at an easy to moderate effort.

THE BENEFIT: Builds your aerobic engine—the foundation upon which all cycling performance is built. Do these on days you don't do intervals.

PIMP IT UP: Start a "garage band." Meet with friends once a week for long trainer sessions. Each week a different "band member" brings the soundtrack. Keep the intensity conversational.

Mix It Up: Your Guide to Cross-Training

When the days grow shorter and colder, there will be times when you can't ride your bike. And honestly, you shouldn't. Your body needs breaks from the bike to straighten up and stretch out. In the end, that off-bike time will make you a better rider, says cyclist and orthopedic surgeon Kevin Stone, MD, of the Stone Clinic in San Francisco.

"Cycling is great for your legs, but it does nothing for your core or upper body," says Stone. Strengthening noncycling muscles with cross-training will help you avoid being sidelined by back, neck or shoulder pain, all common in avid cyclists. You'll also ride stronger because you'll have improved stability and a greater, more comfortable range of motion to turn the pedals and maneuver the bike, both in and out of the saddle. Here are five fun, off-the-bike ways to balance your body.

GO KAYAKING. Paddling is like cycling in reverse. Your legs are planted, providing a platform for your upper body to work against. Each time you rotate your torso and pull the paddle through the water, you build your woefully neglected twisting (oblique) muscles, as well as the postural muscles in your shoulders and along your spine. **BIKE BENEFIT:** You'll strengthen your core, which results in less back pain when you start building your cycling base in spring. Well-conditioned obliques also provide better power transfer from your hands to your feet as you rise out of the saddle and rock your bike up rollers or kick-start a sprint.

RUN A TRAIL. A lot of cyclists despise running, but scampering down a wooded trail is like mountain biking without the wheels—you still get the pleasure of hopping through rock gardens, jumping logs and bounding across streams. Plus, you improve your bone density (something mountain biking doesn't do well), scorch calories and strengthen those underused stabilizing muscles in your hips that help keep you rock-steady in the saddle. **BIKE BENEFIT:** Running uphill, especially off-road, where you need to drive your knees skyward and pick up your feet, develops on-the-bike climbing power in your lower body and conditions your heart and lungs for the battle against gravity.

PLAY SOCCER. Running up and down a big open field with few breaks is tremendous exercise. "You move so much from side to side and develop speed and agility that you lose when you cycle only," says Stone. Being forced to change direction on a dime and brace yourself to kick and head-strike the ball also helps hone core stability. **BIKE BENEFIT:** All that fancy footwork and high kicking improves the dynamic flexibility and range of motion in your hips for a more fluid spin in every pedaling position.

Pro **Tip**

"MY OFF-SEASON IS A SHORT, CHERISHED TIME OF YEAR THAT'S ABOUT SKIING—WHICH I CONSIDER A FLIPPING PRIORITY. I GET MORE ANXIOUS DRIVING UP FOR A POWDER DAY THAN I DO ON A WORLD CHAMPIONSHIP START LINE. IT'S AN INCREDIBLE, DYNAMIC, ANAEROBIC WORKOUT, AND I DON'T DARE COMPARE IT WITH ANYTHING IN A GYM."
—*JAMEY DRISCOLL, PROFESSIONAL ROAD AND CYCLOCROSS RACER*

VISIT THE GYM. Strength training targets and tones every underused muscle. Get your supporting muscles up to speed with the exercises in Chapter 19. "Cyclists also reap terrific benefits from Pilates, because it trains the core to be strong and stable while the limbs are in motion," says Stone. Take a class or buy a DVD. **BIKE BENEFIT:** Strength transforms into speed.

GO FOR A SWIM. Slicing through water is an amazing strengthening and cardio workout because it uses every muscle in your body. "It also lengthens abdominal and hip flexor muscles, which are typically shortened in cyclists," says Stone. "And it strengthens and improves range of motion in your shoulders." **BIKE BENEFIT:** Swimming turbocharges your breathing capacity. Exercising facedown in water demands deep, well-timed breaths that stretch and strengthen your diaphragm and the intercostal muscles between your ribs. It also strengthens the back and shoulder muscles that hold your chest open to allow for maximum airflow.

CHAPTER 19

Get Strong

If you're like most cyclists, you barely have enough hours to ride, let alone strength train. So don't spend your limited gym time mindlessly wandering from contraption to contraption—instead, focus your effort on exercises that will directly benefit your cycling. Here you'll find an off-season strength-building routine, exercises for your core and other important cycling muscles, and, once you've developed a foundation of strength and balance, a plyometric routine to boost your power on the bike. Bonus: Most of the moves can be done in the privacy of your own home.

BUILD OFF-SEASON STRENGTH

To ride a bike really fast, mile after mile, hour after hour, you need whole-body strength. "Think about what gets sore during those first long rides of the season," says Nick Winkelman, performance specialist at Athlete's Performance, in Tempe, Arizona. "It's your neck, back, knees and core. That's because the muscles that support you in the cycling position and provide a platform for your legs to push against aren't prepared."

Get fit fast with this body-preparation routine devised by Winkelman especially for cyclists. Do it every day during the off-season, and you'll roar into the new year.

Forward Lunge, Forearm-to-Instep

Improves flexibility in hips, torso, hamstrings, lower back, groin, hip flexors and quads.

Step forward with your left leg, bend down, and place your right hand on the floor even with your left foot. Bend your left arm and reach the elbow toward the inside of your left foot. Pause. Move your left hand outside your left foot and push your hips toward the ceiling, straightening both legs and pulling your left toe up toward your shin. Repeat on opposite side. Alternate for 5 to 10 lunges.

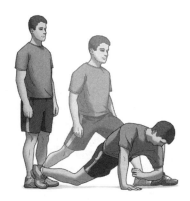

Inverted Hamstring

Improves hamstring flexibility and balance for better range of motion and more power throughout the pedal stroke.

Stand with arms out to the sides, shoulder height. Keeping your right leg extended, lift your left foot behind you and balance on your right leg. Hinge forward from the waist, keeping your body in a straight line from your head through your left heel, until parallel to the floor. Alternate for a set of 10 on each side.

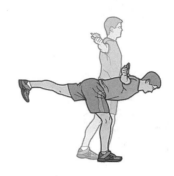

Hand Walk

Lengthens hamstrings, calves, and lower-back muscles for improved range of pedaling motion; more stability in shoulders and core.

Stand with legs straight, bend forward, and place your hands on the floor in front of your feet as close to your toes as comfortably possible (you can bend your knees). Pull your navel toward your spine and walk your hands forward until your body is nearly parallel to the floor. Keeping legs straight, take baby steps to walk your feet back to your hands. Repeat 5 to 10 times.

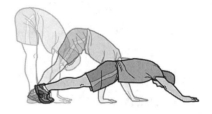

Diagonal Arm Lift

Improves strength and stability through shoulders, upper back, and core, making you rock steady on the bar, even on the roughest rides.

Assume a plank position on your forearms (arms close together, feet far apart), so your body forms a straight line from head to heels. Lift your right arm overhead and out to the side in a half-Y position. Hold for two seconds. Repeat on the opposite side. Alternate for six to 10 lifts per side. As the move becomes easier, place your feet closer together.

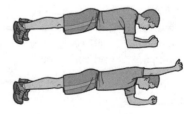

Miniband Walks

Builds a stronger gluteus medius (the outside of your butt),
which in cyclists can be eclipsed by the big gluteus maximus
that propels you forward.

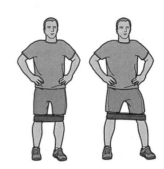

In a standing position, loop a resistance band around your legs
just above your knees. Step laterally to the right while keeping
the left leg planted. Take a small step with the left to return to
start, and continue for 10 steps. Repeat to the left.

WORK YOUR CORE

The simplest, most important thing a cyclist can do to boost power, improve balance and prevent injury takes just 20 minutes. Cross-country pro Jeremy Horgan-Kobelski was coming off the Athens Olympics and the best year of his career when disaster struck: At the 2005 Sea Otter Classic, strong winds pushed him off his line during a high-speed descent. The crash required a helicopter medevac and left him with eight shattered ribs. Robbed of his power and control, he limped through the rest of the season. His wife, fellow pro Heather Irmiger, picked up a yoga-for-athletes video that fall, and the couple began doing yoga together.

Now, both say the core strength and flexibility developed through yoga has improved their riding. "On a supersteep climb, I don't waste energy rocking back and forth," says Irmiger. "The power comes from my core instead." Horgan-Kobelski adds that he has no lower-back pain anymore, and says his newfound core strength has also helped his handling skills.

Cycling is a unique sport in that it fundamentally relies on power from the abdominals and lower back, but does virtually nothing to build or maintain it. In fact, cycling can sap your core strength and actually create problems, says Patty Tomlin, an exercise physiologist certified in Pilates at Colorado's Boulder Center for Sports Medicine. Many of the cyclists she sees have overdeveloped quadriceps muscles and weak hamstrings, a classic problem that is a result of pedaling. Even off the bike, those powerful quads pull the hips forward and down, and the weaker hamstrings can't pull back enough. This leads to poor posture and weak lower-back and abdominal muscles, says Tomlin. On the bike, it translates into a loss of power due to fatigue, and a greater chance of back pain, even injury.

The hamstring link is key. We think of the "core" as abdominals and lower back, but the hamstrings are essential to developing core power, says Dave Farmar, a Baptiste Vinyasa power yoga instructor and mountain biker from Denver. "The tendency is to muscle through a ride with your quads," he says. "In the process, the core isn't engaged and this even prevents it from being used." But if you're flexible enough to engage your hamstrings, he adds, you'll recruit core power and ride faster. Farmar credits regular yoga practice with helping him shave minutes off his 2005 Leadville 100 time, even though he trained less on the bike that year.

Developing core power takes as little as 20 to 25 minutes per session. The following workout, designed for *Bicycling* by Farmar and Tomlin, combines the yoga and Pilates moves cyclists need to strengthen their abs, hips, hamstrings and lower back. It's short and intense, and it will begin to pay dividends in only a few weeks. Start it now, do it two or three times a week, and continue it into the riding season for your most powerful year ever.

Part 1: Warm-Up and Flexibility

Total time: 10 minutes

These yoga poses, though they're also strength moves, will double as stretches to warm up. You'll need a soft surface or yoga mat, a foam support block, and a strap or latex resistance band. Hold each pose for five to 10 breaths (about 30 seconds), remembering to breathe through your nose. After you reach the proper position, says Farmar, concentrate on improving it with each inhalation—flatten your back a little more, stretch your hamstrings a tiny bit farther. When you're done, move to Part 2 without stopping.

Downward-Facing Dog

Start on hands and knees. Lift hips into an upside-down V shape, keeping palms on the floor. "Bend your knees if necessary," says Farmar. "Don't focus on putting your heels on the ground, but rather on flattening your back."

Works: *Lengthens back muscles and hamstrings for more power on the pedal backstroke*

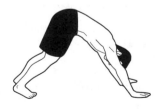

Thunderbolt Pose

From downward dog, walk your feet to your hands and then squat as if you're sitting in a chair. "The tendency here is to have a big C curve in your back," says Farmar. "But you want to engage your core, so pull your belly up and in, and flatten your back." Reach your arms up over your head and roll your shoulders back and down to open your chest.

Works: *Glutes, quads, hamstrings, and lower back; also helps open chest for better breathing*

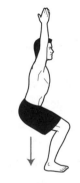

Crescent Lunge

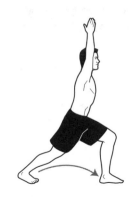

Step one foot forward into a lunge position, arms still raised. Focus on keeping the heel of your back foot as close to the floor as possible and your back leg as straight as possible, and keeping your shoulders aligned over your pelvis. Never push your front knee past your toes, or you'll put undue stress on the joint. Hold for 5 to 10 breaths, then switch.

Works: *Hip flexors, quads, hamstrings*

Half-Pigeon

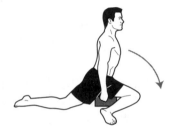

From the crescent lunge, lower yourself to the floor with your forward leg crossed in front of you, rear leg straight out behind. Unless you're ridiculously flexible, use a block under your hip for this pose. Don't worry about how low you go—the important thing is to keep your hips level, without letting one sink to one side. Fold forward, if possible. Hold 5 to 10 breaths, then switch legs.

Works: *Hips. "This leads to less hip rock and less knee rotation while pedaling," says Farmar, so your pedal stroke is more efficient.*

Bridge

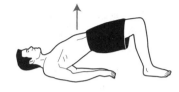

Lie on your back, knees bent with feet planted close to your butt, arms by your sides. Exhale and lift your pelvis up in line with your knees and your sternum toward your chin, keeping shoulder blades and head flat on the floor. Join your hands underneath you. Note: Never turn your head in this pose. If you have a back or neck injury, skip this exercise or do it with extra care, and place a folded towel under your shoulders at the base of your neck.

Works: *Glutes and abdominals; helps strengthen your back and open your chest to make your reach to the handlebar more comfortable*

Recline Hands-to-Toes Pose

Lie on your back and, using a strap looped under one foot, lift that leg up in the air, leaving the other leg flat on the ground. Don't worry about keeping the raised leg perfectly straight if you're not flexible, but do try to pull your heel past your hip. As you hold the stretch, point your toes to the sky and then flex your foot so your heel points skyward. Do this several times; switch legs after 5 to 10 breaths.

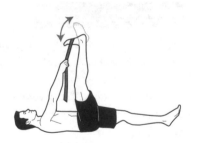

Works: *Hamstrings*

Part 2: Strength Building

Total time: 10 to 15 minutes

As you do these Pilates exercises, remember to breathe deeply from your belly and flow from one to the next without resting. When you're finished, do yourself a favor and cool down by lying flat on your back, arms at your sides, and resting for a couple of minutes to let your mind and body settle.

Unsupported Marching

Lie on your back, hands by your sides. Take a deep belly breath and exhale, pulling in your abdominals. Inhale and bend your left leg 90 degrees at the hip and 90 degrees at the knee. Exhale and raise your right leg to match. Inhale and lower your left leg, then exhale and lower your right leg. Repeat 10 to 20 times total.

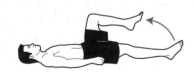

Works: *Hip flexors, transverse abdominus; also trains you to belly breathe*

The Hundred

Do the first half of the unsupported marching exercise, but instead of lowering back down, curl your shoulders toward your legs like a crunch—the focal point of the crunch should be where a heart-rate monitor strap would sit, not your belly. Focus your gaze between your knees, not at the ceiling. Lift your arms off the ground and pump them up and down five times, taking a short, partial inhalation on each pump. Then pump five more times, exhaling one long breath throughout the five count. That's one set; start with three and work your way up to 10.

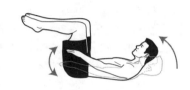

Works: *All abs*

Half Roll Down

Sit with knees bent 90 degrees and feet flat on the floor; place a foam block between your knees for proper form. Lightly place your fingers at the crease in your knee (no pulling), then exhale and slowly roll your torso back until you threaten to tip backward. Keep your feet on the floor, creating a C-curve in your spine that allows you to roll rather than flop. A classic half roll down has you inhale and raise your torso back to the start position, but Tomlin recommends that if you're a beginner, at the tip point you should complete the roll down, then turn onto your side and resume the starting position. Eventually, you'll work up to the full exercise. Do 10 of these.

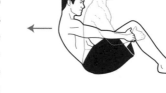

Works: *All abs, hip flexors; increases spinal mobility, so you'll be more flexible on the bike*

Single-Leg Stretch

Starting on your back, lift your feet into the air, toes pointed, then tuck your left leg up against your chest. Inhale and curl your shoulders off the floor, with your right hand on your ankle and the left on your knee. Your other leg stays straight out. Exhale and reverse, extending the left and tucking the right leg. Repeat 5 to 10 times, slowly. (Hint: This looks like slow-motion pedaling.)

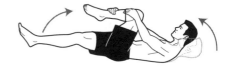

Works: *Obliques, which are stabilizer muscles, so you'll have better control of your bike*

Criss-Cross

On your back, loosely knit your fingers behind your head and bring your knees toward your chest. Inhale, lift your shoulders off the floor and twist to touch your right elbow to your left knee. Extend your right leg simultaneously. Exhale and reverse to tuck the right leg and extend the left. Note: Keep your elbows out wide, and don't pull your head forward, which could strain your neck. Repeat 5 to 10 times, slowly, emphasizing proper form.

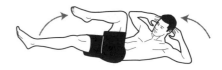

Works: *Rectus abdominus (a.k.a. six-pack abs muscles), obliques*

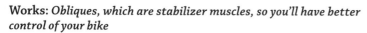

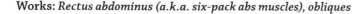

Forward Plank

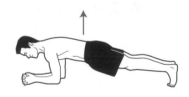

Lie facedown and prop yourself up on your elbows and forearms. Position your shoulders directly above your elbows and rise up on your toes. Envision yourself as a plank and be careful not to let your back sag. Keep your shoulders pulled back, rather than rounded forward. Hold for 30 seconds.

Works: *Lower-back muscles and shoulders; mimics your position on the bike*

BUTT SERIOUSLY . . .

To strengthen your core, you also have to get tough on your rear. The true source of strength on the bike starts where the core ends, in the power generators known as the glutes. They support everything you do, from pedaling your bike to standing up. Cycling builds your booty, but even all that pedal pushing does little to strengthen the outer glutes. And weak outer glutes not only make you less solid in the saddle, they can also contribute to knee pain or injury—a potential nightmare for cyclists whose knees need to track about 5,400 times each hour. "Many persistent aches and pains in our knees, ankles and feet begin with weak glutes," says Andy Pruitt, EdD, director of the Boulder Center for Sports Medicine, in Colorado. "Building strong buns and stable hips means better knee stability and a stronger, healthier pedal stroke." To tap the full power of your glutes, do two to three sets of 15 reps three times a week for a rock-solid butt that looks better in spandex.

Single-Leg Stability Curl

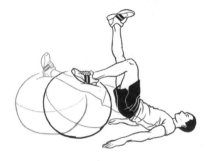

Lie faceup on the floor with your shoulders flat, arms at sides and legs extended, ankles resting on a stability ball. Raise your right foot off the ball. Squeeze your glutes and lift your hips off the floor while bending your left knee and pulling the ball toward your butt with your left heel. Return to start. Repeat for a full set, then switch legs.

Speed Skater

Stand with feet shoulder-width apart, knees slightly bent. Shift your weight onto your right leg, bending it about 45 degrees while sweeping your left leg behind you. In one smooth motion, sweep your left leg back to the left and jump from your right leg to your left, immediately bending into a half squat with your left leg as you sweep your right behind you. Alternate for a full set on each leg.

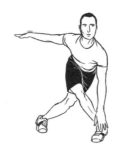

Step Dip

Holding dumbbells, stand on the edge of a 12- to 18-inch step so your right foot is planted and your left leg hangs free. Pull your navel toward your spine and, keeping your chest lifted and back straight, lower until your right leg is bent 45 to 90 degrees. Return to start, keeping your right foot planted on the step. Repeat for a full set, then switch legs.

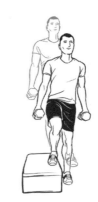

SUPPORT YOUR SUPPORTERS

If you're like most cyclists, your legs aren't the first part of your body to call it quits on a long ride. Chances are it's your back, your neck or even your arms. Use these moves to tune up the supporting muscles, and they won't slow you down. Do two sets of each move once or twice a week.

Lower-Back Muscles

Any force you direct into your pedals also travels up into your torso, particularly your lower back. The muscles running along the lower section of your spine go into overdrive to support you when you pedal hard, especially during long, seated climbs.

They've quit when: You slow down and start veering side to side, as the muscle platform you're pushing against collapses.

Tune 'em up: Assume a push-up position with your hands on a low step directly beneath your shoulders, feet on the floor. Extend your right arm overhead and lift your left foot a few inches off the floor, pointing your toes. Hold for a few seconds, then return to start. Repeat with the opposite arm and leg. That's one rep. Do 10.

Upper-Back Muscles

Your trapezius and rhomboid muscles run along your upper back and into your neck. They hold your head up and shoulders back as you stretch across your top tube in the riding position.

They've quit when: Your neck aches so much you can't get aero without saying, "Ow!"

Tune 'em up: Lie facedown on an exercise ball with your feet planted on the floor shoulder-width apart, and your belly and hips pressed into the ball. Keep your back flat and your chest off the ball so your body forms a straight line from your head to your heels. Drop your arms toward the floor, keeping elbows slightly bent and close to your torso. Squeeze your shoulder blades together and lift your arms out to the sides. Lower and repeat 10 to 12 times.

Triceps

The backs of your arms act as your upper-body shocks, supporting your torso on the bar and absorbing chatter from the road.

They've quit when: You begin straightening your arms, locking your elbows, and taking hits in your shoulders from rough pavement.

Tune 'em up: Sit on the edge of a chair with your feet flat on the floor, knees bent 90 degrees. Grasp the seat on each side of your butt and walk your feet out as you inch off the seat. Extend your legs and plant your heels on the floor. Bend your elbows back and dip your butt toward the ground until your shoulders and elbows are in line. Press back to start. Repeat 10 times.

Abdominals

Your abdominal muscles support your torso. They also pull your legs around the top of the pedal stroke and, with your lower back, provide a stiff platform for your legs to push against as you punch the pedals back down.

They've quit when: You start feeling wobbly on your wheels, just as with your fatigued lower back.

Tune 'em up: Lie on your back, hands behind your head, knees bent. Lift your feet off the floor until your legs form a 90-degree angle, calves parallel to the floor. Pull your navel to your spine, and lift your head and shoulders off the floor. Curl your right shoulder across your body toward your left knee while extending your right leg. Do not draw your left knee into your chest; keep it still. Then, keeping your torso lifted, switch sides, bringing your right leg back to start and curling your left shoulder toward your right knee, while extending your left leg. That's one rep. Do 10.

Forearms

Your arms support about one-third of your body weight when you're perched atop your bike. The muscles in your forearms pull double duty, supporting you but also squeezing the brakes and working the shifters.

They've quit when: Your hands, wrists and forearms fatigue or ache. If you have a lot of pain or tingly, numb fingers, check your position; you may be putting too much weight on your hands.

Tune 'em up: Try wrist extension and flexion. While seated, hold a light weight in your right hand and rest your right forearm on your right leg so your hand dangles toward the floor, palm down. Slowly raise and lower the weight 10 times. Flip your arm over and repeat the move, this time with palm facing up. Repeat with your left hand.

POWER UP WITH PLYOMETRICS

Resistance training will boost your brute force, but unless you convert that strength to cycling-specific fitness, those new muscles will be all show and no go. Because weight lifting tends to be a slow-moving sport, after hundreds of reps and sets, your muscles are finely tuned to move in slo-mo, not hammer down the road at 20 mph. Pick up the pace with plyometrics—jumps, hops and leaps that develop lightning-quick

explosive power, which is exactly what you need to jump to attack, sprint to the finish or crank up steep inclines. Research shows that a twice-weekly plyometric routine can boost power endurance—the ability of your muscles to contract at near max force for a greater amount of time—by 17 percent in just four weeks.

The following program contains three lower-body moves to power up your hips, glutes and legs, and two to target your core. Do one or two sets of eight to 12 reps twice a week, allowing at least one day off between efforts (and avoid these in the few days before a big event). This routine assumes you have good strength and balance. Proper form and technique are essential. Warm up thoroughly, and always land softly by coiling your joints like a spring as you hit the ground. If fatigue is making your form sloppy, stop. Plyometrics work best when you practice quality, not quantity.

Star Jump

From a standing position, crouch toward the floor. Swiftly jump upward and outward, opening your legs wide and moving your arms out, creating a star shape while in the air. As you land, bringing your legs back together and arms to your sides, bend your knees until your hands touch the floor on each side of your feet.

Pedaling Split Jump

Stand with your right leg forward and your left leg behind you. Bend your right knee and dip your left knee toward the floor, so you're in a lunge position. Extend your arms out to the sides. Swiftly jump up, switching legs in midair, driving the back knee up (like the upward pedal stroke) as you bring it forward. Softly land in a lunge position and immediately jump again.

Blast Off

Stand facing a step 8 to 12 inches high. Plant your right foot on the step. Forcefully push off the right foot and jump straight up, swinging your arms forward and up for added momentum. Land with your right foot on the step and immediately push off for the next rep. Complete a set, then switch legs.

Ovation Push-Up

Lie facedown on an exercise ball with both hands on the floor on a cushioned surface or exercise mat. Walk your hands out until the ball is under your thighs, and position your hands directly below your shoulders. Keeping your torso straight, bend your elbows and lower your chest toward the floor until your arms are bent 90 degrees. Push up as hard as you can, clap your hands once, and return to the push-up position before immediately dropping into another repetition.

Toss Crunch

Lie back on an exercise mat, knees open to the sides, soles of your feet together. Hold a light medicine ball (or basketball to start) over your chest with both hands, elbows bent out to the sides. Contract your abs by pulling your navel toward your spine, then quickly lift your head, shoulders and upper back off the floor, tossing the ball straight up toward the ceiling. Hold the up position, catch the ball and return to start.

CHAPTER 20

Your Comeback Starts Now

When an injury, work or family commitments, or just plain laziness keeps you off the bike for an extended period of time, it's easy to feel like your fitness has vanished forever, especially if you're an older athlete. The good news: It's never too late to get back in the saddle. Here's how to put the spring back into your spin, while keeping burnout at bay.

REHAB THE RIGHT WAY

If your layoff is due to injury, the standard recipe for recovery is usually six to eight weeks of rest, ice and Advil. But there are steps you can take to minimize lost saddle time and bounce back to become better than before.

EASY ON THE VITAMIN I. For most of us, the reflex response to pain is to reach for a bottle of ibuprofen to reduce swelling. Killing pain is fine, says Andy Pruitt, director of the Boulder Center for Sports Medicine in Colorado and author of *Andy Pruitt's Medical Guide for Cyclists*, but deflating inflammation during the initial stages of an injury may actually delay healing. Anti-inflammatories inhibit enzymes called prostaglandins, which promote circulation to the injured area and increase tissue permeability, so your body's repair-crew cells can come in and clear out the wreckage. For the first 48 hours, use Tylenol, which is purely a pain reliever, says Pruitt, "so you don't suppress the healing process." After that, anti-inflammatories are fine.

MOVE IT. Resting doesn't mean immobilizing yourself in front of the TV for a *Jersey Shore* marathon. Take it easy on the injured body part, but stay in motion to keep blood flowing, which will help you heal faster and maintain fitness. Try swimming, resistance training, rowing or even riding the trainer.

EAT TO HEAL. You may not be riding, but your body still burns about 10 percent more calories than usual when it's trying to repair an injury. "It's important that you feed your body what it needs to mend," says Liz Applegate, author of *Nutrition Basics for Better Performance*. She recommends boosting your intake of protein, which builds muscle and soft tissues, to 100 to 120 grams a day. Other essential recovery nutrients: iron, which builds blood, and zinc, to speed wound healing; both are found in lean meat, whole grains and fortified cereals. Vitamins A and C help make new skin and collagen, so stock up to help heal road rash. Finally, if you broke a bone, your body needs extra calcium to bridge the gap. Bump your intake to 1,500 milligrams a day.

USE THE ONE-TO-TWO RULE. For each week you couldn't train, spend one to two weeks rebuilding your base before returning to hard riding. So if you were off for three weeks, it could take as many as six before you can tear up the local crit again.

START EN MASSE, FINISH SOLO. During those first weeks back in the saddle, limit group rides, where you'll be tempted to push your pace. If you long for camaraderie, roll out with the group for the first few miles, then spin off to do your own thing when it turns up the heat.

WATCH THE WARNING SIGNS. It's natural to feel little niggling twinges when you saddle up for the first few times. But that discomfort should dim as you warm up. Let pain be your guide: If it flares or stubbornly persists, back off. The single most common cause of reinjury is doing too much too soon, Pruitt says. Likewise, as you come back your body may be particularly vulnerable to overtraining. Now is the time to respect rest and easy days.

ROOT OUT THE CAUSE. If your injury is one of overuse, such as tendonitis, "don't jump right back on the bike without figuring out what went wrong," says Pruitt. Have a professional fitting to ensure your bike is set up to work with your anatomical alignment. Optimum

Reader Tip

"I STARTED OFF WITH TWO MINUTES A DAY FOR THE FIRST WEEK SO I WOULDN'T GET SORE AND QUIT LIKE MOST PEOPLE DO."—*RICK HAYNES, 43, WHO PEDALED AWAY NEARLY 100 POUNDS*

body-to-bike harmony not only prevents chronic aches and pains, but also improves bike handling and performance, which may prevent the more acute injuries that come with hitting the pavement.

GET FASTER AS YOU AGE

It's possible for some cyclists. Chris Carmichael explains why:

Just shy of his 38th birthday, Lance Armstrong won the Leadville 100 mountain bike race in record time. Like so many ultraendurance events, the race tends to be dominated by older athletes. Only five of the 20 fastest riders were younger than 30—and four were over 40. Leadville, then, was a reminder that there are habits and techniques all athletes can learn from the "fast old guys."

Diversity Trumps Specialization

Longtime cyclists all seem to have off-the-bike athletic interests. In fact, participation in other sports enhances your riding—in terms of both quality and longevity. The Leadville 100 happens in mid-August, and already some riders were looking forward to using their skis, or to indoor soccer and ice-hockey leagues.

Why Does My Butt Hurt?

Got an embarrassing case of beginner's butt? There are ways to avoid that soreness. There are at least four layers between your saddle and your sit bones, including your chamois, skin, fat and muscle, says Roger Minkow, MD, an ergonomics consultant and the inventor of Specialized's Body Geometry saddle. "When you ride and get in shape, your muscle tissue gets firmer," Minkow says. "This gives you more muscle mass between your sit bones and your seat," which offers additional protection. But after a few weeks of couch training, a hard ride on soft muscles can leave you feeling bruised for a couple of days. To prevent this, Minkow recommends keeping muscles firm by spending 20 to 40 minutes for three days a week on your trainer or in Spin class if you can't ride outside, or with exercises such as leg presses.

Softer saddles don't necessarily make for comfortable rides, especially if your sit bones sink into the padding, which can compress nerves, leaving you with a numb rear end. "It's fine for short trips," Minkow says. "But you really want to be lifted up, and a firmer saddle of a proper width will provide this."

Riders of all levels should get out of the saddle occasionally to relieve pressure on nerves and bones. Your position on the seat is equally important. "You want your sit bones to be on the wide part of the seat, so they're supported," Minkow says. "If you're on the nose, the saddle goes in between the sit bones and compresses the nerves." When your seat starts to feel more like a slab of cement than an ergonomic component, it may be time to replace it— temperature, humidity and mileage can wear out the foam.

Sleep Is the Best Ergogenic Aid

Because their lives tend to be more settled, with stable careers and families, older athletes often go to bed earlier, and those extra hours of sleep make a huge difference in the quality and rate of postworkout recovery. Over time I've discounted the theory that older athletes need more recovery time than younger ones; this is because of their improved sleep habits.

Go Hard and Go Home

Experience has taught us older folks to be time-efficient. This means 60-minute weekday rides with a short warm-up, some hard intervals, a cool-down, and you're done. High-intensity, low-volume training, as described in my new book, *The Time-Crunched Cyclist*, is emerging in cycling now because for some people it's the only way to attain high-performance fitness without losing your job and family.

Better Recovery Is Free Training

Older athletes tend to be more open to focusing on new recovery tools like compression technology. Many people noticed that Armstrong wore compression socks between Tour de France stages. In the winter I also had him wear pneumatic compression boots. There's still a lot of research to be done here, but the idea is that compression improves recovery by helping to circulate blood and lymph fluids through tired muscles.

Then there's active-recovery footwear from MBT. After I tried a pair for a week in 2008, I partnered with the company and put my coaches in them. The curved sole spreads the pressure of walking along the length of your foot, lessening the impact on your feet, knees, hips and spine. The balance point under the middle of your foot also forces you to constantly engage muscles in your hips and torso as you stand and walk, and lightly engaging muscles on a consistent basis is one of the primary tenets of active recovery.

Don't Always Follow the Leader

Many times you'll have to make a choice between following a young and strong rider, or an older but slower one. The choice is easy. Whether it's avoiding crashes, getting into position to stay out of the wind, or deciding it's time to put on a rain jacket, there are reasons old guys reach the finish line despite lower power outputs and VO_2 max values than racers half their ages.

Training Is Cumulative

Experienced riders need less time than novices to return to optimal fitness. Following six months off the bike, it will take a cyclist who's been riding for two years about 1.5 times as long to return to top fitness as a cyclist who'd been riding consistently for five years. The more years you ride, the greater the advantage. So there's a benefit to continuing to ride at any level—even if your performance drops off for a season or two. After competing in the Leadville 100, Lance said he could imagine racing there when he's 50, at which time I'll be 61. At least there will be a good chance we can both win our age groups.

MAKE YOUR OWN COMEBACK

There's no way to stop the years from ticking by, but you can do what Armstrong did: embark on an athletic renaissance no matter what your age. "We're seeing endurance athletes stay competitive later in life," says Peter Park, Armstrong's personal trainer and the owner of Platinum Fitness, in Santa Barbara, California. Case in point: Constantina Tomescu-Dita, the Romanian who won the women's Olympic marathon in Beijing at age 38. "These days, older athletes believe they can still win—and they do," Park says. Here's how to get back in the game after age 35.

Embrace Resistance

Let nature take its course, and you'll lose about 5 percent of your muscle mass every decade. But athletes can maintain strength and power by adding resistance training to their routine. Yoga, Pilates and weight-lifting are all useful; for Armstrong, Park's program keeps upper-body bulk to a minimum, but strengthens hips, glutes and legs with kettlebell exercises and plyometrics. Park's favorites: planks (holding your body in a modified push-up position for core strength, Bulgarian split squats (with one foot resting on a bench behind you) for glutes and quads, and kettlebell swings (bending low with a weight held between your legs and thrusting it forward using the pelvis) for glutes and hips. Do two days of full-body resistance training per week on the days you ride hardest. "That way, you can use one rest session to recover from both workouts," Park says.

Eight Tips for Starting Over

A new season presents a clean slate, so anything that may have happened last year to keep you from riding like you wanted to—injury, parenthood, romance, or just burn-out—happened last year. It's time for your comeback.

1. Go to the bike shop for inspiration and take your bike along for a much-needed overhaul. While there, buy a jersey, a quality pair of shorts, a shiny helmet or all three—not only because this will jump-start your enthusiasm, but also because time away from your Grateful Dead jersey has made you come to your senses.

2. If you've been injured, follow this equation: The length of time to return to your previous condition should be double the time you were off the bike. If cycling was the cause of your injury, figure out what went wrong and fix it so it doesn't happen again.

3. Ride in street clothes your first time back—like you used to do, to explore other kids' neighborhoods, spend one dollar on 100 Swedish Fish, or see who could lay down the longest skid on the way back from the creek. Now you remember how your bike makes you feel free.

4. Don't immediately throw yourself into a fast group ride where the only things you'll see are everyone's backs and your lunch dripping down the frame. Start solo at your own pace, or with a friend who's slower than you.

5. Every few weeks find a new route, because the unexpected is more exciting than the expected, and because you won't be able to compare your performance to previous rides.

6. Once a week, ride a different type of bike, just for fun.

7. When you feel like your fitness has a long way to go, stop comparing yourself with other cyclists. Go to the mall and compare yourself to the average American. You feel better now, right?

8. Before you set goals, know your personality type. Baby steppers need frequent benchmarks to show incremental improvement. Big dreamers need to jolt themselves into action by signing up for an event well beyond their current abilities and telling all their friends about it so there's no backing down.

Think Quality, Not Quantity

At 40, you can ride just as hard as when you were younger—you just can't do it as often. In fact, building intensity into your regimen is key to attaining high-end fitness, which athletes over 35 can lose unless they regularly redline it. Do one interval workout (hitting 80 to 95 percent of your max heart rate) per week.

Stretch for Speed

Flexibility suffers as you age, and tightness in your hips, hamstrings and lower back slows you down. Stay limber with stretching or yoga, which creates the flexibility required to get low in the saddle. Loose hamstrings let you raise your saddle height for more powerful pedal strokes. Park recommends goblet squats: Stand with your feet slightly wider than your hips, holding a dumbbell or medicine ball close to your chest, and squat to the floor, resting your elbows on your inner knees to urge them outward.

Watch Your Weight

Older athletes have slower metabolisms, which reduce calorie requirements. Weight gain compromises your VO_2 max, which for sedentary people over 25 can decrease as much as 10 percent per decade, Park says. Keep your weight down and you can trim that decline to more like 3 percent.

Opt for Antioxidants

Because antioxidants combat the muscle-munching free radicals produced during tough workouts, they're good for all cyclists. But Park says older athletes in particular benefit from a diet rich in antioxidants, because they improve recovery. Eat at least five daily servings of colorful fruits and vegetables for the widest array of antioxidants, or take a supplement.

CHAPTER 21

Off to the Races

Click into racing and your body and mind will be pushed beyond the boundaries of reason—and you'll love it.

SHOULD YOU RACE?

Yes, you should—at least once. Writer Ben Hewitt explains:

This is what I remember: We were climbing through a farm field, our progress marked by lumbering Jersey cows as they chewed cuds of frost-nipped October grass. It was early, not yet 9 a.m., sunny and cool; maybe 50, maybe a touch warmer. I was on the wheel of my friend Brian Moody, a mop-haired New Englander who likes to laugh, drink beer, and race his mountain bike, in approximately that order.

Being on Moody's wheel was nothing new to me; we'd traded punches all that summer of '98, lining up at races each weekend trying to pretend that the rotation of our own, small worlds didn't depend on which of us crossed the line in front of the other. There were other racers, of course, but Moody and I were pretty much in lockstep and that only intensified our rivalry. Whether you've raced or not, you know exactly what I mean.

I remember, too, that I was feeling like dung, clinging to the backside of Moody's Fat Chance out of sheer pride and the grim knowledge that the pain I felt now was less than only one thing: the agony I'd know if I fell off the pace. This was no small cause for concern; the race was the Vermont 50, which, as its name suggests, is 50 miles long. Go 50 miles in Vermont, and you're pretty much guaranteed to rack up some serious vert—about 10,000 feet in the case of the Vermont 50.

Moody and I were about halfway in when we passed those doe-eyed cows, and all I wanted to do was collapse at their cloven hooves, smear my body into the sun-warm grass, and sleep. My pride had endured 25 miles and 5,000 feet of climbing. The thought of doing it again made crying a distinct possibility.

And then it happened: Moody cracked. Folded. Buckled. Shattered. Blew. I slid by, at first unsure of what was happening. Then the slow dawning—Moody's toast!—gave way to a steady drip of energy and confidence as I fed off his remains, pushing the pedals harder and faster, all focus and resolve now, leaving the cows to plod through their day and Brian Moody to whatever cruel fate waited up the trail.

Years later, I still get a rush thinking about it, which I suppose makes me pathetic, mean or addicted, and quite possibly a little of each. Racing can make you all of these things, in varying amounts and at different times. It can also make you happy, scared, wistful, excited, sad, jealous and angry. And that's just in the head; it is equally capricious when it comes to your body.

I'll be honest. Some of my absolute lowest moments—not only as a cyclist, but as a human being—have come to pass on a bicycle. I have lain next to my bike and fed the Earth with the contents of my stomach. I have ridden through tears—not just little drippy snivels, but real, gushing, bawling tears. I have pulled over to the side of a mountain road, the heat drumming my body, cramps riveting my legs from ass to heel, and simply sat, wanting nothing more than this moment to be gone from my life but almost as scared of the moment to follow.

But for every one of those windows to hell, there's a Brian Moody cracking. There's a sideways glance at my reflection in a window as I ride by, smooth and angular on the bike, body and style honed as only the rigors of competition can hone them. There are the minutes after a race, still flush with the fight, heart seeking level ground, basking in the small triumph of simply finishing. And yes, there are the times

I've climbed a makeshift podium, or been called to the winners' table for a handshake and maybe a check and the confirmation that, for the day at least, I had what everyone else in the race wanted, what everyone else had spent hours and days and weeks and months and maybe even years trying to get. What I had spent years trying to get.

I suppose that's why the memory of that Vermont 50 still gets me: It is the good and evil of the sport, compressed into a 30-second slice of my 38 years. Moments like that can happen only under the microscope of competition, when body and mind are pushed beyond the boundary line of reason. Most people never go there, not by free will, at least, and that is fine. Who am I to say they're not the smart ones? After all, they're not spending their Sundays bleeding sweat onto the top tube of their bike to finish 18th out of 27. Nope, they're the ones lying in bed at 9 on a Sunday morning, thinking about bacon and pancakes and coffee and maybe even sex.

Sleep, food, sex. Good things, sure. Our very survival depends on them, and no one's ever going to say that about bike racing. But the first time you attack a hill out of the saddle and hear the desperate, ragged draws of breath behind you, you'll feel it. The first time you charge a piece of singletrack with no other purpose than to make it pass beneath you as quickly as possible, you'll feel it. The first time you work a break with three other riders hell-bent on making it stick, you'll feel it. And you'll never be the same.

WHAT KIND OF RACE SHOULD YOU DO?

Time Trial

Green light: Simplicity of the discipline (you vs. clock) makes this the easiest way to launch your career. **Red light:** There's not much to distract you from the hurt. And there's a hell of a lot of hurt in time-trialing. **Do it if:** You're not ready to embrace the complexity of racing in a group.

Criterium

Green light: Going balls-out, elbow-to-elbow, around 110-degree, off-camber corners does wonders for handling skills and high-end fitness. **Red light:** Do enough crits, and it's a question of when, not if, you'll eat pavement. **Do it if:** You bet on Ultimate Fighting matches and have stock in Neosporin.

Road Race

Green light: A peloton turned loose on a long stretch of pavement is the essence of bicycle racing. Demands an encyclopedic set of skills: fitness, endurance and tactical savvy. **Red light:** It takes years to master the nuances of road racing. **Do it if:** You seek cycling enlightenment.

Track

Green light: No brakes, no gears and no margin for error. **Red light:** See above. **Do it if:** You have anger-management, or zen, issues.

Mountain Bike Cross-Country

Green light: "Yo dude" vibe makes for a non-intimidating immersion; terrain challenges provide pleasant distraction from the suffering. **Red light:** Are these people serious? Does anyone really talk like that these days? **Do it if:** You're looking for a low-key, friendly scene.

Mountain Bike Downhill

Green light: You can drink all the beer you want the night before. **Red light:** Hangovers suck; a good DH bike will set you back five grand. **Do it if:** You've got all your Metallica concert ticket stubs. In a safe.

Cyclocross

Green light: Short races don't require major training hours; nothing teaches bike handling like cutting through 6 inches of mud on a modified road bike. **Red light:** It's November. It's raining. There's football on the tube and apple pie in the oven. **Do it if:** You have lots of thermal underwear and nothing better to do.

SO YOU'LL NEVER RACE, HUH?

I have this friend. I'll call him Rick—because that's his name. Rick rides his bike a lot. A whole heck of a lot. He's fit. He—is fast. He could kick some butt.

But Rick has never raced. "It's stupid," he says, and I don't take offense because that's just the way Rick is. "Racing is stupid."

Thing is, Rick's lying. Not only to me, but also to himself. That's because Rick is perhaps the most competitive person I know. He frequents a 40-mile out-and-back route over a hilly swath of Vermont tarmac, and he times himself. Not once in a while, like we all do to mark progress, but every friggin' ride. When he pedals elsewhere, he measures the distance to the tenth of a mile, the time to the second, and computes his average speed. He doesn't ride with other people very often; the one time we rode together, he bolted off the front in the first mile and stayed there, bucking the wind, about 100 feet up the road. We didn't speak once during the entire 50 miles. Now, that was a hoot.

Everyone has the right to think racing is stupid. Everyone has the right to decide it's not for him or her. And, of course, sometimes it isn't. My point is this: Before you close that door, take a look at yourself. What's keeping you from trying it just once? Pop psychoanalysis tells me that Rick is so competitive he can't stand the thought of losing. Maybe if he raced, he'd find out that losing is bad, but doesn't kill you. Maybe he'd win.

Try one race. Then you can call it stupid. Here's our no-fail survival guide.

Best Way to Prepare Your Body

It's possible to develop race-worthy fitness on your own, but to learn race tactics and how to feel comfortable jockeying for position, you need to pedal with a group. Become a regular on your local shop's "fast" rides, or join the local club, and you'll get a feel for riding shoulder-to-shoulder at speed, and gain instant access to the insights of more-experienced racers. If you have a race question, they're the ones to ask. Find a club near you by visiting usacycling.org/clubs.

How to Pick Your Race

Scan the race fliers at your local shop; look for a relatively small but established event, such as a weeknight crit series, time trial or cross-country mountain bike race put on by a local club. Not only will entry fees be cheaper than at larger regional events, but you'll also race against a less-crowded, more evenly matched field—experienced racers are much less likely to sandbag when they're lining up against their friends.

Best Way to Screw It All Up

Decide to do the race the night before, and show up with just one hour to the gun, saying, "Where do I sign up?" Register a few weeks, if not months, ahead. Early sign-up will prompt you to train more consistently by giving you a definite goal—and give you time to convince your buddies to sign up for the same event. Even better, you'll have ample time to study the details, such as how to get there, the route, your start time, etc., reducing your chances of slap-to-the-forehead stupid mistakes.

How to Spend the Day Before

Don't do anything major to your bike right before a race, unless a crisis forces your hand.

The Ultimate Clip 'n' Save Race Day Packing Checklist

→ Directions/registration info

→ Bike (including the front wheel if you use a fork-mount rack)

→ Helmet

→ Shoes

→ Shorts

→ Jersey

→ Gloves

→ Sunglasses

→ Sunscreen

→ Socks

→ Other bike clothing, as needed (leg and arm warmers, rain jacket, vest, booties)

→ Water bottles/hydration pack (already full, just in case)

→ Extra water

→ Energy bars/gels

→ Post-race clothes (comfortable, loose fitting) and flip-flops

→ Post-race food and drink

→ Towel and washcloth

→ Extra tube

→ Patch kit

→ Tire levers

→ Minitool

→ Floor pump

→ Minipump/CO_2

→ Lube

→ Keys, wallet (with photo ID and at least $20 cash)

→ Race license, if you have one

But do go over your bike with hex wrenches to ensure everything is appropriately snug. And don't eat anything weird. Or, if all you eat is weird, don't eat anything normal. Point being, don't mess with your diet.

Pack the night before using our fail-safe checklist (above). Remember that small luxuries can salvage a rough day. They include: a cooler packed with beer and sandwiches (for after the race); solar shower (the height of racing savvy, particularly among the mountain bike crowd, who won't mind when you strip naked in the parking lot); camp chair; workstand; fully stocked tool box; a first-aid kit.

Smartest Order of Events

On race day, arrive at least an hour before your start. Then do these things in this sequence, without straying: Pick up your registration packet, which contains your numbers, and purchase your race license, if needed. If it's not obvious by watching other racers, ask an official where you should place your numbers. Pee. Put on your race clothes, and ask a friend to pin your number on securely. Zip-tie your bike number in place, too. Check the pressure in your tires, and pump if necessary. Take a 20-minute or longer warm-up ride; after the first five minutes, add to the intensity, and build to a few bursts of race-pace, adrenaline-pumping effort. (Picture the Tour guys dripping with sweat on their trainers before a TT—that's a warm-up.) Refill your water bottles. Pee again. Roll up to the start line 10 to 15 minutes before race time.

Best Way to Get From Start to Finish

At the start line, listen closely to the instructions; if you have a question, ask. Try to line up in the middle of the pack to avoid getting tangled up in a crash or being caught behind slower riders in the first corners. Mass starts are often chaotic and have an unbelievably high pace, but things will settle down. Try to stay loose on the bike; wiggle your fingers and relax your shoulders. Drink often. Before the finish, look around. Don't sprint if you're alone, but don't get nipped at the line. Savor the moment.

Post-Race Order of Things

After you finish, catch your breath, change your clothes and grab that snack—nothing says newbie like munching post-race goodies while you're still chamoised up. Head back to the finish and, if the schedule works out that way, watch the more-experienced racers compete. Study what they do, where they're positioned, and how they look at the line—and picture yourself doing the same thing at your next race.

HOW TO RACE IN STYLE

These tips won't make you faster—but they'll help you fit in. That'll help calm you down—which just might mean you ride faster. Or something like that.

1. For road races, take off your saddlebag to save weight and show the proper laissez-faire attitude toward breakdowns. For a mountain bike race: If your bench grinder fits into your hydration pack, take it.

2. When you realize your front brake is squealing during warm-ups, do not stop to adjust it. Pedal casually to the nearest car, hide behind it and do the repair. In public, your bike must be impeccable.

3. When registering, don't ask if the officials have safety pins. (They do, in a box right there on the table. Look.) And don't ask, "Where do I put my number?" Display confidence with a question that implies familiarity—"Number on the side, right?"—and which will, when corrected, elicit the information you need.

4. Use no more than four safety pins, one at each corner. Additional pins suggest worry that your number might flap in the wind. Spread out your jersey, flatten the number on it and pin the corners lightly taut. When you put your jersey on, your body will stretch the number to prevent flapping.

5. Don't drive to the race in your bike clothes. Wear civvies. Never change in the Porta Potti, or while squiggling like a pervert in the front seat of your car. Better to discreetly drop trou while facing the open door of your car. Don't fret the backside; everyone's used to seeing booty at a race.

6. Pee the first time you have to. Ignore the next three urges, then indulge your bladder one last time. Never pee more than five times.

7. White shoes? Yes, if you'll be first—or last. Only at either end of the race lies sufficient self-knowledge to sustain them.

TRAIN YOUR BRAIN

When all physical things are equal, it's the most mentally fit rider who finishes first. Yet few of us ever bother training our brain. "Mental strength is what sets you apart as an athlete," says Paige Dunn, former sport psychology consultant for Clif Bar and founder of Xcel Sport Psychology Group, in Oakland, California. Here are her four ways to keep your head in the game and out of the clouds on race day.

BREATHE TO RID STRESS. Racing with unmanaged stress is like riding in a wet suit—your chest feels too strapped to breathe and your muscles too constricted to move. "A little nervous energy is natural and healthy, but too much can cause you to tense up and waste energy," says Dunn. "I have my athletes do 'circle breathing' before a competition or anytime they feel stressed out." Inhale deeply and slowly through your nose, feeling your chest expand from top to bottom, finally allowing your abdomen to push fully outward. Pause. Then steadily exhale through your mouth, pushing out that last bit of breath so your belly empties. Feel your muscles relax. Repeat 5 to 10 times. "It helps you focus," says Dunn. "It's physiologically impossible to freak out while doing it."

REHEARSE RACE DAY. French researchers recently found that athletes who mentally ran through specific steps improved their performance even if they didn't physically practice. Succeeding in your brain without putting time in on your bike won't win races, of course, but the combination could, says Dunn. "Come race day, you're almost on autopilot because you've practiced over and over and over in your mind everything you need to do."

The night before, visualize how race day will go, then write down every detail. Is it dark when

Pro **Tip**

"WHILE TIME-TRIALING, I LIKE TO REPEAT 'CAN YOU GO ANY HARDER? CAN YOU GO ANY HARDER?'"—*KRISTIN ARMSTRONG, 2008 OLYMPIC TIME TRIAL GOLD MEDALIST* you get up? What are you wearing? What should you pack? What type of warm-up will you do? What do your legs feel like? How's your breathing? Are you psyched up? Are you sitting or standing on climbs? Mentally rehearse every aspect before you fall asleep.

BE YOUR OWN CHEERLEADER. As we push through the pain during a race, it's natural to talk to ourselves. It's also natural to have an unpleasant conversation. Studies show that both negative and positive self-talk influence performance—you can guess which works best. "When you say, 'Oh, no. Here comes the hill. This is going to hurt,' it will," says Dunn. "Worse than it would without the negative self-talk." Instead, says Dunn, think, "Hills are hard, but I can hang with the pack." If you can't spin your thoughts as quickly as you spin your wheels, develop a mantra to repeat when you need to block negative thoughts from rushing in. "'Relax' and 'spin fast and easy' are good ones," suggests Dunn. "Or 'smooth, perfect circles.'"

STAY FOCUSED. "People underestimate their pain threshold—and overestimate everyone else's," says Dunn. "Everyone is suffering, not just you. Those who deal with their pain best acknowledge it for what it is and move past it." In other words, when your quads scream, turn your focus to the task at hand: pedaling your bike as fast as possible. "Go back to your breathing and stay in control of your thoughts; you can take more than you think when you keep your mind on your mission," says Dunn.

GIVE TRIATHLONS A TRY

There are plenty of reasons to sign up for a triathlon besides having a masochistic side or an aero equipment fetish. Perhaps you can't stomach the idea of riding the trainer in winter and prefer to keep in shape by running or swimming. Or maybe you want to see how you measure up on the bike without going nose-to-saddle with 50 of your closest friends in a criterium.

But don't just take our word for it. Consider the story of 1990s Tour de France star Laurent Jalabert, who competed in the Ironman world championships—just for the fun of it.

The Transition Man

Before Lance Armstrong began running marathons, there was Laurent Jalabert. The top-ranked cyclist in the world for three years in the 1990s and a beloved French champion, Jalabert retired from pro cycling in 2002 only to reinvent himself as a marathon runner and now a triathlete.

As a bike racer, Jalabert, nicknamed Jaja, French slang for a glass of wine, was seen as his nation's best hope for breaking Miguel Indurain's Tour de France win streak of five wins. He didn't crack Indurain, but Jaja did win multiple sprinter's and climber's jerseys, and maintains the status of a legend in his home country: In Mende, in the south of France, there is a 3-kilometer, 20-percent grade, Montée Jalabert, named after him because he once won a Tour stage there.

These days Jaja is not the world-beater he once was, but he revels in the simple pleasure of being in top shape. For a time after retiring from cycling, he did almost nothing physical. Now that the 41-year-old is nearly as fit and trim as he was in his racing days, he says simply, "You know, I don't think I'll ever let myself go like that again." Bicycling caught up with Jaja in the off-season at his home in Montauban, France, between a bike ride and an evening swim.

So, why do triathlons?

After I retired from cycling I didn't do anything for two years. I gained weight—12 kilos!—and felt the difference. I had trouble climbing stairs even. I started to get a gut and my kids made fun of me. I wasn't really fat, but I didn't recognize myself and I didn't feel good. So I started running. I didn't have any real ambition, but I managed to get my wife and three couples we know to sign up for the New York City Marathon.

It was a lot of fun, but doing an impact sport just killed me. After so many years cycling, which does not beat the body like running, I hurt my knees. I hurt my tendons. I had injuries I never had before. I did three marathons after New York—London, Chicago and Barcelona. But for Chicago I was so injured that I started cycling again because I couldn't run. I basically trained for Chicago on a bike. I would ride three days and run one day.

I was living in Geneva and a friend I rode with who did triathlons encouraged me to do the three disciplines. He said, "You'll see, when you do all three, you are injured less." But, poor me, I didn't swim.

That can be a problem for a triathlete.

Yeah. Just transitioning from one sport to the next was not too hard because the base condition was there. But for me, learning to swim was really difficult. I'm afraid of big open spaces, and I just don't like the water too much. I was bad. Bad! I remember coming home from the first workout and telling my friend, "I think I'm not going to do the triathlon." But he said, "Come on, we'll do it together." And the challenge started there.

In July 2007 you did Ironman Switzerland, in Zurich.

My friend told me that there were 13 places in my age group that qualified for the world championships in Hawaii. In the beginning, I couldn't care less because I didn't want to do Zurich to qualify for something else, but as the race evolved I felt better and better. I finished 10th and then started to think about Hawaii.

It seems you learned to swim. How was it?

In the beginning, I just didn't have the technique. Breathing was hard. My legs were like weights. I remember when I first started I would come home with cramps in the back, in the neck, everywhere.

How do you approach swimming now? Do you work extra hard, or is it more like, "Ah, I'll catch them on the bike"?

Well, I should work harder at it, but here there is one big logistical problem—the pool. We have

Why I Ride

"I do remember when I started, thinking, 'Oh, that's crazy—I'd never do a race that took a month to recover from.' But it's kind of a slippery slope."—KATYA MEYERS, PROFESSIONAL TRIATHLETE, ON IRONMAN RACING

one pool for the entire community. It's just overbooked with all the clubs, the schools and the general population. I can only swim there two days a week, and that's not a lot.

And as I said, it's not a sport I like, though I have to admit it does me good. Sometimes after running, I'm sore here or there, but now that I have some swimming technique, it allows me to forget about all my aches and pains. When I get into the water, all the aches and pains go away.

What's your advice for a cyclist doing his or her first tri?

Don't get on the bike and say, "Now I'm in my domain," and go all out. Because, quite simply, you still have to run afterward.

The other thing that is important is to really work on your transitions in training. When you get off the bike, attack the first couple of kilometers of running. In the beginning, it is important to find your rhythm, and then afterward it gets easier. That's what fascinates me in the triathlon, pacing yourself and really distributing your effort.

What's it like in the bike leg—essentially time trialing surrounded by people who aren't experienced cyclists?

For me it's good, sort of reconciliation. It makes me think about that first session of swimming. I was there with people who were good swimmers, and I was just awful. I was asking myself, "What are you doing here?" And still today, everybody talks about my poor swimming. "Oh lá, lá, he was 1,200th out of the water!" So when I'm passing guys on the bike it's a relief. That's what triathlons are about. We can't be good everywhere.

What are the biggest riding errors you see triathletes make?

I'd say they ride too big of a gear. But I can't say that they are wrong; it's more that I just have the reflexes of a cyclist. I'm in the habit of spinning my legs at 90 rpms, so that's better for me. To me, they put too much emphasis on pushing big gears.

I would also say that often they don't get the most from aero equipment. In Zurich, for example, a lot of guys were riding with disc wheels, but the circuit was really hilly. There was a three-kilometer climb, and riders were just dead stopped. That wasn't the place to use disc wheels, because to get the full benefit you have to be in a situation where you can go around 27 miles per hour.

Jalabert's Typical Ironman Training Week

→ Monday: Morning and evening swim

→ Tuesday: 4-hour ride with a 10-K transition run

→ Wednesday: Morning and evening swim

→ Thursday: 5- to 6-hour ride

→ Friday: Shorter ride with a 10-K transition run

→ Weekend: Long run

→ Total hours: "Between 20 to 25," says Jalabert. "As a pro cyclist, I did about 25 hours per week, sometimes 30. But the best Ironman triathletes do more than that. I've talked with some who are doing 35 to 40 hours per week."

In an Ironman, you're in a time-trial position for about the length of a Tour de France stage—how hard is that?

Really hard. And it is made harder by the fact that you have a marathon waiting for you at the end. I try to find a compromise between a position that is aerodynamic and one that is comfortable. I also spend lots of time training on my time-trial bike.

Have you suffered more on a bike in the Tour de France or at some point in the Ironman?

The pain isn't comparable. In a bike race, you're drafting and reacting to moves—you're always pitted against others. What is unique in triathlons is that you are reacting only to yourself.

You were by far the most accomplished cyclist in the Hawaii Ironman, so why didn't you win the cycling leg?

Simply because I was not the strongest. Cycling is different when you have to run afterward. Obviously you can't be in the red zone for 10 hours, so you are forced to pace yourself differ-

ently. In addition, the guys who beat me are all younger and full-time triathletes.

You seem to have developed quite an obsessive interest in triathlons.

Oui! Back when I was a cyclist, I never would have imagined that I could do one. But I have been happy to rediscover what pleases me in sports—the competition, pushing yourself to the limit, the focus on equipment. As a result, once again I am experiencing sport in the way I did when I first started cycling, just for the passion of it.

Tris: Race Day 101

You might be the strongest cyclist in your age group in a triathlon, but that's no guarantee you'll produce the fastest bike split. Here are five essentials to maximizing your performance.

LEARN THE RULES. You don't want to crush the bike leg only to find out later that you've racked up six minutes in penalties. (Unlike at your Saturday hammerfest, for example, drafting in

Four Tips for First-Timers

Michele Redrow, co-owner of CGI Racing, which hosts the Philadelphia Women's Triathlon, has a few tricks to make your first tri a success.

When you get out of the water in your first race, you're so disoriented that your head is spinning and your legs feel like noodles. Brick training—doing two sports in a single workout—helps avoid that feeling. You train your body to know how to go from one thing to the next without feeling queasy. I practice swimming in the open water and then immediately get out and go for a bike ride or run.

Once you get an aero bar, you'll be addicted to it. If you're new to the bar, try it first on a flat, fast course—it's phenomenal. Don't use the bar on a hilly course, though. You don't want to go down a hill at 30-plus miles an hour on an aero bar until you're comfortable in the position. And I would never suggest getting one three weeks before a race and then using it. You should train on it so you're familiar with it. If you aren't going to race with an aero bar, ride more in your drops to get lower.

A lot of new triathletes blow through the beginning portion of the bike. They're three-quarters of the way into the bike and they totally bonk. They're done. Then they still need to get off and run. Use the first 15 to 20 percent of the bike to allow your body to make the transition. Go at a nice, steady speed, and then start pouring it on.

Take the last mile on the bike a little easy to allow your heart rate to come down. Hopefully you will have done some bike-to-run training and you will be used to the feeling of beginning the run on somewhat shaky legs. After about half a mile they return to normal.

triathlon is almost always illegal.) If you're at all unsure of the things that will cause you to lose time, go to the prerace meeting.

ACE THE TRANSITION. Clear thinking becomes almost impossible in the chaos of the transition area, so "practice your swim-to-bike and bike-to-run transitions at least once before race day," suggests six-time Hawaii Ironman winner Dave Scott. In the first transition, or T1, that means stripping off your wet suit, putting on your helmet and mounting your bike. In T2, you'll dismount your bike, remove your helmet (yes, in that order) and put on your running shoes.

PACE YOURSELF. "Any experienced cyclist knows that when you finish an open 40-K time trial you can hardly walk afterward, much less run a

10-K," says Troy Jacobson, head coach of the Triathlon Academy, in White Hall, Maryland. To run well in a triathlon, you need to control your effort on the bike. "You should be able to say to yourself during the entire bike leg, 'I feel like I should be going faster,'" says Gale Bernhardt, former head coach of the U.S. Olympic triathlon team. After you've done a couple of tris, you'll develop a sense of pace on the bike leg, and if you train properly for the run, you won't have to hold back much at all. "When competitive cyclists get a little triathlon experience, I tell them to go for it on the bike," says Jacobson. "That's their strength. Ride hard and let the run take care of itself."

ASSUME THE POSITION. Work on finding your optimal time-trial position—one that balances

How to Survive a Tri . . .

. . . IF YOU DON'T SWIM

Step number one is to stop fighting the water, says Mikael Hanson, founder of coaching company Enhance Sports. "Cyclists and runners are used to powering through workouts, but in swimming you're much better off starting with form drills to build good habits." You'll make more and faster progress under a coach's watch. Once confident in a pool, think about race day. "A tri swim is disorienting, so you'll need skills to deal with that," says Hanson. To simulate murky open water, go a few strokes in the pool with your eyes closed, then open them, lift your head out of the water, see where you are and correct your course. Race-day swim anxiety can still strike, even for experienced triathletes. Just try to keep moving forward however you can as you calm yourself, Hanson says. "Backstroke, doggie paddle, they're all okay."

. . . IF YOU DON'T BIKE

For a first triathlon, Hanson recommends sticking with your unmodified road bike. "Aero bars take your hands away from the brakes and shifters," he says. "Plus your road bike climbs better and handles better. Just stay in the drops." The key to effective aero riding is core strength and flexibility. "I see people spend tons of money on a tri bike and then ride on the bullhorns because they're not comfortable on the aero bars," he says. The goal is to remain in your aero tuck on flats, though Hanson recommends shifting your position for hills. "Aerodynamics mean very little under 15 miles per hour. It's all about breathing and getting the oxgen you need." So choke up on the extensions or use the base bar for leverage.

. . . IF YOU DON'T RUN

Before you start, buy new shoes at a running-specific store. "It sounds basic, but I have people show up with shoes that are years old and not right for their feet anyway," says Hanson. Begin with a slow, 10-minute run after a ride to let your running muscles take over gradually. From there, slowly build mileage. This is a pounding sport, so be kind to your body. Stick to soft surfaces if you can. Warm up beforehand, even if it's just a few minutes of trotting or walking briskly. Afterward, stretch. "You can get away with not stretching after a swim or ride, but not a run," says Hanson. "It's better to stop your run five minutes early and use the time to stretch than it is to skip stretching."

---

aero gains, comfort and power production—before event day. Stay in that aero position throughout the race except when cornering and descending steep hills, when having your arms in the aero bars is unsafe, and when climbing, because aerodynamics offer no advantage on uphills and power production is everything.

DRINK UP. The bike leg is your best chance to take in fluids and food. "By the time you're done swimming you've expended a lot of energy and experienced some dehydration," explains Jacobson. "And when you run, you can't take in calories like you can on the bike." In sprint- or Olympic-distance tris, there's no need to fuel up with much more than a sports drink: Take a sip every 10 minutes or so throughout the ride. Only in long-distance triathlons (half Ironman and up) does it become necessary to supplement your drinking with gels, bars and real food.

RIDER **RESOURCES**

Keep track of your training with the free log at traininglog.bicycling.com.

Pick up a cycling racing license at usacycling.org; for triathlon licenses, go to usatriathlon.org.

Looking for a race near you? Active.com, bikereg.com, bicycling.com/event_finder and trifind.com are good places to start.

VII

Centuries and Cause Rides

THE CENTURY RIDE—100 MILES IN ONE DAY—IS TO cyclists what the marathon is to runners, except that it's much more fun. (The short-shorts set doesn't usually get to stop for lunch, for one thing.) And with proper preparation, just about anybody can do one.

If you've never ridden a century before, the advice on the following pages will help you not only make it to the finish line, but also enjoy the trip. If you're a long ride veteran, we can help you finish even faster. And if you're one of the hundreds of thousands of cyclists who go the distance each year for charity, we'll help ensure that your fund-raising goes as smoothly as your training.

CHAPTER 22

Your Century Training Plan

Over the past 25 years, more than half a million people have completed a century using Bicycling's simple, 10-week training plans. There are never any guarantees in cycling—you might suffer the seven-flat day, or meet the love of your life munching a PB&J at the first rest stop and abandon all other pursuits on the spot—but these plans are as locked down as you get.

One is for cyclists attempting their first century, for those who currently average 40 to 50 miles per week, or who are by nature more tentative. The second program is designed for riders who want to power through a century, or those whose current weekly mileage exceeds 75. We've also included a five-week plan for shorter events, and three workouts from Chris Carmichael that will prepare you for the big day no matter how fast or far you want to go.

CHRIS CARMICHAEL'S THREE BEST CENTURY TRAINING WORKOUTS

Whether you're pushing your limits to cover 100 miles or hammering to break the five-hour barrier, you'll finish fresher and faster by incorporating the following workouts into your plan. Do them once or twice a week in the six weeks before the big day. When my coaches and I put them into the programs of our cyclists, we see dramatically improved times and happier faces at the finish line.

Fast Pedal Intervals

During a flat century, there are few chances to rest your legs, so a smooth pedal stroke will help you save energy. On a relatively flat road, shift into an easy gear and bring your cadence to about 90 rpm. Then pedal as fast as you can without bouncing in the saddle. Maintain that cadence for five minutes. Start with four five-minute intervals, with five minutes of easy riding between efforts. As you progress, extend the intervals and recovery to 10 minutes each.

Money for Something

For many charity rides, you have to donate to participate. Here are four ways to put the fun in fund-raising.

→**Throw a party or potluck with a door fee.** Everyone gives a little, but everyone also gets something out of it.

→**Have a tag sale and channel the money to the cause.** And let buyers know your motives up front so they don't dicker over prices.

→**Hold an auction.** See if any of your friends would be willing to donate a service—such as massage, dental work, or gift certificates to a restaurant, bar, inn, gym, yoga studio or bike shop—to be bid on. You can combine this with the potluck (above).

→**Work your connections.** What major company in your area already has a charity-line item in its budget this year? It could become your corporate underwriter and earn a special place on the team jerseys. Who's in a band that can play at your fund-raiser? Maybe your local bike or coffee shop would be willing to host your function.

Climbing Repeats

In a hilly hundred, fatigue can set in if climbs repeatedly push you over lactate threshold. This workout helps increase your aerobic power before you reach threshold. Find a climb that's 10 or more minutes long. (If you don't have hills, ride a trainer with your front wheel propped up, or do the intervals into a stiff headwind.) The interval intensity should be an 8 on a scale of 10, or 95 to 97 percent of your time trial (max sustainable) heart rate, or 95 to 100 percent of your TT power output. Beginners should do two 6- to 8-minute intervals,

Fun Fact

The Pan-Mass Challenge ride (pmc.org) has given more money to charity than any other athletic event in the United States. Since 1980, cyclists have raised more than $270 million to fight cancer.

intermediates can try three 8- to 10-minute intervals, and advanced riders get three 12- to 15-minute intervals. Recover between intervals with 10–15 minutes of easy spinning.

Over-Unders

The ability to get into and maintain contact with a group can save you a tremendous amount of energy. When the group surges and a gap opens, you need the power to close it; when the pace picks up toward the top of a climb, you need to be able to keep up. Over-unders include periods above and below lactate threshold, so you develop the ability to ride steady, push, then ride steady again. Pedal for three minutes at 92 to 95 percent of your max sustainable heart rate (85 to 90 percent of time-trial power or an 8 on a 10 scale of exertion). Then pick up the pace for two minutes (95+ percent of time-trial HR and power). After the two minutes, back off to the initial intensity for three minutes, then surge

PLAN 1: TO DO IT

WEEK	MON	TUES	WED	THURS	FRI	SAT	SUN	WEEKLY MILEAGE
	EASY	PACE	BRISK	REST	PACE	PACE	PACE	
1	6	10	12	OFF	10	30	9	77
2	7	11	13	OFF	11	34	10	86
3	8	13	15	OFF	13	38	11	98
4	8	14	17	OFF	14	42	13	108
5	9	15	19	OFF	15	47	14	119
6	11	15	21	OFF	15	53	16	131
7	12	15	24	OFF	15	59	18	143
8	13	15	25	OFF	15	65	20	153
9	15	15	25	OFF	15	65	20	155
10	15	15	25	OFF	10	5 EASY	CENTURY	170

for the final two minutes. Recovery between intervals is 15 minutes of easy spinning. Beginners should aim for two intervals; intermediate riders, three. Advanced riders can do three 12-minute intervals: 2:00 steady/2:00 harder/2:00 steady/2:00 harder/2:00 steady/2:00 harder.

Guide to Plans 1 & 2

Easy = Leisurely ride. If you need to adjust the schedule because of time crunches or other commitments, always make sure the easy day follows a high-mileage or brisk day.

Pace = The average speed you're aiming for on century day.

Brisk = Two to three mph faster than average century speed.

Rest = It's important to take at least one day per week—but no more than two—completely off the bike. (Easy riding helps you recover better than inactivity.)

If your event is on a Saturday, simply shift the last week's schedule back a day. (Take Wednesday off, and ride 10 miles on Thursday and 5 on Friday.)

PLAN 2: TO PUT THE SCREWS TO IT

WEEK	MON	TUES	WED	THURS	FRI	SAT	SUN	WEEKLY MILEAGE
	EASY	PACE	BRISK	REST	PACE	PACE	PACE	
1	10	12	14	OFF	12	40	15	103
2	10	13	15	OFF	13	44	17	112
3	10	15	17	OFF	15	48	18	123
4	11	16	19	OFF	16	53	20	135
5	12	18	20	OFF	18	59	22	149
6	13	19	23	OFF	19	64	24	162
7	14	20	25	OFF	20	71	27	177
8	16	20	27	OFF	20	75	29	187
9	17	20	30	OFF	20	75	32	194
10	19	20	30	OFF	10	5 EASY	CENTURY	184

Stay Loose

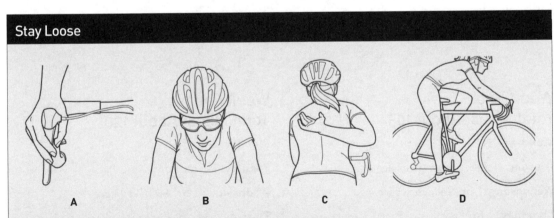

A B C D

Aches and pains crop up during long rides. To minimize them, move.

    A) Periodically change hand positions, keeping your thumbs wrapped around the bar or brake lever for security.

    B) To relieve your neck and shoulders, shrug for 5 to 10 seconds.

    C) On a clear stretch of road, reach one hand up between your shoulders for a few seconds, then swap hands.

    D) Stand up and drop one pedal so your leg is straight. Let your heel sag below the pedal. Hold for 20 seconds, then switch legs.—*Alex Stieda*

Celeb Cyclist

"I'm a little nervous. I don't really know what I'm in for."—PHIL KEOGHAN, HOST OF *THE AMAZING RACE*, WHO RAISED $500,000 FOR THE NATIONAL MS SOCIETY IN 2009 BY RIDING ACROSS THE COUNTRY

PLAN 3: THE HALF CENTURY

Week One
Total Miles: About 90

Monday: Off

Tuesday: 1 hr. Endurance Pace

Wednesday: 1 hr. Endurance Pace

Thursday: 1 hr. Recovery Pace

Friday: Off

Saturday: 2 hr.

Sunday: 1 hr. Recovery Pace

Week Two
Total Miles: About 105

Monday: Off

Tuesday: 1.5 hr. Endurance Pace

Wednesday: 1 hr. Recovery Pace

Thursday: 1 hr. Endurance Pace

Friday: Off

Saturday: 2.5 hr.

Sunday: 1 hr. Endurance Pace

Week Three
Total Miles: About 128

Monday: Off

Tuesday: 1.5 hr. Endurance Pace

Wednesday: 1 hr. Recovery Pace

Thursday: 1.5 hr. Endurance Pace

Friday: Off

Saturday: 3 hr.

Sunday: 1.5 hr. Endurance Pace

Week Four
Total Miles: About 120

Monday: Off

Tuesday: 1.5 hr. Endurance Pace

Wednesday: 1 hr. Recovery Pace

Thursday: 1.5 hr. Endurance Pace

Friday: Off

Saturday: 3 hr.

Sunday: 1 hr. Recovery Pace

Why I Ride

"The saddest part is seeing a family member standing next to a wreath along the route . . . no one utters a word. It's an amazing thing to listen to 400 people just spinning their wheels. You can almost hear people's thoughts: 'What if that were my child?'"

—KATE W. ALCOTT, PARTICIPANT, RIDE FOR MISSING CHILDREN

Week Five
Total Miles: About 100

Monday: Off

Tuesday: 1.5 hr. Endurance Pace w/Intervals

Wednesday: 1 hr. Recovery Pace

Thursday: 1 hr. Recovery Pace

Friday: Off

Saturday: EVENT

Sunday: Off

Guide to the Half Century Plan

Off: Take a break from riding; do some weight work or yoga.

Recovery Pace: Rate of perceived exertion (RPE) 1 to 4. A very slow pace; you're able to hold a conversation.

Endurance Pace: RPE 5 to 6. A pace that you can endure and still speak; typical Saturday ride effort.

Intervals: 4x6-minute intervals at RPE 9. A pace at which you can't speak, but not quite all out.

CHAPTER 23

The Final Countdown . . . to the Big Day

The good news: The time for hard training is over, and it's time to enjoy the rewards of all your hard work. The bad news: It doesn't take much (a forgotten shoe, a pre-ride taco craving) to mess things up. So in this section you'll find time-tested tips on how to eat, dress, pace yourself and keep calm before or during your event. And if you're pedaling more for scenery than speed, Chris Carmichael has some special advice for you.

EATING FOR 100

It's important to know what and what not to put into your body the week before a big event. **LEAD WITH CARBS.** The days of restricting carbohydrate then bingeing on pasta are over, but carbs still rule the week prior to a big event. Glycogen—what a carbohydrate turns into in

the body—fuels your engine. "In our carb-phobic society, I don't like to tell people to carbo-load," says sports nutritionist Molly Kimball, RD. "Instead, I say to let carbs take center stage." Consume 3 to 5 grams (g) of carbs per day for each pound of your body weight (about 600g for a 150-pound cyclist), suggests Kimball. "It's not just pasta and rice. Fruit yogurt, apples, even chocolate milk are great sources."

Also, let your guard down. "Before an event, your body can use some of those refined carbs that you usually avoid," says Kimball. "This is your chance to indulge."

DON'T SKIMP ON CALORIES. You may cut back on training, but don't cut food. "Cyclists in a

Pro **Tip**

"IF YOU HAVE TO OPEN YOUR MOUTH TO GET ENOUGH AIR, YOU'RE GOING TOO HARD FOR A FIVE- TO SIX-HOUR RIDE."—*ALEC DONAHUE, SENIOR ASSOCIATE COACH FOR CYCLE-SMART AND A FORMER PRO ROAD AND MOUNTAIN BIKE RACER* taper will feel just as hungry because of all the hard work they've put in over the previous weeks," says Nancy Clark, RD, a sports dietitian and author of *The Cyclist's Food Guide: Fueling for the Distance*. Eating during the taper phase keeps your tank full. "Expect to gain two to four pounds in the days before the big event," says Clark. "You'll need it—and lose it—during the race." See Clark's sample menu on page 198.

EAT OFTEN, AND REFUEL QUICKLY. To keep your blood sugar from dipping, eat every three hours and refuel within 20 minutes of exercise. "These guidelines are especially important during the seven days before your event because you don't want to give your body any reason to tap into energy stores," says Kim-

ball. "Plus, cells are most receptive to recovering glycogen and muscle immediately after activity."

Eat protein, too—it helps muscle cells repair and recover. "Use a 4:1 carb-to-protein ratio," says Kimball. For example, a cup of low-fat yogurt, with about 30g of carbs and 6g of protein, is an ideal snack.

STAY TRIED AND TRUE. The time for experimenting with new gels, sports drinks and other foods is over. "What worked for you during your early weeks of training is what you need to stick with now," says Kimball. This goes for all food on your daily menu. Avoid eating new foods, foods you eat infrequently, or foods that upset your system.

Eight Things to Take Care of Before the Ride

→ Practice riding in a group—the bigger the better. You'll be less nervous and far safer than if your first ride in a pack is on event day.

→ Prevent "Oh $%&#!" moments on event day by taking your bike to the shop for a check-up at least two weeks before your ride.

→ Find out what food will be available. If you have special dietary needs, bring your own drink powder and food.

→ If your ride falls on a Sunday, pack on Thursday. That gives you time to remember items you might forget if you're rushed.

→ Don't party the night before. Instead, prehydrate, eat a nice meal, put your legs up, rest and go to bed early. Celebrate after the ride.

→ Dress for success. Technical cycling apparel exists for a reason. Don't have the right duds? Your friendly bike dealer will explain what you need. And remember rain gear as well.

→ Be prepared: Pack a little cash and a credit card in a plastic bag.

→ Arrive early. Leave time to sign in, change and hit the restroom.

Experts: Alex Stieda; Richard Fries, professional race announcer; Renee Nicholas, director of the Livestrong Challenge series; Marty Rosen, coordinator, Empire State AIDS Ride

YOUR CENTURY TAPER MENU

FOOD	CALORIES	CARBS
BREAKFAST		
OATMEAL, 1 CUP DRY, COOKED IN	300	55
MILK, 1% FAT, 1 CUP, WITH	200	25
RAISINS, ¼ CUP, AND	130	30
BROWN SUGAR, 1½ TBSP	50	12
APPLE JUICE, 8 OZ	120	30
SNACK		
CANNED PEACHES IN SYRUP, 1 CUP	200	48
LUNCH		
SUB SANDWICH ROLL, 6-INCH (4 OZ)	320	60
LEAN MEAT, 4 OZ	200	—
FRUIT YOGURT, 8 OZ	240	40
GRAPE JUICE, 12 OZ	220	55
SNACK		
FIG NEWTONS, 6	330	65
JELLY BEANS, 15 LARGE	150	38
DINNER		
SPAGHETTI, 2 CUPS COOKED	400	80
PREGO SPAGHETTI SAUCE, 1 CUP	250	40
ITALIAN BREAD, 2 SLICES	150	30
ROOT BEER, 12 OZ	140	38
DAY TOTAL	3,400	646

CHRIS CARMICHAEL'S PERFECT BACK-OF-THE-PACK CENTURY

My colleague Jim was driving to the Santa Fe Century in New Mexico when his car sputtered and died at the side of the highway. He managed to get it going again, but by the time he got to the start, most of the riders were already miles up the road. As a result, Jim, who normally finishes a century in 5½ hours, had the opportunity to ride with slower cyclists and experience a hundred from the back of the pack. Upon his return he pointed out that slower riders and late starters face different challenges than the fast riders and early birds. Learning from his experience, here are tips to help you get through a long day in the saddle.

CARRY EXTRA FOOD. Fast century riders and early birds have a secret they're keeping from the rest of the century-riding crowd: The first people to the rest stops get the best food. Despite organizers' best intentions, by the time the back-of-the-packers arrive, the rest stops are likely to be picked clean of the best choices. Shoving a few more snacks into your pockets at the start or at an early rest stop means carrying a bit more weight, but it'll be well worth it a few hours later when you pull into a rest stop at mile 80 that has only pretzels and orange slices left. Carry cash as well, in case the route passes a convenience store.

STUDY WEATHER.COM. Late starters and riders heading for eight-hour-plus finishing times need to be prepared to ride the majority of their century in the heat of the day. That means consuming more fluids—aim for two-and-a-half to three bottles an hour instead of two—and plenty of foods rich in electrolytes to avoid dehydration. Sports drinks, bars and gels are good ways to ensure you're getting enough sodium; try to have sports drink in one out of every two or three bottles you drink. A later finish also means more sunscreen, which breaks down in intense sun and needs to be reapplied every two hours.

Riding into the afternoon also increases your chances of encountering stronger winds or storms. In many parts of New Mexico and Colorado, for instance, calm mornings typically give way to windy afternoons, with thunderstorms sometime between 1 and 3 p.m. Check weather patterns in the days prior to your event, and ask the locals how the weather normally works this time of year. If a shower rolls in most afternoons, stuff a rain jacket into your pocket—even if there's not a cloud in the sky when you start.

SKIP THE EARLY REST STOP. The first few rest stops on many century rides quickly become overcrowded. If you're a mid-packer, late-starter, or simply don't like crowds, begin the ride with plenty of food and fluid so you can bypass the early rest stop. You shouldn't need to refill bottles for at least 20 miles, and you won't need to stop for calories in the first 30 to 40 miles of the ride. Skipping the first stop can save time and give you a jump on a lot of other riders, which means better food choices and smaller crowds when you pull into the later stops.

The Path to Mid-Ride Nirvana

→The buddy system builds camaraderie and offers a safety net if something goes wrong. Riding by yourself can be disconcerting if you are lost or exhausted.

→Divide the ride into three more or less equal distances. The first segment should feel easy, just spinning along. During the second, you should start to feel your muscles working. If you have any jam left, show it in the last third.

→Don't spend more than 10 minutes at rest stations. It's much harder to ride that last 20 miles if you've been sitting around for a half hour beforehand, stiffening up. Go steady, and keep going.

→A bonk is real. Sometimes that Snickers bar in your pocket will help, but sometimes when you're done, you're done. Trying to push through could lead to injury.

→Aim to drink one bottle of water or sports drink per hour, depending on heat and exertion level. Out of fluids? Ask a rider who has extra. Don't be ashamed. And don't go without; knock on a stranger's door if you have to.

→If you're riding with your kids, make sure they're having a good time. Drop out when it stops being fun. It's not about finishing or accomplishing something grueling or scary, it's about doing something great as a family.

DON'T MAKE UP FOR LOST TIME. Even experienced cyclists make mistakes, and there's a lesson we can all learn from Jim's performance in Santa Fe. Because he got a late start, he tried to make up time by pushing harder than normal in the first few hours. About 30 miles from the finish, he cracked and was passed by a 54-year-old grandmother—a wise woman who rode sensibly, knew her pace and stuck to it. If you're a six-hour century rider, you're not going to become a five-hour finisher just because you started late. Digging too deep catches up with you. The same applies to riders who start out clinging to a group of riders faster than they are; eventually they will have to pay the high cost of keeping up. Stick with the pace you can sustain, and you'll finish strong; ride above your level, and you risk falling apart in the last third of the ride and crawling across the finish line.

CHAPTER 24

Roll Your Own Ride

Once you've experienced the camaraderie of a cause ride, you might decide that you'd like to organize your own. These tips will go a long way toward making things run smoothly—and helping you keep your sanity.

ROUTE IT, THEN RIDE IT. Roads with the least traffic make for a safer experience—and are also key to healthy long-term community relations, particularly if the event includes large numbers of riders. Full road closure for cyclists is rare (and costly), so work with local police in advance to align expectations. Use those officials to help create a plan for covering every intersection with signage, a volunteer marshal or police. Remember that each turn is a potential traffic friction point, as well as a chance for participants to steer off course and get lost.

DELEGATE DUTIES. Managing everything solo will stretch you thinner than worn-out spandex. You'll need a committee that includes expertise in fund-raising, public relations and event planning. For labor, tap friends, family, riding buddies and community organizations. Then divvy up the duties and assign a chief to each: registration, course setup, food wrangling, money management, mechanical support

and so on. The key is having leaders who know their line of work and can quickly train their volunteers.

SPREAD THE WORD. There's no such thing as too much preride buzz. Several months before your event, e-mail a press release to local media. Follow up with additional notices one month and one week before the big day. Call your media targets to make sure they saw the releases and to answer questions. Hook potential sponsors using a brochure that describes your event and the benefits they'll reap from supporting it—their logos on your T-shirts, for example. Companies are often willing to donate products or services—a good way to get postride food. Even better: Recruit someone from the media and a local business owner to be on your planning committee. They'll be conversant and well connected in their fields and will open doors you alone cannot.

MAKE A GOOD FIRST IMPRESSION. The registration and start areas are the face of the event.

Cycling Celeb

"You can draw a parallel between biking and fighting cancer. There are good days, bad days, days you're winning and days you're losing. Cycling is a great metaphor for whatever challenge you're facing." —PATRICK DEMPSEY, ACTOR AND FOUNDER OF THE DEMPSEY CHALLENGE FUND-RAISING RIDE (DEMPSEYCHALLENGE.ORG)

An indoor space, such as a school gym, keeps volunteers comfortable. Make sure there are more than enough portable toilets stationed in the parking lot to accommodate the preride nervous urination that runs rampant among participants: We know of one event that abruptly ended its 20-year run when a cyclist was spotted watering a town selectman's lawn. To keep chaos and confusion in check, set up a PA system for announcements and instructions, and stream music to provide a festive atmosphere.

SCREW UP AND MOVE ON. Even the Tour de France occasionally sends a rider off course. Don't fret about things you can't control, such as rain. Most cycling events run regardless of weather, except in extreme cases. Strive for perfection, but accept that there will be hiccups along the way and learn from them to make next year's event even better.

RIDER **RESOURCES**

Find hundreds of mass rides of various distances—along with races, skills clinics, and bike swaps—at Bicycling.com/event_finder.

Charity evaluator charitynavigator.org helps you find out how much of your hard-earned donation actually goes to fighting disease, saving the baby seals, or whatever cause you've chosen.

Pedaling with a team? Let the world know with custom matching jerseys. The following companies accept small orders:

AK Apparel (akapparel.com)

Atac Sportswear (bikeatac.com)

VIII

Nutrition for Cyclists

WANT TO RIDE BETTER WITHOUT PUTTING MORE hours in the saddle? The solution could be as easy as changing what—or when—you eat. On the following pages, we'll help you choose the fuel you need to ride well without feeling deprived, whether you're training for a century, recovering from a race, or just bellying up to the bar at the office holiday party.

CHAPTER 25

The Foods You Need

As a cyclist, chances are you already know the basics of healthy eating: apples, good; apple fritters, not so much. You probably also know you need carbohydrate and protein—exactly how much of each depends in part on whether you're trying to lose weight (Chapter 26) or training for a big ride (Chapter 22). Beyond that, here's how to round out your daily diet so you can ride—and feel—your best.

CHOOSE HEALTHY FATS

Fat helps us absorb essential antioxidant vitamins such as A, D, E and beta-carotene, as well as vitamin K. Our bodies use it to build nerve tissue and to produce hormones such as estrogen and testosterone. Without enough fat, we'd be sickly and slow. Too much, however, especially the wrong kind, can also make us sickly and slow.

"Endurance athletes, such as cyclists, are very efficient at using the fat stored in their muscles, so keeping those stores stocked is essential for performance and recovery," says Carmichael Training Systems sports nutritionist Kathy Zawadzki, coauthor of *Food for Fitness: Eat Right to Train Right.* But, she says, you don't want to eat so much calorie-rich, fatty food that you start putting it away in other places—like your gut. Also, not all fats are created equal, and when it comes to health and exercise performance the quality of fat you eat is just as, if not more, important than the quantity. Heart-healthy fats keep your cholesterol in check, and may even raise your protective HDL ("good" cholesterol) levels, while others increase "bad" LDL cholesterol and clog your circulatory system.

Your goal: Eat enough of the right kinds of fat to stock your muscles without getting it stuck in your arteries or around your waist. Here they are, from best to worst.

Unsaturated

The fats that come from plants and fish are good. They slide through your arteries without gunking up the works. There are two varieties.

Three Important Nutrients for Cyclists

Cyclists in particular should eat a diet rich in iron, vitamin B12 and folic acid, says University of Utah dietitian Nanna Meyer, RD, who works with cyclists from the recreational to the elite level. These nutrients help form healthy red blood cells, which cyclists need to enhance endurance. To get all three in one meal, Meyer suggests a veggie-and-beef stir-fry. Stir-fry beef is low in fat, and because the dish cooks quickly, few nutrients are lost from the vegetables.

Your number-one choice is monounsaturated fats, or MUFAs. These fats lower LDL cholesterol while raising or maintaining HDL. Evidence shows that they may also improve your fat-burning metabolism and shrink your midsection. In one study, Harvard researchers put 101 men and women on either a low-fat or moderate-fat diet that included about 20 percent of calories from MUFAs. After 18 months, the MUFA-eating group dropped an average of nine pounds and shed nearly 3 inches from their waists, compared with the low-fat group, which gained an average of six pounds and added nearly an inch around their middles. This is important because high levels of belly fat, even in people who are otherwise a healthy weight, have been linked to a host of diseases including heart disease, diabetes and even Alzheimer's. Great sources of MUFAs include nuts, avocados, olive and canola oils, and dark chocolate.

Polyunsaturated fats are also generally healthy, but they slightly lower HDL levels, so they're considered a small step down. Prime sources: seeds, most vegetable oils (corn, sunflower, soy) and fatty fish such as salmon. Omega fatty acids (omega-3 and omega-6) fall into this category. Most health experts agree that we get too much omega-6 (mostly from vegetable oils) and not enough omega-3 (fish and flaxseed), which fights the inflammation that omega-6 creates. So go easy on foods from the fryer and eat more from the sea. Choose cold-water fish known to contain less mercury, such as Alaska wild salmon, herring and sardines.

Saturated

These fats are less healthy, but not all bad. Mainly animal fats, they're found in meats and dairy foods such as burgers, butter, lard and cheese. (Coconut oil is saturated, too, but scientists say for unknown reasons it acts more like an unsaturated fat in your body.) Some saturated fatty acids may actually improve your cholesterol profile, but on the whole they tend to raise your heart-disease risk, so it's best to keep your consumption of them in check.

Trans Fats

Evil. Forget the "there are no bad foods" BS and get these out of your diet. Trans fats occur in very small amounts in nature (mostly in animal foods), but for the most part are a product of food processing that solidifies vegetable oils. Trans fats are found in fried, processed and packaged foods such as crackers, cookies and chips, as well as in shortening and margarine, and have been linked to heart disease. Read your labels and steer clear of buying or eating foods that contain trans fats. Note: A food can contain up to half a gram of trans fat and still be labeled as containing zero. To know if you're about to buy or eat something evil, look for the words "hydrogenated" or "partially hydrogenated" on the ingredient list. And as a general rule, avoid eating these foods as much as possible.

Fishing for Fatty Acids

There are some good omega-3-fortified foods (like grass-fed beef) and other natural sources. But if you want to increase your intake of omega-3 fatty acids, you'd better learn to love fish. Here's how some common food sources stack up. Leslie Bonci, MPH, RD, director of sports nutrition at the University of Pittsburgh Medical Center, recommends aiming for 1,000 to 2,000 milligrams (mg) of omega-3 a day.

FOOD	OMEGA-3S
SALMON	1,830MG
ANCHOVIES	1,750MG
TUNA	1,280MG
MACKEREL	1,020MG
LEAN BEEF (3 OZ, GRASS FED)	136MG
EGGS (2, OMEGA-3 FORTIFIED)	114MG

EAT YOUR IBUPROFEN: 3 FOODS THAT FIGHT INFLAMMATION

BLACK OR GREEN TEA. Sports scientists at Rutgers University found that a nine-day supplement of black-tea extract decreased delayed-onset muscle soreness after cycling intervals.

Recharge: "Add four bags of decaffeinated tea to 32 ounces of cold water, and steep in the refrigerator overnight," suggests Barbara Lewin, RD, a sports nutritionist who owns Sports-Nutritionist.com. Drink tea in place of water before, during and after rides.

SOYBEANS AND TOFU. Research published in *The Nutrition Journal* found that both soy and whey proteins build lean muscle mass, but soy protein also prevents exercise-induced inflammation. You don't want to consume excess amounts; some researchers think superhigh soy intake might trigger some cancers. But scientists agree that two to three servings—about 25 grams (g)—of soy foods, such as soy milk, soy burgers and tofu, are safe.

Recharge: "Chocolate soy milk makes an excellent recovery drink," says Lewin. Also, keep soy nuts in the car or at the office for a great protein-rich snack.

CHERRIES AND BERRIES. In a study at the University of Vermont, students who were given 12 ounces of tart cherry juice before and after strenuous exercises suffered only a four percent reduction in muscle strength the next day compared with a 22 percent loss found in subjects given a placebo. "Antioxidants and anti-inflammatory molecules in tart cherries suppress and treat the micro-tears in muscles," says Declan Connolly, PhD. These molecules are also found in blackberries, raspberries and strawberries.

Recharge: Stock up on frozen berries, and add them to smoothies, yogurt and cereal. Or defrost a few in the microwave for a sweet postride snack.

FILL UP WITH FIBER

Fiber is the indigestible part of plants: It travels through the digestive system intact and flushes out the plumbing "like nature's scrub brush," says Amy Jamieson-Petonic, RD, director of wellness coaching at the Cleveland Clinic and a spokesperson for the American Dietetic Association. Because fiber swells in the stomach and intestinal tract, it helps you feel fuller longer, so you eat less: Tufts University researchers found that adding 14g of fiber a day to their diets helped people eat about 10 percent fewer calories and lose five pounds over four months. But beyond keeping you regular, fiber-rich fruits and vegetables often contain vitamins and minerals that cyclists need for energy and recovery. By targeting fiber, you're indirectly upping your nutrient density, Jamieson-Petonic says. "Plus, research indicates that a high-fiber diet reduces your risk for cardiovascular disease, cancer and diabetes," she says.

But don't overdo it. Experts recommend 25 to 38g of fiber per day—any more and you'll likely experience gastrointestinal distress. To avoid that, Jamieson-Petonic recommends cyclists gradually increase their fiber intake while also increasing water consumption. "Fiber draws water from the intestinal lining, so you'll need additional fluids to help move things along," she says.

There's also the question of timing. Fiber's filling properties are great—except when you're sprinting or cranking up a hill. That's when you want ready fuel, not bulk that cuts down on how fast you can tap into food's energy. "Fiber slows digestion and the release of sugar into the system," says Coni Francis, RD, senior manager for scientific and government affairs at GTC Nutrition. That's why high-fiber foods tend to score low on the glycemic index (GI).

So low-GI foods that are high in fiber (like beans, apples and whole grains) aren't a smart fuel choice during your ride. It's also best to limit fiber right afterward, when recovering muscles require the immediate replenishment of high-GI foods. Instead, eat fiber-rich carbohydrates (such as rolled oats or brown rice) before your workout: They'll provide sustained energy and keep you from bonking. And enjoy fiber-rich fruits and vegetables as snacks and additions to regular meals.

CHOOSE A RAINBOW OF FRUITS AND VEGETABLES

A plate of brown chow spells trouble if you're aiming for optimum nutrition. That's because colorful foods deliver concentrated amounts of the vitamins, minerals and antioxidants cyclists need for peak performance: "The more colors in a meal, the more nutritious it is," says Amy Jamieson-Petonic, RD.

Brown foods include carbohydrate and protein, which are essential for fueling workouts and building muscle. But colorful foods contain phytochemicals—compounds credited with health benefits that range from fighting inflammation to preventing cancer. Some phytochemicals, known as antioxidants, have particular value for cyclists: Because exercise produces free radicals that cause oxidative damage to muscle cells, "cyclists want to make sure they're consuming antioxidant-rich fruits and vegetables that help repair those cells," explains Jamieson-Petonic.

Go easy on colorful foods just before a big ride or race, advises registered dietitian Shawn Dolan, PhD. They tend to be high in fiber, which can cause stomach upset during exercise. But in between workouts, go crazy with color.

Red

Red foods such as tomatoes, watermelon and pink grapefruit contain lycopene, which may help protect the skin from the sun's damaging UV rays. Red cherries contain compounds called anthocyanins that appear to ease postexercise pain and inflammation: One study published in the *British Journal of Sports Medicine* concluded that drinking cherry juice preserved muscle strength and reduced inflammation after workouts.

Orange and Yellow

Orange and yellow foods such as carrots, sweet potatoes and yellow peppers get their color from carotenoids, compounds that boost the immune system. "Longer-duration training can compromise the immune system," says Dolan, so eat yellows and oranges to fend off the colds and respiratory infections that can plague endurance cyclists. Carotenoids are also converted into nutrients such as vitamin A, which helps prevent anemia by helping the body absorb iron.

Green

"Athletes tend to eat more green than other colors," says Dolan. That's a good habit: Broccoli and kale rank among the world's most nutritious foods, and spinach and chard are high in folate, a B vitamin that helps build the red blood cells required to deliver oxygen to exercising muscles. Because the body can't store folate in large amounts, it's smart to eat greens often. By doing so, you'll also enjoy impressive amounts of vitamins A, C and K, plus minerals such as calcium, potassium and magnesium, which play a vital role in muscle contraction.

Blue and Violet

Blueberries, beets, blackberries and red cabbage derive their rich colors from anthocyanidins, anti-inflammatory compounds that promote healthy circulation. Swirl blues and purples into a smoothie for a postride recovery drink that's loaded with muscle-repairing

antioxidants. Top salads with red onions, which contain a potent antioxidant called quercetin that boosts alertness much like caffeine does.

Pro **Tip**

"EAT THINGS THAT HAVE BEEN AROUND FOR 10,000 YEARS, BECAUSE YOUR BODY KNOWS WHAT TO DO WITH THEM OR YOU WOULDN'T STILL BE IN THE GENE POOL."—*JOHN STAMSTAD, HOLDER OF THE ULTRA-MARATHON CYCLING ASSOCIATION 24 HOUR OFF-ROAD WORLD RECORD OF 352 MILES*

BUT EAT YOUR PALE VEGGIES, TOO

If broccoli and spinach are the rock stars of the vegetable world, then corn and celery are the stagehands, working hard outside the limelight. For years we've dismissed these pale staples as nutritionally barren, focusing our attention on their brighter, more colorful kin. Today we know better.

"We've done a disservice to a lot of common vegetables," says Liz Applegate, PhD. "All vegetables have nutritional value. And every vegetable contains potent chemicals that help it survive. When you eat them, you get those chemicals. We are always discovering new phytochemicals that may fight cancer and heart disease, so it's wise to eat a large variety of vegetables every day." Here are seven underrated foods that do much more than fill space in the salad bowl.

Iceberg Lettuce

It's always been: An inexpensive way for restaurants to offer a salad with every meal.

It's also: A source of vitamin K (one serving provides up to 20 percent of your daily needs), which helps your body build new bone. In a study of women ages 38 to 74, researchers found that those who ate lettuce once or twice a day had a 45 percent lower risk of hip fracture than peers who ate lettuce one or fewer times per week.

Mushroom (white button)

It's always been: A fungus that doubles as a pizza topping and smothers a New York strip.

It's also: A good source of B vitamins that help convert food into energy. Mushrooms are also rich in the antioxidant selenium, and contain potent anti-tumor compounds called triterpenoids. Little wonder mushrooms have long been revered for their medicinal properties.

Radish

It's always been: A spicy garnish that gets thrown out with the parsley and kale.

It's also: Part of the cruciferous vegetable family, which means it contains cancer-protective properties. It's also an excellent source of vitamin C and heart-healthy potassium and folate, plus the trace mineral molybdenum, which assists energy production in the cells.

Cucumber

It's always been: A refreshing addition to a summer salad and a cool treat for tired eyes.

It's also: A good source of caffeic acid, which helps soothe skin irritation, and silica, an essential building block of connective tissue like muscle, tendons and ligaments, and bone. The flesh contains vitamin C, and the skin is rich in potassium and magnesium.

Onion

It's always been: An ingredient that turns up the flavor volume in any dish it's added to.

It's also: "One of the richest sources of flavonoids in the human diet," according to researchers at Cornell University. Flavonoids are plant compounds that fight bacteria, viruses and inflammation, and help reduce the risk of heart disease, cancer and diabetes.

Celery

It's always been: A low-calorie weight-loss standby and a stick that holds peanut butter.

It's also: A good source of energy-converting B vitamins such as riboflavin, B6 and pantothenic acid, as well as bone-building calcium and magnesium. It's also a good source of fiber, antioxidants, vitamins A and C, folate, potassium and blood-and-bone-preserving vitamin K.

Corn

It's always been: A buttery, salty backyard BBQ favorite and a reason to buy cob holders.

It's also: Rich in fiber as well as B vitamins thiamin and folate. Maybe more important, each kernel is brimming with ferulic acid, a known cancer-fighting phytochemical. Research shows the longer you cook it, the more potent it becomes. So fire up the coals and let it roast.

FIND A NEW FAVORITE FRUIT

Apples and oranges have held down major real estate in our produce aisles for decades. But there's a whole world of fruit out there—and some come with hype involving their health benefits. But are these fruits better than apples and oranges? "In some cases, these so-called super-fruits are higher in nutrients," says Molly Kimball, RD, sports nutritionist at Ochsner's Elmwood Fitness Center, in New Orleans. But the secret to benefiting from fruits, says Kimball, is to eat a rich variety. Here are some of the rising stars in the fruit bowl.

ACAI. A dark purple Brazilian berry rich in essential fatty acids and fiber, the fruit also boasts powerful antioxidants such as anthocyanins and flavonoids, which protect your cells from damage and may reduce the risk of heart disease and cancer.

ACEROLA. This sweet fruit is apple-like in flavor and rich in vitamin C. It contains as much immunity-boosting vitamin A as a similar-size serving of carrots.

BLOOD ORANGE. The deep color of this sweet, tart orange comes from anthocyanin, an antioxidant that's been shown to help fight cancer, inflammation and diabetes.

CHERIMOYA. Mark Twain once characterized this complex tropical fruit as "deliciousness itself." It can be sliced or scooped like an avocado and has a similar velvety texture. One fruit provides 7g of protein and 15 percent of your daily value of iron.

GOJI BERRY. Most commonly found in dried form, this Asian fruit has been used in traditional medicine for years to enhance health and longevity. It packs a massive nutritional punch, including beta-carotene, vitamin C, iron, protein, trace minerals and B vitamins.

GUAVA. According to USDA researchers, this fruit may be the highest of them all in antioxidants. One cup delivers 8,500 micrograms of cancer-fighting lycopene and serves up as many of the free-radical fighters as one serving of broccoli.

PAPAYA. Rich in immunity-building vitamin A and papain, an enzyme that aids digestion, papaya is a delicious addition to salads and stir-fries.

PASSION FRUIT. This egg-shaped, intensely sweet tropical fruit is rich in cancer-fighting carotenoids and polyphenols. It also delivers an appetite-satisfying 12g of fiber per fruit.

POMEGRANATE. The tangy seeds of this fruit are rich in polyphenols, plant chemicals that fight inflammation and may fend off cancer and heart disease.

PRICKLY PEAR. The pulp of this cactus fruit is mild and sweet (reminiscent of watermelon), rich in potassium, and delivers 10 percent of your daily calcium requirement in one cup.

STAR FRUIT. Each fruit contains 4g of fiber and fewer than 40 calories, and is rich in potassium and vitamin C.

Women and Iron

Female riders should remember to get enough iron, especially if your training program represents a significant increase in training load. A premenopausal woman's daily requirement for iron is 18mg, more than double that of a man's, and balloons to 33mg for premenopausal vegetarian women. Iron is a crucial component of oxygen-carrying hemoglobin, and fortunately it's easy to get without resorting to supplements. Foods rich in iron include:

Tofu: 13mg in ½ cup of firm style

Fortified breakfast cereals: 5 to 16mg in a ¾-cup serving, depending on the brand

Beans: 5 to 7mg per cup, depending on the bean

Lean beef: roughly 1mg per ounce

Vitamin C increases iron absorption, while tea hinders it. Fish and white-meat poultry are lower in iron, but shellfish, especially clams, are good sources.

UGLI FRUIT. The lumpy, bumpy exterior of this milder-tasting cousin of the grapefruit gives this food its name. It's rich in vitamins C and A as well as potassium, and is low in calories.

SPICE UP YOUR LIFE

Spices make up an all-natural arsenal that scientists say can fight infection, ease tummy troubles and keep you rolling strong right through cycling season.

"Spices are one of the fastest-growing areas of research in nutrition as we realize the tremendous health benefits they provide," says sports nutritionist James Russell Stevens, RD, visiting assistant professor of nutrition at Metropolitan State College of Denver. The following flavor enhancers are a few of his favorites.

PEPPERMINT. This herb may minimize bronchial spasms that lead to coughing and help open clogged sinuses and clear respiratory passages. As a bonus, it also soothes indigestion. Because the vapors provide much of the healing effect, add peppermint to hot beverages such as tea and cocoa.

WASABI. There's a reason this green paste is served with raw-fish dishes such as sushi. It's a potent antimicrobial, so it's like Raid for your food—it kills bugs dead, including H. pylori, a bacteria that's been linked to stomach ulcers.

CINNAMON. Government testing suggests that a teaspoon of cinnamon a day may lower blood sugar, triglycerides (dangerous blood fats) and the "bad" LDL cholesterol that gunks up your arteries. Sprinkle it on oatmeal, bake it into cookies and add it to hot drinks such as cocoa and mulled cider.

TURMERIC. A super free-radical fighter, this member of the ginger family has antioxidant powers that some believe may lower the risk for certain cancers. Because stress, alcohol, tobacco smoke and even strenuous exercise generate free radicals, you need all the protection you can get. Use it to turn up the heat in curries, stews and soups.

FENNEL. The aromatic seeds of the fennel plant are Mother Nature's Gas-X, offering relief from bloating, cramping and other GI unpleasantries. You can chew them on their own—they taste like licorice—or toast them in a dry pan on the stovetop and grind them up as a seasoning for meat and poultry dishes.

GINGER. A classic for quelling nausea and calming a busy tummy, ginger also stimulates immunity. Slice a piece of gingerroot into slivers and add them to green tea. Let it steep for five minutes for an antioxidant-rich, immunity-boosting brew. Ginger also livens up stir-fries and adds zing to beans and rice dishes.

GET JUICED WITH ELECTROLYTES

If carbohydrate is your body's fuel, electrolytes are the spark plugs, motor oil and engine coolant. These minerals, such as sodium and potassium, form electrically charged particles in the body that work together to regulate nerve transmission, muscle contraction and fluid balance. When their levels run low, your internal dash lights up with warning signals in the form of fatigue, cramping, nausea and a cadence that slows to a crawl.

"Whenever you sweat, you lose electrolytes," says Cindy Dallow, PhD, RD, of Partners in Nutrition, in Loveland, Colorado. When it's hot, you easily sweat out two pounds an hour, so it's important to replenish more than just fluid. Here's how to stock up to stay strong.

SODIUM. Salt is two electrolytes, sodium and chlorine, bound together. Sodium is the most talked about because of the volume lost during exercise—450mg, or 20 percent of the recommended daily value, per pound of sweat—but both minerals are needed to maintain fluid balance inside the cells. **Replenish Rx:** Most sports drinks have 120 to 200mg per bottle, enough for most cyclists, says Dallow. If you end rides with salt crust on your jersey or will be out all day, take a drink such as Gatorade Endurance or PowerBar Endurance with twice the sodium of a typical drink. "If you're on an easy ride with food available, there's no need to take a sodium-heavy drink," Dallow says.

POTASSIUM. Potassium helps maintain the body's water balance and regulates sodium levels. Deficiency is very uncommon, but can leave you with a racing heart rate and muscle weakness. **Replenish Rx:** Most sports drinks provide plenty, and too much can harm your heart, so doctors caution against supplementing beyond that.

CALCIUM. It builds bone, but calcium also aids muscle contraction and helps convert stored fuel into energy. You should get at least 1,000mg a day, especially if you put in big miles: When your body doesn't have enough, it steals the mineral from your skeleton. During long, intense efforts, you blow through 150 to 300mg per hour. **Replenish Rx:** Replacing calcium on

Drink Up

Electrolyte beverages replenish key minerals lost during exercise, as sports drinks do, but they supply few if any calories. If you're skipping the sports drink but still want a drink with electrolyte-boosting benefits, these may hit the spot.

Elete. Electro-boost: sodium, 125mg; potassium, 130mg; magnesium, 45mg

Made from seawater concentrates, these drops provide no calcium. Add to water as recommended. eletewater.com

Hammer Nutrition Endurolytes Powder. Electro-boost: sodium, 40mg; potassium, 25mg; calcium, 50mg; magnesium, 25mg

Add a scoop (or more) to your bottle as needed. Available as capsules, too. hammernutrition.com

Nuun. Electro-boost: sodium, 360mg; potassium, 100mg; calcium, 12.5mg; magnesium, 25mg

Drop a tablet into your bottle and go. In six flavors; the Kona cola one has caffeine. nuun.com

---

the bike is less vital than getting it in your daily diet. Just one cup of yogurt will get you nearly a third of the way to the recommended daily value.

MAGNESIUM. Working with calcium to enable smooth muscle contraction, magnesium also lends a hand to energy production. You lose only 10mg per pound of sweat, more during exercise.

Replenish Rx: Magnesium is easy to get in your daily diet. Nuts, leafy greens and whole grains are great sources.

HYDRATE PROPERLY

Cyclists, like all athletes, need plenty of liquids. But beyond that basic tenet, things get murky fast—and for years, riders have heard conflicting reports about what, when and how much to drink. We tapped our best resources, from the latest research to sports nutrition expert Monique Ryan, RD, author of *Sports Nutrition*

for Endurance Athletes, to separate the facts from the fiction.

HYPE: REPLACE EVERY LOST OUNCE. For years cyclists have been told to drink enough on the bike so they weigh the same after the ride as they did beforehand. The truth is, your body can't absorb fluids as fast as it loses them, and not every ounce of weight is lost through sweat anyway.

TRUTH: KEEP UP WITH SWEAT LOSS—MOSTLY. Replace about 75 percent of lost sweat during a long ride. "To do that, you need to know your sweat rate," says Ryan, who recently coached a heavy-sweating triathlete who routinely lost 40 ounces of fluid an hour. To determine your sweat rate, weigh yourself before and after a short ride. "An hour ride is a good indicator of what you're losing through sweat alone," Ryan says.

HYPE: OVERFLOW BEFOREHAND. Guzzling gallons of fluids before a ride or race will do little more than send you searching for rest stops.

TRUTH: TOP OFF AS YOU GO. Sip a 16-ounce sports drink an hour or two before you saddle up. That's enough time for your body to absorb what it needs and eliminate what it doesn't. Then take in about six to eight ounces (two to three gulps) every 15 to 20 minutes while you ride.

HYPE: CAFFEINE WILL DEHYDRATE YOU. Caffeine has long been demonized as a diuretic. On paper, that means it should lead to dehydration and heat stress, especially when you consider that it also raises your heart rate and increases your metabolism.

TRUTH: CAFFEINE IMPROVES CARB BURNING. A review of ongoing research recently revealed that caffeinated drinks don't make you pee that much more than equal amounts of beverages without the buzz. The stimulant also doesn't worsen the effects of summertime heat. In fact, caffeine makes you feel better. Numerous studies have shown that it lowers your rate of perceived exertion while improving your strength, endurance and mental performance. Even better, researchers from the University of Birmingham, in England, found that riders who drank a caffeinated sports beverage burned the drink's carbs 26 percent faster than those who consumed a noncaffeinated sports drink, likely because caffeine speeds glucose absorption in the intestine.

HYPE: YOU NEED MORE PROTEIN. Initially, carbohydrates were the essential building blocks of the sports beverage. Then protein muscled its way onto the scene, after early studies showed that carb-protein blends seemed to shoot into the bloodstream and enhance endurance cycling performance better than carb-only beverages.

TRUTH: YOU NEED A LITTLE PROTEIN . . . MAYBE. Recent research on 10 trained cyclists performing an 80-K trial showed that riders drinking carb-only beverages did just as well as those drinking carb-protein beverages, and both groups did better than those consuming flavored water. However, the International Society of Sports Nutrition recently reported that taking in branched-chain amino acids (BCAAs) during vigorous aerobic exercise can decrease muscle damage and depletion. "If you're on a long ride where you're also eating, you'll be taking in protein already," says Ryan, "so it's likely not necessary to also have it in your drink."

HYPE: HYDRATION DURING EXERCISE IS THE BE-ALL AND END-ALL. Big beverage companies would have you grabbing your sports drink during every ride, no matter how long or short the effort, lest you suffer the ill effects of dehydration.

TRUTH: DRINKING EVERY DAY IS ESSENTIAL. "Your first priority should be staying on top of your daily hydration," says Ryan. Research on gym-goers found that nearly half began their workouts in a dehydrated state. "Many people don't consume enough fluids during the day," Ryan says. "If you hydrate properly on a regular basis, you won't need to worry as much about getting dehydrated during a typical moderate ride." The old eight-glasses-a-day dictum is a good guidepost.

SPEAKING OF DRINKING. . .

We're still waiting for the study that says booze makes us better bicyclists. Until then, it's best to stick to the usual advice: If you're going to drink alcohol, enjoy antioxidant-rich red wine, and skip the fat-laden spiked eggnog. But not all drinks between those bookends are equally good choices. Here's how to minimize diet damage at your next celebration.

The Office Party

Drink: Tom Collins

Gin, club soda, lemon juice and a pinch of sugar rack up only 120 calories for a half pint (eight ounces). The ally for such drinks is sparkling water, which you can add to taste without offending the drink—make a tall glass for long, slow sipping.

Skip: Margarita

Often delivered in supersized portions with three drinks' worth of alcohol, some of the 12-ounce vats served at restaurants tally more than 700 calories. We're not sure what the nutritional value of the tequila worm is, but we doubt it's good.

Pro Tip

"IF YOU DRINK ALCOHOL WHILE YOU'RE IN TRAINING, CONSUME 16 OUNCES OF WATER FOR EVERY ALCOHOLIC DRINK YOU HAVE." —*CHRIS CARMICHAEL*

Postride Football Game

Drink: Guinness Draught

It's surprising but true: The stout variety—not the extra stout—of this classic, dark Irish brew packs only 125 calories for 12 ounces. That's barely more than pale, flavorless 100-calorie light beers.

Skip: Molson XXX

At 7.3 percent alcohol, a 12-ounce bottle packs 213 calories. With weak, bland malts and hops, it's little more than a conduit for delivering a buzz. Call it Canada's Colt 45.

Holiday Brunch

Drink: Bloody Mary

This classic vodka mixture gets a thumbs-up for tomato juice, which packs in vitamins A, C and B6, and has only one-third the calories of orange or pineapple juice, making Mary quite svelte at 120 calories for a regular five-ounce cocktail.

Skip: Sex on the Beach

Not only does this vodka mixer include other calorie-rich booze like schnapps and rum, but sometimes fat- and cholesterol-laden heavy cream is also used. Count on a minimum of 300 calories for a 4-ounce cocktail.

Happy Hour

Drink: Mojito

With rum, mint, a little sugar, a lot of lime juice and fizzy water, it's a simple drink that's not loaded with cloying syrups. Even an eight-ounce glass has only 210 calories. Bonus for literary types: The mojito was enjoyed by Ernest Hemingway, a lover of bicycles.

Skip: Mai Tai

The drink usually includes two kinds of rum (light and dark) and curaçao liqueur, plus orgeat syrup (almonds, sugar and orange-flower water). A four-and-a-half-ounce drink has more than 300 calories, with the only hint of goodness coming from a squeeze of lime juice.

CHAPTER 26

The Cyclist's Guide to Weight Loss

It's no secret that losing weight can help your cycling—improving your power-to-weight ratio will make you ride faster and climb better. However, athletes who want to drop pounds must do so carefully: Cut too many calories too quickly, and you could be losing muscle as well as fat, not to mention depriving your body of the nutrients it needs to perform at its best. But with this advice from Bicycling's *weight-loss experts, you won't just get lean. You'll also be able to ride longer on less food—and never bonk.*

THE SEVEN BIGGEST WEIGHT LOSS MYTHS

Cyclists typically turn to the same trusty old sources for fuel. (Linguini, anyone?) But the latest research is clear: Not all carbs and fat are created equal. Here, Selene Yeager presents a surprising new approach to losing weight and keeping it off—and riding longer and stronger than ever.

One of the long-enduring traditions at bike events of all stripes is the pasta dinner the evening before the big ride. After all, who doesn't believe in the hearty, turbo-fueling quality of a whopping plate of spaghetti with tomato sauce? As it turns out, the nonbelievers include a number of highly informed people, including physiologist Allen Lim, PhD, the brains behind

much of Team RadioShack's training and race preparation. "There's nothing nutritious about that," Lim says. In fact, when Lim worked with the Garmin-Slipstream team from 2007 through 2009, he eliminated all processed wheat from the team's diet, and at races replaced traditional starchy foods with balanced, whole-food fuel such as rice cakes made with eggs, olive oil, prosciutto and liquid amino acids. If this creates the impression that Lim knows something you don't, well, that's probably true. His job is to make sure that, unlike the rest of us, his riders don't blithely adhere to old, counterproductive eating habits—habits that can lead to unnecessary weight fluctuation and diminished performance. Here's the good news. We've tapped into this new school of food science led by the likes of Lim to correct popular misconceptions about food, particularly about carbs and fat. Proponents of this new approach believe, for example, that a diet heavy in starch causes your body to burn sugar instead of fat, so you bonk more easily, often eat too much and end up overweight rather than properly fueled. Even coach Joe Friel, who relentlessly advocated carbohydrates in his Training Bible series of books, has done a 180, turning his back on starches and relying instead on vegetables, fruits and lean meats as fuel. Consider this our effort to correct myths and misconceptions you've been exposed to over the years.

Fallacy #1

A CALORIE IS A CALORIE. This might be the biggest weight-loss misunderstanding in existence. For years we've been told that weight loss is a simple calories-in, calories-out equation, and 3,500 excess calories will put on a pound whether they come from soybeans or banana cream pie. That's simply not true.

"There are three key types of calories: carbohydrate, protein and fat," says sports nutritionist Cynthia Sass, MPH, RD, CSSD, creator and coauthor of *The Flat Belly Diet* (published by Rodale, *Bicycling's* parent company and the publisher of this book). "They're as different as gasoline, motor oil and brake fluid in terms of the roles they play in keeping your body operating optimally." Sass says that many of her clients might eat the perfect number of calories, but they have cut their fat intake too much. So

the jobs that fat does, such as repairing cell membranes and optimizing hormones, go undone, and the surplus carbs are stored as fat. By correcting her clients' balance of carbs, protein and fat without changing their calorie intake, she says, she has helped them lose weight, improve their immune systems, gain muscle and boost energy.

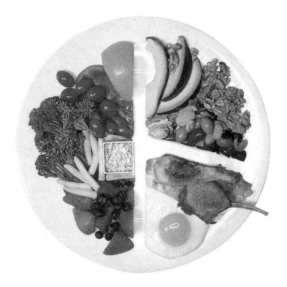

The Get-Lean Fix: Eat a representative of each macronutrient group at every meal. Sass recommends getting 50 to 55 percent of your calories from carbs (fill half your plate with vegetables, fruits and some whole grains), 25 to 30 percent from fats (olive oil, avocado and so on), and 15 to 20 percent from protein (lean meats, fish, eggs and poultry). "Just be sure to skew your preworkout meals or snacks to be heavier in carbs and lower in fat and protein to fuel up properly and avoid cramps," says Sass.

Fallacy #2

STARCHES ARE SENSIBLE FUEL. At some point, starch became synonymous with carbohydrate. While pasta and bagels are carbohydrates, and you do need carbs for fuel, they're often not the best sources, especially if you're trying to keep weight off. Starchy carbs are easy to overeat, and any surplus goes to your fat stores. "Your brain operates on sugar, and when you eat bagels or potatoes, your body turns them into sugar and delivers them to your cells quickly, which makes your brain happy and leaves you wanting more," says Friel. So in this case, you shouldn't listen to your body.

Fruits and vegetables, by contrast, are rich in carbs but often lower in calories and also digest more slowly. You're less likely to plow through so many berries and carrots that you end up with more fuel than you need. As a bonus, plant foods are loaded with vitamins, minerals and immunity-boosting phytonutrients that make you healthier and stronger, so you can ride better and burn more calories.

The Get-Lean Fix: Choose carbs wisely. Eat starchy, quick-digesting carbs only during and right before and after training rides or races, when it's important to get food that can be quickly digested and converted to fuel. Otherwise, get your carbs from fruits and vegetables.

How much is enough? If you're eating considerably more than Sass's recommended 50 to 55 percent, especially from starchy sources, then you risk changing your metabolism, says Friel. "When I see someone who has started eating lots of starch," he says, "they not only have

> ## Pro **Tip**
>
> "WHEN YOU WEIGH LESS, YOU NEED FEWER CALORIES TO MAINTAIN THAT WEIGHT. IT'S A CRUEL REWARD."—*JAMES RUSSELL STEVENS, NUTRITIONIST AT THE METROPOLITAN STATE COLLEGE OF DENVER*

gained fat, they've also changed their metabolism from fat-burning to sugar-burning." It doesn't happen over one plate of pasta, but the body is adaptable. "Over the course of a few months," Friel says, "it will switch over to burn whatever you're feeding it most."

When possible, pair your carbs with some protein. Lean meats, nut butters, fish and eggs slow digestion, so you feel full sooner, get a steadier supply of energy from your meals and stay full longer. The amino acids in protein also help repair, build and maintain muscle tissue.

It's no coincidence that Americans got heavier as fat consumption went down. For years, the government preached low-fat, carb-heavy diets. "This wasn't only misguided; it was flat-out wrong," Friel says.

Fallacy #3

ALL FAT MAKES YOU FAT. As your body becomes more conditioned, you become a better fat burner. You need ample amounts of healthy fat, which, contrary to widely held belief, won't make you fat. In fact, starchy foods turn to stored fat far more quickly. What's more, evidence is stacking up that healthy unsaturated fats are essential for firing up your fat-burning metabolism. In a study of 101 men and women, Harvard researchers put half the group on a low-fat diet and half on a diet that included about 20 percent of calories from monounsaturated fatty acids (MUFAs). After 18 months, the MUFA-eating group had dropped 11 pounds; its low-fat-eating peers had shed only six. Fat is also slower to digest than carbs, so it helps you stay hunger-free longer.

Fat will help you ride longer so you can burn more calories, says Friel. Research shows that athletes who get about 50-plus percent of their diet from fat produce better average times to exhaustion in exercise tests than those eating typical low-fat, high-carb diets.

The Get-Lean Fix: Add healthy fats to every meal. Sass recommends getting about 20 percent of your calories from MUFAs, or about 55g per day at 2,500 calories, which is what most cyclists eat as training ramps up. "Because most athletes don't have time to count fat grams, the simpler message is: Include small portions of good fats, like almonds, avocado and olive oil, with all meals and snacks," she says. Try nuts and seeds, olive-based tapenades and even the occasional chunk of dark chocolate. Some healthy portions to shoot for:

→**Nuts and seeds.** Everything from pecans to pine nuts, almond butter to tahini. A serving size is 2 tablespoons.

→**Olives**. Black, green, mixed or blended in a spreadable tapenade. A serving is 10 large olives or 2 tablespoons of spread.

→**Oils**. Canola, flaxseed, peanut, safflower, walnut, sunflower, sesame or olive. Cook with them; drizzle them; eat them in pesto. One serving is 1 tablespoon.

→**Avocado.** As guacamole or just slice and serve. One-quarter cup equals one serving.

→**Dark chocolate.** Go for one-quarter cup of dark or semisweet, or about 2 ounces.

Fallacy #4

FOOD COMES FROM A BOX. Many cyclists who think they're eating healthfully often consume far more sugar and sodium than they realize because they eat so much pasta, cereals, energy bars and other processed foods. "The vast majority of grocery-store foods are packaged junk," says sports nutritionist and exercise physiologist Tavis Piattoly, RD, LD, of Elmwood Fitness Center, in New Orleans. Some items also contain trans fats—the kinds of fats you want to avoid. The sugar is also troublesome for weight loss because it causes the body to step up its production of insulin, which in turn blocks hormones that control appetite. As a result, the food you eat is quickly stored as fat—and still, you're always hungry.

The Get-Lean Fix: Eat mostly whole foods that are part of an animal or plant, Piattoly says. Fill most of your cart with foods from the grocery store's perimeter first; that's where the fresh produce, meats, fish and other whole foods are found. Then go down the center aisles to fill in the rest. That should reflect the proportion of processed foods you include in your diet.

Fallacy #5

SKIPPING BREAKFAST IS FINE IF YOU NEED TO DROP A FEW POUNDS. Eat breakfast. That bit of essential advice is food gospel. Still, according to a survey by the International Food Information Council Foundation, fewer than half of us eat a morning meal.

Breakfast is the key that starts your fat-burning metabolism. Without it, you go into an energy deficit that not only leaves you ravenous (and more likely to overeat) later, but also suppresses your calorie-burning furnace, so what you do eat is more likely to go into storage. Research shows that people who skip breakfast are 4½ times more likely to be overweight than those who don't. "It's one of the biggest fueling mistakes almost everyone makes," says Piattoly.

The Get-Lean Fix: Because you have a whole day of activity—usually including a ride—ahead of you, try to eat about 25 percent of your daily calories at your morning meal. That meal should include protein, healthy fat and fiber-rich carbs like fruit. A British study found that exercisers who ate a breakfast high in fiber burned twice as much fat during workouts later in the day as those who ate less fibrous foods.

For a power breakfast that'll sustain you well into the day, try two eggs any style; half a cup of whole oats, cooked; 1 cup of yogurt; a cup of mixed berries; coffee; and orange juice.

SMART SWAPS

INSTEAD OF:	GO FOR:
CREAM CHEESE	AVOCADO SPREAD
PASTA	SWEET POTATO
SALMON SALAD ON BREAD	SALMON SALAD IN A ROMAINE LETTUCE WRAP
MAYO	PESTO
DOUGHNUT	DARK CHOCOLATE
CHIPS AND PRETZELS	MIXED NUTS AND DRIED FRUIT
RISOTTO	MIXED SAUTÉED VEGETABLES

Fallacy #6

YOU CAN EAT THE SAME AT AGE 40 AS AGE 20. Muscle is the engine that powers your pedals, but it also drives your calorie-burning metabolism. The more lean tissue you have, the more calories you burn and the leaner you stay. As we age, we naturally lose muscle and thus gain fat. Cycling and strength training help stem that loss, but the right foods are more important for muscle maintenance than most people realize.

Because of age-related kidney changes, our blood becomes more acidic and we excrete nitrogen, an essential component of muscle protein, faster than we take it in, Friel says. "Essentially we end up peeing away our muscles," he says. And with a net loss of nitrogen, you can't form new muscle.

The Get-Lean Fix: Turn the tide on nitrogen loss and preserve muscle mass by increasing the alkalinity of your blood to neutralize the acidity, says Friel. One way is with supplements like Acid Zapper, but you can also eat foods that enhance alkaline. Fruits and veggies are the only foods that offer a net increase, says Friel. Fats and oils are neutral. All other foods, including grains, legumes and meats, have an acid-producing effect. If you don't get most of your carbs from fruits and vegetables, Friel says, you're losing muscle mass as well as calcium from your bones, which also gets leached away in an acidic environment as you age.

Fallacy #7

YOU'RE NEVER HUNGRY. . . OR YOU'RE ALWAYS HUNGRY. Most diets treat hunger as the enemy. But it's actually your closest ally, says Piattoly. "Once you start the fat-reduction process, you'll be a little hungry, but not starving," he says. "The trick is balancing the two, so you're losing weight but not setting yourself up for a binge."

The Get-Lean Fix: Try to eat every three to four hours, says Piattoly. "Eat breakfast, then wait until you feel hungry and eat just until you're no longer hungry," he says. "That's where people usually go wrong. They eat past the point of satisfaction until they're 'full.' Eat only until you're no longer hungry. If you don't feel hungry again in three to four hours, you ate too much earlier." Once you get the hang of it, weight loss and maintenance is much easier.

Step on It

Body-fat scales ($40–$150) use a technology called bioelectrical impedance, in which the device sends a weak electrical current through your body and measures the degree to which your tissues resist it. Muscle impedes the current more than fat. "This method is not quite as accurate as more-involved ways to estimate body fat," says dietitian Paul Goldberg. "But what body-fat scales lack in precision they make up for in consistency." In *Bicycling's* experience, these scales tend to measure high, but are useful for tracking changes—you don't necessarily get an accurate value, but you'll know if you're making progress.

Be sure to buy one with an "athlete" mode, which uses a slightly more accurate calculation for people who are already fairly lean. Goldberg recommends the Tanita Ironman line of body-fat scales, all of which are tuned for athletes. In addition to body-fat percentage, higher-end scales such as the Ironman BC-549 (tanita.com) also estimate your hydration level, bone mass, basal metabolic rate and visceral fat.

THE GET-LEAN MEAL PLAN

This sample menu from sports-nutrition expert John Berardi, an adjunct associate professor of exercise science at the University of Texas, assumes a rider weight of 165 pounds and a two-hour ride. It supplies 2,500 to 3,000 calories, depending on portion sizes, so adjust portions up or down based on differences in your weight or workout time.

Breakfast

Omelet with 2 whole eggs and 2 egg whites

½ cup oatmeal with ½ cup fruit and ½ cup mixed nuts

1 cup coffee or green tea

Large glass of water

Snack

Smoothie made with 1 cup low-fat or unsweetened soy milk, 1 scoop vanilla protein powder, ½ cup fresh or frozen berries, 1 cup spinach, 1 Tbsp flaxseed

Lunch

Chicken salad with two 4-oz chicken breasts, spinach and a variety of other vegetables, plus olive oil and vinegar dressing

1 piece of fruit

Large glass of water

Snack

1 slice whole-grain bread with 1 Tbsp all-natural peanut butter

1 cup baby carrots

Large glass of water

Dinner

6-oz piece of fish such as salmon or orange roughy

½ cup wild rice

2 cups steamed veggies

Large glass of water

Postworkout Recovery

Drink or snack containing 50g carbohydrate and 25g protein

Omega-3s: Supplement your diet with 3,000mg of fish oil daily with meals, says Berardi.

Fun **Fact**

To lose 1 pound, you need to burn 3,500 more calories than you take in. Here is why cycling is the best sport in the world: A 180-pound cyclist pedaling at a moderate pace for just 1 hour can zap as many as 820 calories.

Where the Carbs Are

FRUITS AND VEGETABLES:
(They're a more substantial source of carbohydrate than most people realize.)

SUCCOTASH, cooked (1 cup) 47g

SWEET POTATO, baked w/skin (large) 44g

RAISINS, seedless (¼ cup) 32g

BANANA (medium) 30g

SQUASH, winter, acorn, cooked (1 cup) 30g

PEAS, cooked (1 cup) 25g

PEACH (large) 17g

CANTALOUPE (1 cup) 15g

ORANGE (1 medium) 14g

ARTICHOKE, cooked (1 medium) 13g

COLLARD GREENS, cooked (1 cup) 12g

STRAWBERRIES (1 cup) 11g

WATERMELON (1 cup) 11g

GREEN PEPPER (1 cup) 10g

CARROTS, cooked (½ cup) 8g

BRUSSELS SPROUTS, cooked (½ cup) 7g

CORN, sweet, cooked (1 ounce) 7g

SPINACH, cooked (1 cup) 7g

BROCCOLI, raw (1 cup) 4g

PASTA & GRAINS:

LONG-GRAIN WHITE RICE (1 cup) 45g

TAGLIATELLE (1 cup) 44g

SPAGHETTI (1 cup) 40g

SHORT-GRAIN WHITE RICE (1 cup) 37g

SPAGHETTI, whole wheat (1 cup) 37g

PITA BREAD, WHITE (6-inch diameter) 33g

FRENCH BREAD (5 inches) 18g

RYE BREAD (1 slice) 15g

WHEAT BREAD (1 slice) 12g

MIXED-GRAIN BREAD (1 large slice) 5g

SEVEN FAT-BURNING FOODS

The key to weight loss is taking in fewer calories than you burn, but what you eat can give you a tremendous advantage. "We really are what we eat," says Samantha Heller, RD, senior clinical nutritionist at New York University Medical Center. "Food is nothing but a bunch of chemicals that unravels during digestion and becomes part of your body." The key is to eat foods that help your bodily systems run smoothly and optimally, so your energy and metabolism stay set to high. Here are seven to stock up on.

ORANGE JUICE. New research reveals that your body has a harder time burning fat without adequate levels of vitamin C—the star nutrient in OJ. Some experts estimate that up to one-third of Americans routinely run low on this important antioxidant. Why? Because we're still not eating enough fresh fruits and vegetables.

Strawberries, kiwi, red bell peppers, tomatoes, citrus fruits and spinach are all excellent sources. **Good to know:** Fresh orange juice is brimming with C. (It delivers 80mg or more per cup, above the Daily Value of 60mg.) But vitamin C degrades with exposure to oxygen and light. Within a month every trace of C disappears from the juice, leaving you with nothing but a carton of orange-colored calories. "By the time you reach the expiration date, the C is lost," says vitamin C researcher Carol Johnston, PhD, RD, professor of nutrition at Arizona State University in Mesa. "Skip the gallon jug. Buy smaller containers instead and drink it within a week."

SALMON. People who eat fish three or four times a week have higher levels of leptin, a hormone that is believed to control appetite and promote fat loss. One recent study showed that 73 dieters who were given leptin injections lost about four times as much weight (15 pounds versus 3½), most of it from fat, during a six-month period as

Pick the Perfect Portion

Weighing and measuring food is a sure way to monitor portion sizes, but it isn't always practical. Use these equations recommended by the United States Department of Agriculture to estimate portions.

1 deck of cards = 3 oz meat, fish or poultry or one slice of bread

1 Ping-Pong ball = 2 tablespoons peanut butter or 1 ounce nuts

4 stacked dice = 1.5 ounces cheese

1 die = 1 teaspoon butter or margarine

1 baseball = 1 cup cooked rice or pasta

½ baseball = ½ cup ice cream

those who didn't receive leptin. Fish are also rich in omega-3 fatty acids, which help to regulate the body's blood-sugar levels, keeping hunger at bay. Most Americans get only about 15 percent of the recommended daily amount (650mg) of omega-3s. **Good to know:** Canned tuna contains fewer omega-3s than salmon, and it has recently come under fire for its high mercury content, which limits the amount of tuna you should eat. Buy canned salmon instead. Twelve ounces a week, or four 3-ounce cans, deliver all the omega-3s you need, plus it's low in calories (80 per can) and high in protein. Toss it in salads, mix it with pasta, or just serve it up with a little mayo in a salmon sub.

SIRLOIN. Lean meats, such as sirloin steak, as well as turkey, chicken, tuna, lentils and fortified cereals, are rich in iron, the mineral that's responsible for forming hemoglobin and carrying oxygen in your red blood cells. Without enough oxygen-carrying hemoglobin, your energy flags and your metabolism falls, says Heller. "Because they're so active, athletes such as cyclists may need about 30 percent more iron than the general population." Supplementing iron can be risky, so it's best to get it from food, she says. **Good to know:** Cook in cast iron. "The mineral leaches from the pot or pan into the food," says Heller. Acidic foods work best. One study showed that the iron content of three ounces of spaghetti sauce skyrocketed from 0.6mg to 5.7mg of iron after being cooked in a cast iron pot.

EGGS. If you want to burn fat, nothing beats breakfast. The morning meal fires up your metabolism and increases your energy to tackle the day—and hopefully the ride—ahead. Eat eggs. Research shows that egg eaters consume fewer calories than non-egg eaters in the hours following breakfast. **Good to know:** Almost 80 percent of people who lose and keep off large amounts of weight eat breakfast daily, according to the National Weight Control Registry.

WATER. There's a reason every weight-loss plan recommends guzzling plenty of water. It helps keep off the pounds. When German researchers gave 14 men and women two cups of water, they found that the subjects' metabolism began to rise within 10 minutes of their final sip. After 40 minutes, their average calorie-burning rate was 30 percent higher and stayed elevated for more than an hour. What's more, water quenches your thirst and helps prevent dehydration, which can slow your metabolism. **Good to know:** Part of the increased calorie burn occurs as your body warms the liquid to your body temperature, so if you're aiming for max burn, dump ice cubes into a 16-ounce water bottle and fill it to the brim with water.

MILK. Sure, milk delivers bone-building calcium, and some studies suggest that calcium promotes fat burning, but that's not the whole story, or perhaps even the most important part. Milk is also an important source of vitamin D, otherwise known as the sunshine vitamin. Researchers are now discovering that vitamin D is an important player in metabolism, as well as bone development. The problem is that up to 70 percent of us routinely get less than we need. If you live in the northern states (any above the

Find Your Burn Rate

How many calories do you need each day to maintain your weight? For a rough idea, use this formula.

STEP 1: Calculate your resting metabolic rate (RMR), or the number of calories your body needs just to function at rest.

Female: 655 + (4.35 x weight in pounds) + (4.7 x height in inches)—(4.7 x age)

Male: 66 + (6.23 x weight in pounds) + (12.7 x height in inches)—(6.8 x age)

STEP 2: Multiply your RMR by your activity factor to find the number of calories you burn daily.

Sedentary (no exercise): 1.2

Light activity (exercising one to three days per week): 1.3 to 1.4

Moderate activity (three to five days per week): 1.5

Very active (six or seven days per week): 1.6 to 1.7

Extreme activity (training twice a day, or doing a physical job plus exercise): 2.0 to 2.4

line from New York City to Northern California), the sun is strong enough for your body to make the vitamin only from May to September. What's more, sunblock with an SPF higher than 8 will block the UV rays necessary to make vitamin D. **Good to know:** Three cups of milk a day deliver your daily dose of calcium and about 75 percent of your vitamin D needs (400 IU a day). For the rest, hang out in the sunshine for about five minutes a day to get some light on your hands, face and arms. Other good food sources include eggs, and fish such as salmon, sardines and herring.

ALMONDS. Adding a handful of almonds to your oatmeal in the morning may help you shed pounds. A study of 65 overweight adults found that even when the dieters ate identical amounts of calories, those who were given three ounces of almonds every day lost consid-

erably more weight (18 percent versus an 11 percent weight loss) and more inches off their waistlines than those who did not eat nuts. Almonds seem to help stabilize blood sugar, which wards off hunger. **Good to know:** Nuts are high in calories, so don't go too nuts. A handful a day should be enough to help keep hunger away.

Cut the Clutter: Chris Carmichael's Five Foods to Avoid

The trouble with a diet is that when you're on it, you're on a diet. That means that, at some point, you'll go off the diet and, hence, off-track again. Instead, strive for a new way of eating and exercising that can integrate so seamlessly into your life that it's easier to stick with the changes than to go back to old habits. Many cyclists may already be very close to eating a powerful diet of whole grains, fruits, vegetables, lean meats and dairy products. They just need to cut the clutter out of what they eat. What's clutter? Fried pork rinds and snack cakes obviously have no nutritional value. But there are also empty calorie sources you don't think about, as well as deceptive junk, foods that started out as high quality but experienced a nutritional hijacking along the way. I'm talking about fruit juices with added sugar, flavorings and preservatives, or breads and crackers that say "whole grain" on the front, but also "high-fructose corn syrup" on the back. Here are the five biggest clutter offenders, and how to avoid them.

SODA. The average American drinks 55 gallons of sweetened soda each year. That's nearly one 20-ounce bottle of soda and 250 calories from sugar every day. Simply cutting out soda would drop an average of 1,750 calories and a half pound each week.

CORN SYRUP. Corn syrup and its evil twin, high-fructose corn syrup (HFCS), are cheap sweeteners used in thousands of products, from colas to condiments to most commercial baked goods, including some whole-wheat breads. Not only is HFCS a concentrated source of empty calories, but it also might convert more easily to body fat than other types of simple sugar, such as those derived from cane or beets, suggests recent research from the University of California, Davis. During exercise, simple sugars can be quite beneficial to performance—energy bars and gels are filled with them. But beware of them as an empty calorie source in your regular diet: In 1966, Americans ate no HFCS, but by 2001 HFCS made up 42 percent—a full 63 pounds—of the 147 pounds of sugar eaten by the average American annually. Check food labels to avoid products with corn syrup and HFCS, and instead look for cereal, juices, pasta sauce, salad dressings and so on that have no added sugar.

TRANS FAT. Man-made trans fat is a product of the food industry, which, to increase shelf life and reduce cost, takes heart-healthy unsaturated fats and chemically corrupts them into molecules that are more harmful to your health than the saturated fat dripping off the greasy bacon in a back-alley diner. For years, partially hydrogenated oils, which contain trans fat, have been used in commercial baked goods, chips and fast food. Trans fat not only increases LDL cholesterol levels (which can contribute to the stiffening of arteries), but also lowers blood levels of beneficial HDL cholesterol, the kind that helps strip plaque off your artery walls. The FDA now requires all manufacturers to list trans fat separately on nutrition labels, and because of bad publicity many food companies have eliminated trans fat from their products. Still, beware: The law allows a label to say zero grams per serving if the food contains 0.5g or less of trans fat. Your best bet is to look for "partially hydrogenated" anything in a food's ingredient list and, if you find it, put the package back on the shelf.

How Lean Should I Be?

Your optimal body-fat level depends on many factors, including gender, age, genetic makeup and your starting point. To find your ideal level, eat right and train smart, then see where you end up. Based on testing large numbers of people, this table, adapted from John Berardi's Precision Nutrition, a multi-media nutrition kit for athletes (precisionnutrition.com), can serve as a rough guideline. Most cyclists should aim to be within the athletic range, at least. Not everyone can reach the elite range.

MEN

Age: 25-30
Elite: < 9%
Athletic: 9-12%
Average: 13-16%
High Fat: 17-19%
Overfat: 20%+

Age: 31-40
Elite: < 11%
Athletic: 11-13%
Average: 14-17%
High Fat: 18-22%
Overfat: 23%+

Age: 41-50
Elite: < 12%
Athletic: 12-15%
Average: 16-20%
High Fat: 21-25%
Overfat: 26%+

Age: 50+
Elite: < 13%
Athletic: 13-16%
Average: 17-21%
High Fat: 22-27%
Overfat: 28%+

WOMEN

Age: 25-30
Elite: < 17%
Athletic: 17-20%
Average: 21-23%
High Fat: 24-27%
Overfat: 28%+

Age: 31-40
Elite: < 18%
Athletic: 18-21%
Average: 22-25%
High Fat: 26-29%
Overfat: 30%+

Age: 41-50
Elite: < 20%
Athletic: 20-23%
Average: 24-27%
High Fat: 28-31%
Overfat: 32%+

Age: 50+
Elite: < 21%
Athletic: 21-24%
Average: 25-28%
High Fat: 29-35%
Overfat: 36%+

ALCOHOL. People don't realize the calorie content of alcohol: Seven useless calories lurk in every gram, or about 98 in each 1.5-ounce shot of spirits such as vodka or whiskey. Liqueurs and cocktails have even more calories per shot because of added sugar. And beer and wine aren't much better. Besides being a source of empty calories, alcoholic beverages are diuretics and contribute to dehydration, even if you have only one or two. Hangover symptoms—the pounding in your head, lethargy and cottonmouth—are primarily due to dehydration. You don't have to go cold turkey, but I recommend no more than four drinks per week.

FANCY COFFEE DRINKS. Recent research confirms what we have believed for decades: Caffeine improves physical and mental performance, including short-term memory. I spent years living in Europe where, on a typical morning, I'd have coffee with milk or a four- to six-ounce latte with breakfast; if I had coffee later in the day, it was a double shot of espresso. Meeting for coffee was about trading stories with a friend; the coffee was small and just an excuse to go for a walk. Coffee itself has virtually no calories. But in America, having coffee means it's possible to drink 700 to 1,000 calories in a single giant cup, thanks to the milk, cream and sugar dumped in. I'm not saying go without coffee. I'm saying go with espresso or a small, fat-free cappuccino or latte—and skip the fancy coffee drinks.

LAST BUT NOT LEAST: SIX SIMPLE WEIGHT-LOSS TIPS

→Beware scale obsession. Weight should come off slowly—a half pound to one pound per week—as a result of cutting junk calories while fueling your body properly for riding and recovery. Think of your body as a high-performance engine: Raise the octane of the fuel you use and stop filling when the tank is full.

→Stay hydrated: Oftentimes cyclists mistake dehydration for hunger.

→Spend a week writing down everything you eat—it's the best way to evaluate what and how much you consume. It also lets you identify troublesome patterns.

→Make foods look bigger: Transfer snacks to a smaller baggie, and eat meals on small plates. A 2005 study in the *Journal of the American Medical Association* found that people ate 56 percent more when they were served meals in large bowls.

Fun **Fact**

Use a napkin to sop up the glistening puddles of grease on pizza, and you can soak up 5g of fat and 45 calories from two slices.

→One of the most overlooked ways to eat less is to slow down. Take smaller bites. Put down your fork between each bite and take a drink. Your body will have time to register what you're consuming, and you'll want less.

→Don't finish your kid's dinner: Nibbling your little one's leftovers sneaks calories that can easily add up to several pounds a year.

CHAPTER 27

Eating for Performance

A balanced daily diet goes a long way toward helping you ride stronger and longer. But when it's time for a big ride, you sometimes need to bend (or break) the rules. Even the most carb-phobic cyclist can benefit from some extra pasta before a century. Five-alarm chili, while nutritious, does not a pre-race meal make. Mid-ride snacks often come in gel form, but a baked potato could work just as well. And sometimes a little sugar is exactly what you need after a killer workout (hello jellybeans, I've missed you). Here's how to fuel properly before, during and after a hard race or ride—without packing on the pounds.

CHRIS CARMICHAEL'S PRE-RIDE EATING PLAN

"What should I eat to ride my best?" is the question I hear most frequently from riders gearing up for a race or century. The 24 hours before a big event are a special occasion. You're going to be blowing through a lot of energy on your ride, and you need to stock your body with the carbs and protein it needs to help you ride strong. It's one of those rare times when you'll want to eat more than your typical amount of daily calories—enjoy, but pay special attention to the foods you're choosing for peak performance. Here's a 24-hour pre-race eating strategy to ensure you'll be ready for any challenging ride.

THE DAY BEFORE. Losing as little as 2 percent of your body weight due to dehydration can lead to a 10 percent drop in athletic performance. Because the majority of Americans, including athletes, are chronically dehydrated, you may be two percent dehydrated before you even start working out. So focusing on fluids is vital. Throughout the day before a big event, I like to see athletes drink around 96 to 128 ounces of fluid, or 12 to 16 eight-ounce glasses. It may seem like a lot, but when you spread it across meals and snacks, it's easily achievable and will help you feel ready to ride. Start first thing. When you get out of bed, drink 16 to 20 ounces of water; it's a simple way to jump-start your hydration. With meals, drink at least 20 ounces of water, and between meals drink another 16 to 20 ounces. By lunch, you'll already have about 60 ounces down the hatch.

Breakfast should be rich in carbohydrate and contain moderate amounts of protein and fat. This means oatmeal, granola or whole-wheat pancakes for carbs, and eggs, yogurt or maybe tofu for protein. Skip the breakfast meats. They're typically higher in saturated fat and sodium, and we're looking for "cleaner" sources of energy in this crucial time period.

As for between-meal snacks, they're a good way to moderately increase the amount of carbs you consume the day before a big event without going through the sometimes-disruptive process of carbo-loading. (If you're experienced with carbo-loading, you're welcome to do it, but now is not the time to experiment.) Again, think clean sources of carbohydrate and protein, like whole-grain bread and peanut butter, or yogurt and granola, hummus with cut vegetables, or an energy bar with balanced carbs and protein. Repeat with a similar snack between lunch and dinner.

Speaking of lunch, skip the all-you-can-eat Indian buffet and have a sandwich, which lets you build your own meal of high-quality carbohydrate and protein. Make it a big one: This is your opportunity to chow down on thick slices of multigrain bread, lean turkey breast, firm tofu or hummus, and plenty of fresh veggies. Add a salad and a side of rice, pasta or potatoes for extra carbs that are easy on the stomach.

Pro Tip

"MY TRACK COACH TOLD ME TO EAT PIZZA THE NIGHT BEFORE A BIG EVENT. HE CLAIMED THAT IT BREAKS DOWN SLOWLY IN THE STOMACH AND WILL KEEP YOUR BODY FEEDING WHILE YOU SLEEP FOR UP TO EIGHT HOURS. I DO IT AND I ALWAYS FEEL GOOD THE NEXT DAY."—*MARK WEIR, DOWNHILL, CROSS-COUNTRY AND 24-HOUR MARATHON RACER*

THE NIGHT BEFORE. While a lot of people automatically go for the heaping bowl of pasta, a meal that's rich in carbohydrate—but not overloaded—gets the job done and is less likely to sit heavily in your gut all night. Grilled fish served on a bed of brown rice, with a big salad and baked potato, works very well. Eat until you're satisfied, but there's no benefit in gorging yourself. Continue consuming fluids throughout the evening, and save the booze for after your ride.

IN THE MORNING. This is where your tried-and-true habits take precedence over science. Lance Armstrong was a cornflake guy. He liked them and found he rode well after eating them, so he started his breakfast there, and often moved on to an omelet and some risotto afterward for some satisfying protein and complex carbs. You want to replenish the carbohydrate stores you burned while you slept, but it's important to eat foods you know will treat you well when you start riding. Two to three hours before the start, eat what you like, aiming for some complex carbs and protein, and skipping heavy foods

24-Hour Pre-Race Meal Plan

Total calories are roughly 3,500 and will vary slightly depending on the vegetables you choose. Servings are based on a 170-pound man who normally consumes about 3,000 calories per day, so adjust up or down according to your size or caloric needs.

BREAKFAST
Two cups of multigrain cereal with one cup of skim milk and a large banana, two scrambled eggs, two slices of whole-wheat toast, coffee and OJ

MORNING SNACK
One-half cup of hummus with one whole-grain pita and one cup of veggies of your choice

LUNCH
Turkey sandwich with three ounces of sliced turkey, mustard, whole-wheat bread and a pile of veggies; on the side: one-and-a-half cups of brown or wild rice, and a garden side salad with two tablespoons of dressing

AFTERNOON SNACK
A couple of handfuls of almonds, a piece of fruit and a cup of coffee or espresso

DINNER
Three ounces of grilled salmon (a smaller piece than you think); two cups of pasta with fresh basil, a drizzle of olive oil and an ounce of Parmesan cheese; one cup of oven-roasted vegetables (zucchini, squash, onion, mushrooms with a little olive oil and spices)

BREAKFAST
One cup of oatmeal with walnuts and raisins or cranberries mixed in, two scrambled eggs, two slices of whole-wheat toast with two tablespoons of peanut butter, plus coffee and OJ

---

like breakfast meats or dairy if you know they don't agree with you before a ride.

TOP OFF THE TANK. In the hours between your final pre-event meal and the main event, have a bottle of sports drink in order to continue hydrating and to top off your carbohydrate stores. Have an energy bar or light carbohydrate snack available in case you feel a hunger pang in the hour before the start.

EATING ON THE ROLL

In 2009, Alberto Contador said he planned to win every race he entered that year—but his dream dissolved by March, when attacking riders left him in the dust at Paris-Nice, seizing the leader's jersey. His show of weakness came not from heavy legs or a superior field; he simply forgot to refuel and bonked hard. It was a rare mistake for an established champion.

Three Eating Tips for Long Rides

→If you're riding all day long, don't try to subsist on energy gels, sports drinks and bars, which consist primarily of processed sugar and aren't meant for sustained energy. A savory snack, such as a turkey sandwich, provides a break for the palette and the stomach (remember, at lunchtime it's expecting a meal), as well as some needed protein and fat.

→Test new foods on shorter rides before eating them on epics. Designate one day a week as "new foods day." You'll never discover your ideal fuel combos until you mix things up a bit.

→Drafting behind other riders can fool you into thinking you don't need to refuel. To make sure you get enough energy on long rides, fill your bottle with a sports beverage rather than water and set your watch alarm to remind you to sip every 15 minutes. Make a game out of eating all the snacks you've stashed in your jersey: End the ride with uneaten food, and you lose.

As Contador demonstrated, failing to fill your glycemic gas tank will quickly ruin a ride. A smooth snack break requires specific bike-handling skills to deliver the proper type and amount of food from your pocket to your mouth, says Sam Callan, USA Cycling's coaching education manager.

STAY ON SCHEDULE. Make timing your nutrition a priority. Take hits from your water bottle after 30 minutes and every 15 minutes thereafter, Callan says. For rides longer than 45 minutes, follow the American College of Sports Medicine's guidelines and eat the equivalent of 1 gram (g) of carbohydrate for each additional minute (gels have about 25g and bars have 40 to 45).

BUILD BALANCE. Holding your handlebar with one hand and eating with the other sounds easy enough. What's not so simple: continuing a perfect line while barreling down a busy road and digging through your back pocket. Practice by riding one-handed along parking-space lines. Then ride the lines while mimicking a snack break. "Just keep pulling food from your pocket, bringing it to your handlebar, and returning it," Callan says. When your support hand is on the brake hoods or the side of the bar, every body motion is exaggerated and transferred to the front wheel. For optimal balance (though reduced braking ability), hold your handlebar next to the stem with your dominant hand.

EAT SAFELY. Hyperawareness during refueling will help keep you—and the people riding with you—safe. First, scan the road for traffic in case you swerve. Then look out for other obstacles. "Potholes and debris can sneak up quickly, even when you're rolling along at a leisurely pace," Callan says.

DIVERSIFY. Blowing through an entire case of Strawberry Blast gels can become tedious, and when you grow tired of a specific flavor, you're less likely to eat. Buy a variety of gels, bars and chewy supplements; most energy foods have a six-month or longer shelf life. When you can, carry unprocessed fare such as bananas and sandwiches.

PREP YOUR FOOD. Avoid an on-bike fight with your food wrapper—and the resulting smashed snack—by partially opening the packaging before you roll out. Another option: Repack your food into a Ziplock bag, which doubles as a used gel-packet depository.

CHOOSE WISELY. The muffin you crave at the pre-ride coffee shop may look delicious, but it is likely to crumble into hard-to-eat bran meal in your jersey pocket. Stick with easy-to-manage foods, says Callan, like a peanut-butter-and-banana sandwich cut into quarters.

THE MOVING FEAST

One of the first things a new cyclist learns is that without on-bike food and fluids, you can't pedal very far or very fast. Here's what Chris Carmichael suggests eating and drinking on rides of various lengths:

Ride Duration: 1 hour or less
Primary concern: Fluid replenishment
What to drink: Plain water
What to eat: Most people start with enough stored energy for a 60-minute workout, but

Pro Tip

"RESERVE CAFFEINATED GELS OR DRINKS FOR LATER IN LONG TRAINING SESSIONS, BECAUSE IF YOU START WITH A STIMULANT EARLY ON, YOU WON'T BE ABLE TO GET A BOOST LATER IN THE RIDE WHEN YOU REALLY NEED ONE."—*CHRIS CARMICHAEL*

carry one energy gel, which has about 27g of carbs and 200 milligrams (mg) of sodium, just in case

Bonus tip: For optimal recovery, eat a full meal within an hour of finishing an intense workout.

Ride Duration: 1 to 3 hours
Primary concern: Carbohydrate replenishment
What to drink: 1 bottle water and 1 bottle sports drink per hour, at least
What to eat: 30–60g of carb per hour from bars, gels and sports drinks—up to 80g if you're consuming glucose and fructose together, as your body can process this combination more efficiently.
Bonus tip: Don't dilute the sports drinks—your body absorbs them most efficiently at their correct concentrations.

Ride Duration: 3 hours or more
Primary concern: Carbohydrate and electrolyte replenishment; food boredom
What to drink: 1 bottle water and 1 bottle sports drink per hour, at least
What to eat: 30–60g of carbs per hour, total. Digestion can get harder as rides get longer, so eat more solids at the beginning of the ride, and rely on gels for quick energy in the last third of the ride.
Bonus tip: Supplement bars and gels with carb-rich, low-protein, moderate-fat "real" foods. Don't worry about specific amounts of protein or fat; just eat what tastes good so you keep eating.

The Ultimate On-Bike Snack

Potatoes are an abundant source of potassium, sodium, fluid and carbohydrates, says Allen Lim, physiologist for Team RadioShack. Here's how he prepares them for his athletes to eat on the fly.

→Boil a handful of new potatoes. "I skin them for the team because pro riders take in so many calories, the extra fiber could upset their stomachs," he says. "But it doesn't really matter for most people."

→Drizzle the potatoes with olive oil and add a pinch of salt.

→Grate Parmesan cheese onto the potatoes to taste.

→Wrap in foil using Lim's technique, which gives easy access while keeping hands and jersey pockets clean:

Use paper aluminum foil, often used at fast-food restaurants. Stores in Europe sell it, but in the United States Lim buys wholesale or bargains with a fry jockey for a stack.

Cut a 5-inch-wide strip of foil and place your food in the center.

Fold one long edge over, and then back again halfway.

Repeat with the other long edge, creating a seam.

Tightly wrap the outer edges around the back, leaving the seam exposed.

Store in a jersey pocket. When hunger strikes, you can easily rip half the foil off at the seam and take a bite.

 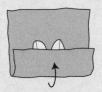 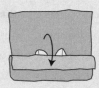

Fig. 1: Fold one edge and double back.

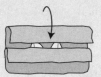 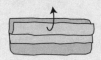

Fig. 2: Fold again to make a seam.

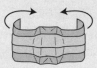

Fig. 3: Wrap outer edges; rip open to eat.

EATING FOR RECOVERY

When you return from a ride, don't feel guilty about chowing down before you shower. Eat within 30 to 60 minutes of ending your workout, and your body fast-tracks those nutrients to muscle repair and glycogen replacement. (After that, you'll still benefit—just not as much.) Put off eating, and you're more likely to feel tired from the effort, not stronger for the next one.

Chances are, the ideal formula for recovery is already sitting in your fridge.

Over the past decade, sports-nutrition companies have begun selling recovery drinks or powders to help you bounce back faster. They work because they serve up the right blend of carbs and protein to restock glycogen stores and to jump-start muscle repair. "They're convenient, too, but real food works just as well," says Monique Ryan, RD, author of *Sports Nutrition for Endurance Athletes*. Plus, real food tastes better, so you may be more likely to eat it. For optimal muscle recovery, aim for 75 to 80g of carbs and 15 to 20g of protein (based on a 150-pound rider) after short, hard rides or rides longer than 90 minutes. These standard-serving combos serve up the right blend while also helping to replenish fluids.

CEREAL WITH SLICED BANANA. Try one cup of Kashi GoLean Crunch! with half of a sliced banana and a half-cup of skim milk, washed down with a small glass of orange juice, which is a good source of carbs as well as immunity-boosting vitamin C. Delivers: 75g carbs and 20g protein

EGG SALAD ON A BAGEL. Eggs are packed with protein and, though bagels get a bad rap from low-carb fanatics, their carbs are exactly what you need after a hard ride. Add a glass of cranberry juice for bonus carbs and cell-repairing antioxidants. Delivers: 82g carbs and 21g protein

SPAGHETTI WITH MEAT SAUCE, AND GRAPES. This classic carbo-loader also makes a great reloader. A serving of pasta refills glycogen stores fast, while red meat sauce provides protein. Add a side of juicy grapes for extra fluid, carbs and antioxidants, and it's a complete meal. Delivers: 76g carbs and 17g protein

HUMMUS, CARROTS AND APPLE, IN A PITA. Made from chickpeas and sesame-seed paste, hummus delivers protein, heart-healthy fats and immunity-boosting antioxidants. Shred the carrots and add apple slices for sweet crunch and extra vitamins. Delivers: 80g carbs and 15g protein

SMOOTHIE. Smoothies help you rehydrate as they replenish, and they go down easy even if you have trouble eating after a sweltering ride. Any variation of this recipe will give you what you need: 1 cup milk (skim or soy), half of a frozen banana, 1 cup yogurt (try lemon or other light flavor), 1 cup of fruit (preferably frozen) and honey to taste. Delivers: 83g carbs and 19g protein

Pro **Tip**

"IMMEDIATELY AFTER EXERCISE IS THE ONLY TIME I LET MY GUYS EAT VERY SWEET FOODS. SIMPLE SUGARS ABSORB INTO YOUR SYSTEM FAST."—*ALLEN LIM, PHYSIOLOGIST FOR TEAM RADIOSHACK*

WAFFLES, YOGURT AND BLACKBERRIES. Crisp waffles with silky yogurt make a meal worth riding an extra mile for. Blackberries top the list of foods with the highest antioxidant levels—just what dinged-up muscles need to mend. Delivers: 76g carbs and 18g protein

RECIPES FOR REFUELING

When 24-hour racer and cookbook writer David Joachim comes in from a grinding two-hour ride in the rocky Pennsylvania hills he calls home, he has roughly 15 minutes to clean up, refuel and head out the door to his son's soccer practice. He could slam a recovery drink and an energy bar, but Joachim demands real food—like good Italian or Mexican. "I want to put nutrients back into my muscles, but I also want a hearty meal to satisfy my stomach," says Joachim, author of *The Tailgater's Cookbook.*

With the right ingredients in the pantry, you can have a hot, healthy meal in about 10 minutes, Joachim says. "Canned fish and beans are great staples because they're versatile, easy to store, and provide lots of protein for muscle repair."

TUNA SOPRANOS

(canned fish, canned tomatoes and canned beans)

* *3 Tbsp olive oil*

* *1 oz canned, rolled anchovies with capers, drained*

* *3 garlic cloves, minced*

* *1 15-oz can Italian-style diced tomatoes, undrained*

* *$1/4$ c dry white wine (or warm water)*

* *1 6-oz can low-sodium chunk white tuna in water, drained*

* *$1/2$ 15-oz can small white beans, drained and rinsed*

* *3 Tbsp chopped parsley*

* *$1/8$ tsp black pepper*

* *8 oz linguine, cooked according to package directions (prepare in advance to save time)*

Put the oil, anchovies with capers, and garlic into a shallow, 2-quart glass dish and nuke for 3 minutes. Mash up the anchovies and capers with a fork until broken into tiny pieces. Stir in the tomatoes with juice and the wine (or water). Nuke for 10 minutes, or until the sauce thickens a little. Mix in the tuna and beans, and nuke 1 minute or until heated through. Stir in the parsley and pepper. Serve over the pasta. Makes 3 servings.

HOT BLACK BEAN DIP

(canned beans and cheese)

* *1 16-oz can refried black beans*

* *1 4-oz can chopped mild green chiles or hot jalapeños, drained*

* 1 8-oz container reduced-fat sour cream

* ¼ tsp ground cumin

* ¼ tsp dried oregano

* 1 cup chunky salsa

* 1 cup finely shredded, reduced-fat sharp
   cheddar or pepper Jack cheese

* Tortilla chips or soft tortillas

Mix beans, chiles, sour cream, cumin, and oregano in a shallow, 1-quart glass dish or pie plate. Nuke for 3 minutes, or until hot. Top with salsa and cheese, mix, then nuke for 5 minutes, or until the cheese melts. Serve with chips or, for a handheld meal, leave out the salsa and sour cream, let the dip cool to lukewarm, then slather onto a tortilla and roll burrito-style. Makes 12 ¼-cup servings.

FAST FISH TACOS

(canned fish, canned tomatoes and cheese)

* 1 Tbsp canola oil

* 1 garlic clove, minced

* ¼ tsp ground cumin

* ½ tsp dried oregano

* 1 15-oz can diced tomatoes with zesty
   jalapeños, well drained in a colander

* 2 6-oz cans low-sodium chunk white tuna,
   drained and flaked

* Juice of ½ lime

* ¼–½ tsp hot pepper sauce

* 4 8-in flour tortillas

* 1 c shredded low-fat sharp cheddar or
   Monterey Jack cheese

Mix the oil, garlic, cumin, and oregano in a shallow, 1-quart glass dish and nuke for 1 minute, or until sizzling. Stir in the tomatoes, tuna, lime juice and hot pepper sauce. Nuke for 2 minutes, or until heated through. Nuke the tortillas on a plate for 10 seconds, or until warm. Spoon the hot filling down the middle of the tortillas, top with the cheese, and fold up. Makes 4 soft tacos.

Pastabilities Galore

One helpful hint for recovery meals in minutes: Keep a tightly sealed container of plain, cooked pasta in the refrigerator. It lasts about 3 days and provides a ready-to-eat base for dozens of dishes.

Pro Tip

TOO OFTEN, CYCLISTS STOP DRINKING WHEN THE RIDE STOPS. BUT BECAUSE IT'S ALMOST IMPOSSIBLE TO TAKE IN ENOUGH FLUIDS WHILE RIDING TO FULLY REPLACE WHAT YOU'VE LOST, CYCLISTS END WORKOUTS DEHYDRATED, WHICH COMPROMISES RECOVERY. REFILL YOUR BOTTLE AFTER YOUR RIDE AND DOWN THE CONTENTS WITHIN AN HOUR. —SUZANNE GIRARD EBERLE, AUTHOR OF ENDURANCE SPORTS NUTRITION

For Your Pantry

Stock up on these convenient foods to make recovery-meal magic:

Canned beans (refried, white, black, kidney, pinto, etc.)

Canned tomatoes (with green chiles, jalapeños, etc.)

Canned fish (salmon, tuna, anchovies, etc.)

Cheese (Colby, cheddar, mozzarella, etc.)

PREVENT THE GORGE

Brian Wansink, author of *Mindless Eating* and director of Cornell University's Food and Brand Lab, knows you're ravenous after a ride—and offers tips to stop you from cramming excess calories down your throat without thinking.

The most important thing you can do is hydrate—a lot more than you think you should, especially in winter. Cyclists often mistake dehydration for hunger.

If you know there's not a chance on earth you're going to exercise self-control, I have one word for you: prepackage. Figure out how many calories you're going to burn, put that amount of food on a plate, and sock it away. When you

raid the fridge, let that plate be the only thing you grab.

I tell athletes that they have license to go home and gorge on as much fruit as they want. No one can pack away 1,000 calories of fruit in 5 minutes.

It can be hard to visually calculate calories, but it's easy to eyeball a portion size. If you equate one handful of anything with 250 calories, you may think twice before going back for seconds.

Doing a 4-hour ride doesn't mean you can reward yourself by taking third helpings at the dinner table. Replenishing the calories you lose through riding with a recovery snack and then making wise eating decisions the rest of the time is the key to not going overboard.

Sometimes you may not feel like eating right after a workout, but have something anyway. You'll stave off the tidal wave of hunger that usually comes later.

RIDER **RESOURCES**

Find out how many calories you burned on your last ride with Bicycling.com's Calorie Counter (bicycling.com/caloriemain).

Look up calorie counts for more than 50,000 fresh, brand-name and generic foods at calorieking.com/foods.

Feeling guilty about a diet slipup? Don't despair: It could have been much, much worse. For a good laugh—or cringe—check out the delicacies displayed at thisiswhyyourefat.com (bacon-wrapped, deep-fried Girl Scout cookies, anyone?).

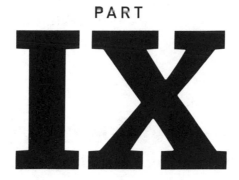

PART

IX

Touring and Travel

WE KNOW, WE KNOW: TECHNICALLY, ANY BIKE RIDE, from an urban cruise to an all-day century, involves travel. But sometimes you may want to take—or ride—your bike even farther away.

CHAPTER 28

Plan Your Next Adventure

The word "touring" means different things to different cyclists. For some, it's carrying all your worldly goods for the week (or month) on two wheels. Others prefer to write a check and let someone else take care of the itinerary—which typically includes sumptuous meals, off-bike excursions and maybe even the chance to watch a major cycling race. Then there's "credit-card touring," where you're essentially self-supported but make liberal use of hotels and restaurants along the way. For an in-depth guide to bike travel, check out Bicycling Magazine's Guide to Bike Touring. *Here, we cover some of the basics: getting your bike and body ready for a trip; packing tips; and, of course, deciding where to go.*

TIPS FROM A TOUR OPERATOR

Mountain Bike Hall of Famer Ashley Korenblat, co-owner of Western Spirit Cycling Adventures (westernspirit.com), shares how to get the most out of your next cycling vacation.

→Here's why to take a guided trip: You know you are riding the best roads and trails for you, hassle-free. And when you're not riding, you'll have the opportunity to hike, fish, boat or explore ruins. Who wants to spend their vacation dealing with logistics? On Mexican night on our trips, we serve the biggest bowl of fresh guacamole you've ever seen, followed by beef and chicken fajitas, and finish up with chocolate-peanut-butter brownies. And, of course, there's a cocktail hour.

→Mountain bike trips take about two to four years for us to design and create. We visit the same place numerous times, talk to all the rangers and ride all possible trail combinations before deciding on the right itinerary. Then, of course, we have to get all the necessary permits. Road trips are a little easier to design. The biggest challenge is to find the right lodging, so we can connect the very best riding routes while minimizing the shuttle times.

→Solo, unguided trips can be exciting. But you need to plan carefully, and be prepared to face that unexpected 4,000-foot climb. And you have to carry and make your own dinner.

→If you've never gone on an organized biking vacation, the best advice I can give is to talk to the guides in the office before choosing a trip. An experienced guide is so much more helpful than a brochure when deciding which adventure is right for you. Some people get hooked on a certain location and only later find out that it doesn't fit into their time frame—snow doesn't melt in Telluride until July, and Moab's too hot in August.

→The best tour companies won't just let you sign up for a trip without asking anything about you—have you been riding for years and need something hard-core, or are you just getting started and want to improve your skills?

→As long as you've chosen a good tour company, you shouldn't worry about the level of the other riders. Most trips are designed with either advanced or beginner riders in mind. It's very rare that we mix different riding levels on the same trip. However, some trips are specifically created to accommodate various levels of experience. On those trips everyone might ride together in the morning, then have a choice of hard singletrack or an easy road cruise in the afternoon.

→Ask the tour operator what type of bikes they supply. If your bike is newer, lighter or just plain better than the rental bikes available, you should bring your own. If not, renting is convenient, and it gives you a chance to try out a new ride.

→And always bring a waterproof coat and pants. If you have those two little things, you will be invincible.

GOING IT ALONE

Here are some no-fail packing tips for self-supported touring.

Ride: The perfect bike is less about weight than fit; perfect ergonomics lead to ache-free long days in the saddle. For any trip short of a global assault, panniers and a rear rack are all you need.

Sleep: A bivy sack is simply too hardcore for most. With a tent and bag/pad combo, you'll sleep better, stay dry and avoid unwanted nocturnal intrusions.

Cook: An ultralight Jetboil stove (jetboil.com) is easy to use, but its full-blast flame limits cooking options; you'll want to supplement with bought treats (or haul a more versatile stove).

Dress: Three rules apply. 1. You need less than you think, so once you pack, go through and purge. You'll be grateful for the saved weight. 2. In camp, stick with natural fibers such as wool, which works in a wide range of temperatures and smells fresh for days. 3. Never, ever forget cheap sandals, a warm beanie and a waterproof shell.

Live: No one needs to haul a virtual Best Buy worth of gadgetry, but allow yourself that which you love most. If you're a birder, pack binoculars; if you can't breathe without The Pixies, take the iPod.

THE UNFRIENDLY SKIES

When trying to decide whether to rent a bicycle on a trip or bring your own, make sure to consider the cost of flying with a bike. The Bureau of Transportation Statistics reported that airline baggage-fee revenue jumped 275 percent from 2008 (when charges for normal-size bags were introduced) to 2009. Unfortunately, some of these new charges end up gouging cyclists. Airlines generally allow a bike case that measures no more than 62 dimensional inches (length plus width plus height) and weighs less than 50 pounds to fly as regular checked baggage. Beyond that, you'll pay extra—as much as $300 each way. Here's how to minimize the damage—both to your wallet and to your bike.

Tips for Beating Bag Fees

→Join an airline mileage rewards program. Once you reach preferred-customer status, you get expedited check-in and a higher weight allowance for checked bags. Several frequent flyers we spoke to said that their status has helped them avoid bike fees almost entirely.

→Agents at smaller airports that don't handle lots of oversize luggage don't always charge the fees, says 2008 U.S. mountain bike national champion Adam Craig, who estimates he flies 70,000 miles a year, much of it with a custom two-bike case from Pika Packworks. If you can fly out of such an airport, he says, "it's suddenly fiscally responsible to spend $75 more on a ticket to save $175 on baggage fees."

→Read your airline's policy carefully. United, for example, will not take packed bikes over 50 pounds, period. They also charge extra on flights to Japan and Brazil. Some carriers have seasonal bans on oversize baggage. And check your aircraft—regional jets have smaller holds and may not be able to take bikes all the time.

→Shipping your ride may be cheaper, depending on your route and airline.

→Some carriers assess lower charges for oversize bags than for bikes. "As soon as you say anything that has to do with a bike, you're done," says pro racer Tim Johnson. Instead, he replies "exercise equipment" when asked what's in the bag. (To make this work, don't check in with your helmet clipped to your carry-on.) Other less-than-honest yet effective answers: massage table, art supplies, trade-show booth. But if your bike is damaged and wasn't declared as a bike, you might forfeit liability payments.

→If challenged, calmly state facts: The package is only X linear inches over the basic baggage

Pro Tip

"EVEN IF SAFELY STOWED, YOUR BIKE MAY NOT ARRIVE WHEN YOU DO. AS INSURANCE, PACK CYCLING SHOES, PEDALS, YOUR HELMET AND A SET OF CLOTHES IN YOUR CARRY-ON. IF YOUR BIKE IS DELAYED, YOU CAN BORROW OR RENT ONE AND USE YOUR OWN GEAR—AT LEAST YOU'LL BE RIDING."—*ALEX STIEDA*

limit; when you checked a few days earlier, the baggage allowance for Premier Exec status was more generous. But always smile and be pleasant.

→ Do your research: If tickets to London are the same price on British Airways and Lufthansa, British Airways is the better deal, because it charges $50 each way for your bike, compared to Lufthansa's $200.

How to Pack Smart

→ Don't use the bike bag as your suitcase. Some carriers assess both oversize and overweight charges.

→ We hesitate to say this, but with increasingly stringent dimensional and weight restrictions, hard-shell cases are looking like a poor idea. While their protection is superb, most weigh more than 30 pounds empty. That said, some carriers require liability release forms for soft-side cases.

→ CO_2 cartridges are prohibited in all checked bags and carry-ons.

→ Checked bag liability usually tops out at $3,300 for domestic flights. Damage must be proved. Check your homeowner's policy to see if it covers items damaged in travel.

→ Finally, it's an urban myth that your tires will burst in the cargo hold—there's no need to deflate them.

Box Your Bike in Nine Easy Steps

Whether you're packing your bike for air travel or shipping it to your destination, here's how to make sure it's still ridable when it arrives.

1. Take out the seatpost with the seat attached.

2. Take cables out of stops. Create slack in brake cables by undoing the releases on the arms (V-brakes, cantis and Shimano road brakes) or at the levers (Campy). Slacken shifter cables by putting the chain in the big ring/big cog combo and then, without pedaling, shifting down. Removing the cables gives you room to remove and position the handlebar.

3. Remove stem, handlebar and front brake. Loop the bar around the fork and pack the computer in the small parts box.

4. Spin off the pedals: Right pedal counterclockwise, left pedal clockwise.

5. Remove quick-releases and put them in the small-parts box.

6. Take off front wheel and slip a piece of wood or plastic block between the drops to keep the fork legs from bending if something heavy is placed on them.*

7. Wrap tubes, fork and crankarms with insulation, bubble wrap or many sheets of newspaper.

8. Zip-tie the stem to the top tube.

9. Slip it all into the box and pad, pad, pad. Use rags, clothing or cardboard to pad places where metal and equipment will rub together. Pad the ends of your hubs so they don't poke through the box.

*If your box is so small that you have to remove the rear wheel as well, insert a quick-release through a spare hub and clamp it between the rear dropouts to protect them from bending.

Supplies you'll need:

→Hex wrenches

→Pedal wrench

→Duct tape

→Wrapping material: bubble wrap, newspaper or pipe insulation

→One or two rolls of 2-inch-wide packing tape

→Fork spacer

→Knife

→Black marker to address and cross out old addresses

→String or zip-ties

→Bike box

→Small-parts box thin enough to fit into bike box

Four Ways to Protect Your Fork

1. Wood block: Cut a 1-inch by 1-inch by 4-inch stock that slides snugly between the fork blades and slip drywall screws and washers into the drops.

2. Old hub: Recycle your old hub by slipping it into the drops with a quick-release.

3. Bolt & nuts: Hit the hardware store for a bolt thin enough to slip into the dropouts and long enough to extend about ½ inch past each side of the dropouts. Hand-tighten two nuts on either side of both drops.

4. Plastic packing stuff: Manufacturers include plastic stocks when they ship bikes to shops. Ask your favorite mechanic for one, then treasure it dearly.

Put this stuff in the small-parts box:

→computer

→quick-releases

→pedals

→tools

→pump

→water bottle

→lock

→seat and seatpost

→extra tape for return-trip packing

Riding High

"Avoid the temptation to train too hard prior to heading to altitude," says Terry Chiplin, who trains cyclists at his coaching facility near Rocky Mountain National Park, in Colorado. "Many people come to a high-altitude environment already depleted and take longer to acclimate as a result."

Riders traveling from lowlands to destinations higher than 5,000 feet face at least a 10 percent reduction in their cardiac capacity (the rate they turn oxygen into energy). Ride the 12,183-foot-high Trail Ridge Road above Chiplin's facility just after arriving from the East Coast, and you'll feel like you've lost a quarter of your aerobic fitness.

Chiplin offers the following guidelines to increase your red-blood-cell density and stockpile glycogen in your legs, which will help your body get ready to perform at altitude.

Weeks to altitude: Eight

Do: More sprints—add them to your normal riding routine

Eat: Complete proteins (meat and dairy)

Weeks to altitude: Three

Do: Less riding—reduce your overall exercise volume by 20 percent

Eat: Carbohydrate

Weeks to altitude: One

Do: More reading—reduce your overall exercise volume from your norm by 65 percent

Eat: Water-soluble vitamins (C, D, E and B12)

RIDE STRONG— DAY AFTER DAY

Follow these recovery techniques from Chris Carmichael to stay strong during training camps and bike tours.

I've been running cycling camps for more than 15 years, first for the U.S. national team, then pros, and now amateur racers and enthusiasts. No matter the group, there's a constant: Someone digs too deep on Day One and runs out of steam before the final ride.

It almost happened to Cliff Valentin at a spring CTS training camp in Asheville, North Carolina. Cliff pushed hard the first two days, and by noon on Saturday he was looking pretty haggard. Sunday was the big Carolina Crusher ride everyone looks forward to. The race was on: We had 18 hours to pump life back into those tired legs and glassy eyes. I know a lot of cyclists can relate to Cliff's situation. Here's how to get your fresh legs back.

Nutrition

This topic is covered a lot, because it's important: Have a recovery drink immediately after the ride, followed by a balanced meal within an hour. Your goal is to consume 1.5 grams (g) of carbohydrate per kilogram (kg) of body weight postride. (That would come to 112.5g for a 75-kg, or 165-pound, athlete.) No need to cram it all in right away. I'd rather you eat the full amount over four hours than stuff yourself in the first hour but get only two-thirds of what you need.

Nap

If you can snooze for even an hour, you'll ride better tomorrow. It doesn't restore like a full night's sleep, but a nap does increase an athlete's attention to detail for the remainder of the day. People who are dead on their feet don't continue drinking and barely touch their dinner, and they go to bed without the fuel to recharge overnight.

Spin

It may seem counterintuitive to put your sore behind back on a saddle, but a 15- to 45-minute spin in the evening works miracles for recovery. Stay in a light gear and keep your cadence above 90 rpm; you should be able to talk easily the entire time. It seems that the old story about flushing lactic acid isn't accurate, but increasing circulation does help move other metabolic waste out of your muscles and bring in more oxygenated blood and nutrients. This ride also helps keep your muscles supple and elongated, so you'll be less stiff tomorrow.

Massage

A restorative rub works for some and not for others; if you've never had a massage, two days into a four-day tour is not the time to try it. If you do go for one, you want a sports-massage therapist or soigneur who understands athletes, ideally cyclists, and knows what you did today and plan to do tomorrow. A relaxing spa massage won't help you ride better, and this is not the time for deep-tissue work.

When you take care of yourself, you can ride four or more days in a row and feel great; you may not even see a decrease in sustainable power or performance on climbs if your fitness is decent. And you can bring yourself back from the brink: Cliff rode powerfully on the Carolina Crusher and went home with confidence for his next challenge.

THE MUST-RIDES

If you've ever pleaded for help, or a merciful end to your suffering, midway through one of those "easy" training rides that closes in on you like an iron maiden, you know that cyclists need a patron saint. If you've ever been climbing the local cloud-tickler and lost track once again of how many turns you've already made, and thus how many turns are left, you know that we cyclists could really use numbered corners on our legendary ascents. And if your hard-riding body has ever craved a feast when you power it solely with high-carb fuel, you know that even for cyclists, meals should matter as much as wheels. Here are seven great riding spots that

Chris Carmichael's 45-Minute Hotel-Bike Workout

If you're going on a long trip and can't bring your bike, try to book at a hotel with highly adjustable spin bikes instead of those big plastic exercise bikes. Pack riding shorts, and maybe even your shoes and pedals (you might be able to sneak your pedals onto the bike if you bring the right tool, but don't blame me if you wreck the hotel's bike in the process). Here's the perfect on-the-go workout, no heart rate or power meter needed.

Warm-up: 8 minutes	Harder: 1 minute
Fast pedal: 1 minute	Easy spin: 6 minutes
Recovery: 30 seconds	Hard effort: 2 minutes
Fast pedal: 1 minute	Harder: 1 minute
Recovery: 30 seconds	Hard effort: 2 minutes
Hard effort (7 on a 1 to 10 scale): 2 minutes	Harder: 1 minute
Harder (9 effort): 1 minute	Hard effort: 2 minutes
Hard effort: 2 minutes	Harder: 1 minute
Harder: 1 minute	Cool-down: 10 minutes
Hard effort: 2 minutes	

deliver these, and other, necessary pleasures of cycling: pedaling paradises that combine amazing roads and trails with surprising delights and the riches of the world that lies beyond our handlebars. As you plan your next vacation, set aside a few days—or weeks—to pedal around one—or all—of these cycling wonderlands.

Tuscany

Simply put, this region of Italy is bicycling heaven. The cuisine—including the wine—can't be beat anywhere in the world, and the lightly traveled roads offer every option a cyclist could want: rollers, speedy flats, famous climbs, tree-shaded lanes, farm paths, traditional training routes with bike-friendly populations, epicurean meanders and anything else you can imagine. You can't go wrong, but you'll go most right in Volterra and Siena, and on the incredible Isle of Elba. **Best Time to Go:** Late spring and early fall are optimal. Serious hedonists might want to observe the grape and olive harvests in late September through early October. **It's Most Fun If You're This Fit:** Novice to pro will find the rides they desire. **Get There With:** Andy Hampsten, the first and still the only American to win the Giro d'Italia, lives in Tuscany and shares its pleasures with guests on Cinghiale Cycling Tours (cinghiale.com).

Crested Butte

When the rides start at 9,000 feet and go up, you know you're in a special place. The routes surrounding this Colorado town, called CB by locals, take you on singletrack through groves of aspens, on wide-open trails through meadows of skunk cabbage and sage, and over rocky mining roads across the Continental Divide. Trail

401 and Trail 403 are not to be missed, and the descent of Teocali Ridge is one of the best mountain bike rides in the world. For those looking for an epic experience, try riding from CB to Aspen and back. And don't miss the Mountain Bike Hall of Fame in town. **Best Time to Go:** Summer, especially for Fat Tire Bike Week, the world's oldest mountain bike festival, at the end of June. But be prepared for afternoon thunderstorms. **It's Most Fun If You're This Fit:** High-volume lungs will be able to make the most of the high-mountain paths, but fun, short, non-technical trails loop around town for novices. **Get There With:** Crested Butte Mountain Guides (crestedbutteguides.com).

Madonna di Ghisallo

In 1948, a modest chapel on the shores of Italy's Lago di Como was christened in honor of the Madonna di Ghisallo, a saint dedicated to the safety and well-being of cyclists. Since then, this tiny sanctuary has become a museum of those who have sought its blessings: Leader jerseys from the Giro d'Italia and Tour de France (as well as those left by amateurs) adorn the walls, and all around are vintage bicycles from legends such as Fausto Coppi, Gino Bartali and Eddy Merckx. There's even a bike from Alfonsina Strada, the first and only woman to ride in the Giro. The surrounding roads are spectacular, but the highlight might be the Wall of Sormano, a gnarly stretch of tarmac whose 1.5 miles of 18-percent grade was used to sort the champions from the fodder in the sport's earliest races. **Best Time to Go:** Moderate elevation and climate make this a year-round destination, but the Tour of Lombardy passes by in early October. **It's Most Fun If You're This Fit:** Moderately fit, riding at least three times a week and prepared to climb. The ascent from Bellagio to the church is about 3 miles at 9–10 percent. **Get There With:** Breaking Away Bicycle Tours (breakingaway.com).

Alpe d'Huez

Since its first inclusion in the Tour de France, in 1952, when Italian *campionissimo* Fausto Coppi climbed to victory, a win atop this 21-switchback ascent has become the most coveted prize in the Grand Tours. It's also the most manic stage of any Tour de France in which it's included. Each turn has a sign commemorating one of the stage winners. (Coppi and Armstrong share a spot on switchback 21.) So popular is this 8-mile climb that photographers stake out the road every day in the summer to sell photos to passing riders. **Best Time to Go:** Late spring through early fall for riding—but if you're into crowds, bring camping gear or rent a van and arrive days early to secure a site to watch the Tour. **It's Most Fun If You're This Fit:** With an average grade of only about 8 percent, this Alp isn't crushing—it's the storied battles between pros that give it notoriety. If you're not trying to race up it at 15 mph, even a moderately fit recreational rider should enjoy summiting. **Get There With:** Discover France (discoverfrance.com).

Napa & Sonoma Valleys

Perhaps because pasta, the cornerstone of the cycling diet, virtually demands to be enjoyed with wine, these adjacent wine-country regions in northern California have become synonymous with good riding—so much so that if you live in the U.S. you might be surprised at how popular our native vineyards have become with foreign cyclists. Napa and Sonoma are not merely local favorites; they're legitimate international must-rides. The varied terrain can satisfy everyone from the flat-seeking novice to the hard-core hammerhead. The roads are lightly traveled. The cuisine maintains its gourmet appeal while ranging in price from cheap basics to outrageously expensive feasts. And there's a wine tasting, it seems, on every mile. **Best Time to Go:** Anytime—that's the beauty of it. **It's Most Fun If You're This Fit:** With the variety of terrain available, readiness to eat and drink is more important than cycling preparedness. Climbs such as Spring Mountain, Skagg's Springs and Oakville Grade will turn sinewy steel bands of muscle into tapioca. West Dry Creek Road, River Road and Silverado Trail are relaxing rambles. **Get There With:** Backroads California wine-country tours (backroads.com).

Moab

The iconic status of this small town in Utah can be explained in one word: slickrock. Cyclists can do things on slickrock that they just can't do anywhere else. The traction is so great that even neophytes can scale walls, bomb down chutes, and thread through sections too technical to walk. The challenges are so great in both scale and in number, and the chance of riding them so real, that it's not uncommon for riders to experience quantum leaps in their skill levels on a single ride. At the same time, cleaning the entire Slickrock Trail is an accomplishment held in high regard around the world. And the stakes are high—and real. Getting lost on Porcupine Rim and dabbing on Negro Bill Canyon have resulted in fatalities. **Best Time to Go:** Spring and fall. The annual Fat Tyre Festival is usually held at the end of October. **It's Most Fun If You're This Fit:** Expect only expert riders to handle everything, but novices will find plenty to keep them motivated. **Get There With:** Rim Tours (rimtours.com).

Bormio

This northern Italian hamlet lies at the core of a trio of legendary climbs, the Gavia, Stelvio and Mortirolo Passes. The Gavia is where, in 1988, Andy Hampsten battled a fierce snowstorm on his way to winning the Giro d'Italia. The treacherous south side was mostly dirt back then, but it's now paved, with a tunnel circumventing the most dangerous section. The plateau on top of the pass was the scene of the fierce fighting in WWI described in Ernest Hemingway's *A Farewell to Arms*. Among European cyclists, the Stelvio, Europe's third-highest continuously paved pass, ranks as the most popular Alpine ascent. It's not the most difficult, but the 48 numbered switchbacks plastered on its improbable-looking north side make it unique. On top, you can purchase a certificate commemorating your ascent and get your picture taken next to the Fausto Coppi memorial. The savage Mortirolo rises 4,000 feet in 7 miles—an average gradient of over 10 percent. **Best Time to Go:** The high passes are clear only in the summer months. **It's Most Fun If**

You're This Fit: Mountain goats only—or those as stubborn as goats. **Get There With:** Granfondo Cycling Tours (granfondoracingtours.com).

EIGHT GREAT FOREIGN CITIES TO VISIT BY BIKE

The next time your travels take you to one of these urban destinations, the best way to get around might be on two wheels.

Amsterdam, The Netherlands

The Netherlands is the Promised Land for cyclists, with flat roads, more than 300 miles of bike paths and lanes, bicycle-only tunnels and bridges, and underground bike parking. It's no wonder that 37 percent of all trips there are made by bike. Another great reason to pedal: the *frites*, or French fries—served in a paper cone with mayonnaise—are to die for.

Copenhagen, Denmark

Perhaps the only major city to rival Amsterdam in terms of the extent to which bikes permeate everyday life, Copenhagen is known, among other nicknames, as "the city of bikes." According to city stats, 36 percent of residents commute by bike daily (only 27 percent drive). And tourists get a free ride: Deposit a 20-kroner ($4) coin into one of the 125 city bike-parking racks to unlock a bike and explore the compact city bike zone, which includes the National Museum, Strøget shopping district, Amalienborg Palace and hippie enclave Christiana town. When you lock the bike at a rack, you get your coin back.

Melbourne, Australia

Follow Melbourne's Capital City Trail, which showcases a dozen areas of interest over 20 miles. The trail travels through a park that creates a circle around the city center, which keeps cyclists away from cars. Each stop on the trail could easily take up a day; Southbank, for instance, is the hub of Melbourne's entertainment district. Almost all streets in Melbourne have bike lanes, and those that don't will in the near future, so it's easy to find all of the city's sights on two wheels.

Montreal

Bicycling named Montreal the best cycling city in North America in 1999, and since then, conditions for cyclists have only improved in Quebec's largest city. The historic—and quintessentially Montreal—Plateau-Mont-Royal neighborhood now provides a fleet of 20 communal bicycles, free of charge, at the Mont-Royal metro station and at La Capitale. Each bike even comes with a VIP card offering special discounts at dozens of businesses on Mont-Royal Avenue.

Bogotá, Colombia

Bad news first: Colombia remains on the U.S. Department of State's list of dangerous countries for tourists. Most of the danger there, however, is limited to rural areas. According to travel.state.gov, "Violence has continued to decrease markedly in most urban areas, including Bogotá"—so don't let it stop you from pedaling one of the most extensive bike-path systems in the world. The 188-mile network stretches from north to south, east to west, allowing tourists easy access to the city's museums, art galleries, monuments, churches and restaurants.

Paris

Do as the French, and join Le Velorution, the bike revolution. Since July 2007, 1,450 bike-rental stations have popped up throughout the city as part of the community bike program Vélib—that's one station every 250 yards. The program logged 2 million trips in its first 40 days. Rental rates encourage short trips (the first 30 minutes are free), so if you stop to visit a museum or snap photos, return your bike to a station and grab a new one when you finish. Paris boasts 195 miles of bike lanes, so nearly the entire city is safely accessible on a bicycle.

Barcelona, Spain

The city introduced Bicing, a community bicycle program, in March 2007, placing 1,500 rental bikes at 25 stations. Now, with 3,000 bikes at nearly 200 stations, Bicing has 100,000 subscribers who use the bikes for short trips around the downtown center. While the official line is that Bicing is for locals, not visitors, you can register on the program's website for a week-long pass (bicing.com). To reach some of the most spectacular spots outside the city center, such as the Gaudi-designed wonderland Parc Guell, you should rent a bike.

Berlin

Starting in the city center, 12 bike routes radiate out in a star-shaped network linked by eight circular routes, with new paths continually being planned and built. Visitors can pick up bikes at one of the numerous rental offices across the city and pick up maps with directions to museums, restaurants and parks. The Traffic Management Centre's online route planner makes navigating Berlin by bike even easier (vmzberlin.de). Plug in your start and end addresses and it will generate several possible biking routes.

RIDER **RESOURCES**

The Adventure Cycling Association (adventurecycling.org) offers tours all over the United States as well as an extensive collection of routes, maps and other resources for cyclists.

Find a frequently updated list of airline bike policies on the International Bicycle Fund's website (ibike.org). To increase the chance that your bike will be accepted as a regular checked bag, check out sandsmachine.com. The company, which makes couplings that let you easily take apart your frame, keeps a list of builders who stock coupling-equipped bikes and/or perform retrofits.

Read about *Bicycling's* favorite 50 U.S. cities at bicycling.com/topbikefriendlycities.

The site crazyguyonabike.com boasts more than 4,000 rider-submitted travel journals—and more than half a million photos. You can read about others' trips and get travel tips.

PART

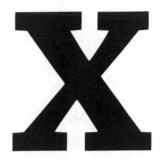

Getting Dirty: Riding Off-Road

WHETHER YOU'RE JUST GETTING STARTED ON DIRT or want to learn how to rail berms like the pros, our experts will help you become a better mountain biker. For tips on buying a bike, see Chapter 2.

CHAPTER 29

From Roadie to Mountain Biker

There's a lot to be said for taking your bike off the pavement and into the woods every once in awhile. You don't have to worry about cars—although you might encounter a kamikaze chipmunk. You'll develop power and handling skills that can translate to your road riding. And if you're a guy, you won't ever be pressured to shave your legs. To help you make the transition, Selene Yeager offers tips on thinking like a trail rider, while Alex Stieda demystifies the sport of cyclocross.

GET OFF-ROAD READY

As cyclists begin racking their road bikes in the fall and heading for the trails, they carry with them the notion that pushing fat tires up technical terrain is harder work than gliding across smooth pavement on skinnies. But "it's a misconception that the mountain is harder than the road," says Dean Golich, a Carmichael Training Systems coach. "Mountain bikes just go up more unforgiving terrain that slows you down and forces you to work a different way. If you try to ride the mountain like you do the road, you'll end up miserable." Here are Golich's off-road-riding tips.

RIDE ACCORDINGLY. While roads are graded to accommodate vehicles, nature's climbs can go straight up. And unlike road riding, off-road downhills tend to be technical, so they don't offer much recovery, says Golich. "People are so shattered by the time they get to the top, they end up crashing on the descents because they're too fatigued to concentrate and hold on," he says. Instead of muscling up climbs, spin and meter out your effort just as you would on the road. If your legs are burning and you are gasping, you're going too hard.

PRACTICE FOR POWER. Though you should hold a steady pace, there will be times when you need to power through a technical section or up a steep pitch. These little surges can wear you out if you're not conditioned for them. If you know you'll be doing long, technical rides, do big-gear intervals, where you practice surging in a difficult gear for 15 to 30 seconds. Do that about 10 times with three to five minutes' recovery between each surge to get used to the accelerations. Practice often.

RELAX—FROM HEAD TO TOE. Some scenarios in mountain biking require more energy than you think, such as crouching over the saddle and bracing the bike over rough terrain. "Don't waste more energy by putting a death grip on the handlebar or tensing up your arms and legs," says Golich. That not only saps you, but it also makes the bike harder to control. Practice progressive relaxation, where you loosen your hands, then arms, shoulders, and all the way down through your legs.

PLAN YOUR MOVE. Off-road riding is like a game of chess: You have to look three steps ahead if you don't want to get checked. On the trail, "you must keep your head up and [your eyes focused on] where you want to go instead of on the obstacles right in front of your wheel," says Golich. For difficult sections, get off your bike and scout ahead to get a sense of the best lines.

STRENGTHEN YOUR CORE. Though Golich is no fan of weight workouts for pro cyclists, he does acknowledge that a strong core is important for general health and fitness. It will also make you less prone to injury as well as a stronger rider. Go to bicycling.com/fitcore for a cycling-specific core workout that includes planks, hip bridges and more.

CYCLOCROSS: THE GATEWAY MUD

Ah, cyclocross: the sport where roadies and mountain bikers meet. Held during the fall and winter, 'cross events usually take place on a closed, mostly grass circuit of 1 to 3 miles. Race distances vary by skill category, with the best riders usually racing for an hour. Courses include barriers such as wooden hurdles and sand pits, which force racers to dismount their bikes. Rowdy spectators, cowbells and beer hand-ups are all encouraged. To find local 'cross races, check the website of your state's cycling association or ask at bike shops. Once you've taken the plunge and signed up, here's what you need to know.

GEAR UP. Serious 'cross riders will ride purpose-built bikes with wider, knobby road tires and an open frame to help shoulder the bike. However, some events allow first-timers to use mountain bikes.

HOP OFF. When an obstacle forces you off the bike, always dismount on the left side, opposite the chain. As you approach the barrier, coast with your left pedal down, unclip the right foot [A] and swing it over the bike [B]. As you get close to the dismount point, brake gently, place your right foot on the ground [C] and unclip your left foot. You should do all this without stopping, which will allow you to maintain your momentum as you lift your bike over the obstacle.

CARRY ON. As you dismount, you should have your left hand on the handlebar and the right one on the top tube [D], so you can easily lift

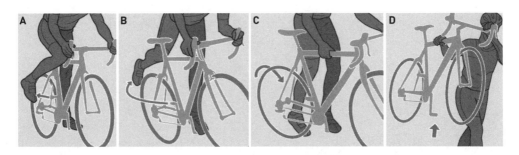

the frame and run over the obstacle. On long climbs that you can't ride, carry the bike on your right shoulder. This is why you dismount on the left, so the drivetrain won't dig into you as you hoist the bike.

SADDLE UP. Remounting the bike on the fly is tricky, but once you learn, it's a beautiful thing. Ask for hands-on advice at your club or shop, or go to bicycling.com/howtocross for a tutorial.

TAKE IT SLOW(ER). Feeling your tires slide on a loose surface can be unnerving, but over time you'll learn how to correct your braking and steering. Squeeze both brakes when descending a steep pitch, the rear brake while slowing in a corner and the front brake while dismounting.

GO DOWN GRACEFULLY. At some point, you will crash—but because you'll usually be on a soft surface, you should be fine. In fact, 'cross presents a great opportunity to learn to roll with the fall and lessen the impact. Plus, as you hone your cyclocross skills, you'll also become a better road rider.

CHAPTER 30

Mountain Biking Essentials

Learn how to climb, descend, turn and tackle obstacles with confidence—along with first-aid tips to use when things go south. Then find out how to help make sure your favorite mountain bike playground stays open.

CLEARING LOGS— BIG AND SMALL

It takes two seconds to ride over a log. It takes 10 more to slow down, stop, dismount, swear, drag your bike over the obstacle, remount and catch your friends who have vanished around the bend. With the right technique, you can clear logs faster than a real estate developer and keep sailing down the trail. "It's all about maintaining momentum," says professional freerider and mountain bike coach Jay Hoots, of British Columbia, who offers clinics and instruction through Hoots Inc. (hoots.ca). Here's what he recommends.

Practice in Your 'Hood

CLEAR CURBS. You won't clear a twig if you can't control your front wheel. "You need to be able to lift your front wheel onto the obstacle you're trying to clear," says Hoots. The easiest place to hone your skills is on a curb, because you can practice lifting without worrying about what's on the other side. Here's how: Roll toward a curb. When you're a few feet away, stand on level pedals, keeping your elbows and knees slightly bent and ready for action. When you're almost there (within about a foot), compress the front end and immediately pull up on the bar to place the wheel onto the curb.

HIT THE PARKING LOT. Lifting the rear wheel is where most riders fizzle, because it feels unnatural at first. In a deserted parking lot, practice by lifting back and up with your feet as you thrust your shoulders forward. "The motion is similar to an eagle swooping down and grabbing a fish in its talons," says Hoots. Your feet come around the pedal stroke, "grab" the pedals, and kick back to lift the rear end. "Don't do the 'humper pumper move' and try to pump just your hips down to generate the lift," cautions Hoots. "All that does is force your body weight down into the bike instead of up and over the obstacles."

Take Your Skills to the Trail

PUSH THE FRONT OVER. This step happens simultaneously with the next, but it's important not to skip it if you don't want to take a trip over your bar. Using your curb-jumping technique, pull your front wheel up and onto the log. When your front wheel starts to roll over the top of the log, push through with your bar—with your butt back and hovering over the saddle—to keep your momentum moving forward. Do not touch your brakes—it'll wreck your momentum.

PULL UP THE REAR. You will bash your chainring into the log a few times as you practice lifting the back end. Just keep pedaling and pushing the bike forward as you normally would, and you'll be able to dig in and ratchet up and over the log without stalling out. Remember to keep your weight centered as you bring up the rear to avoid going over the bar. Follow through once you've made it over. If you stop mid-log, you'll tip over.

Two Helpful Tips

SEE YOUR FUTURE. Look ahead to where you want your front tire to go, not down at the log. The bigger the logs get, the more important this tip is.

LEARN TO FLY. As you become more comfortable rolling over logs, you can graduate to jumping them. The motion is the same, but instead of lifting the front tire onto the log, aim to clear it. Then push forward and out, and lift with the rear as before. "When you get

good at that, you can clear any obstacle at any speed without losing momentum," says Hoots.

BLAST UPHILL OBSTACLES

If you want to learn to climb technical terrain—fast—just get on Georgia Gould's wheel. Or try to, anyway. In 2007, Gould became the second woman ever (Juli Furtado was the first) to sweep the National Mountain Bike Series, often by blasting the competition right from the start. Simply put, Gould is fast, regardless of the terrain. And chances are, it's because she's so aware of what it takes to climb well: practice. "I still have things I work on," Gould says, "and I think I always will. It's part of growing as a rider."

If you're interested in growing your uphill-riding prowess, follow Gould's advice for tackling the technical sections that often bring hard-charging climbers to a halt...as well as the best way to restart if you do get stalled on a climb. If it works for Gould, it's gotta be gold.

ROLL OVER ROCKS. On rock-strewn climbs, shift into a harder gear. It will prevent you from spinning out, and provide extra power for clearing bigger obstacles, says Gould. "Plus," she says, "it boosts your speed, which keeps you from getting snagged on smaller stuff." The downside: The increased effort will spike your heart rate, making it tough to sustain for long periods. When the trail smoothes out, spin in an easier gear to ease your suffering.

LOFT OVER LOGS. The trick here, says Gould, is learning to throw your bike forward. "I get my front wheel on top of the log first," she says, "and then push my momentum into the bike to get it over." Start from a seated position (again, in a big gear). As you approach the log, give your forward pedal a stab and lean back quickly but slightly to pull the wheel into the air and onto the log. As the front wheel hits, stand on the pedals as you push the bike forward with your hands and let the saddle move forward under you. The front wheel should just touch the log before proceeding; you'll end up over the log, pedaling from a standing position, slightly behind the saddle.

GROOVE OVER GRAVEL. Use that same harder gear, but position your weight on the rear so it doesn't slip while keeping enough weight on the front that it doesn't wander. "I move forward on the saddle and drop my torso so I'm closer to the bar," Gould says. "You end up in this perched position that's halfway between seated and standing; it lets you keep pushing the pedals and still shift your weight."

START OVER MID-CLIMB. So you had to put a foot down, and now you're trying to get going again. Keep it simple: Without changing gears, point the bike up the trail, sit on the saddle, clip one foot in for that first powerful stroke up, and go for it. Don't start from standing, and don't worry about clipping in the other foot. "If you're standing, there's a good chance you'll just spin out when you try to start," says Gould. As

for the unclipped foot? "I don't even worry about it until I'm back in a rhythm and climbing smoothly."

Pro **Tip**

"YOU NEED TO COMMIT COMPLETELY TO WHAT YOU'RE DOING ON THE TRAIL. IF YOU HAVE ANY DOUBTS, THAT NEW JUMP OR ROCK SECTION PROBABLY ISN'T GOING TO WORK OUT FOR THE BEST."—*SAM HILL, 2007 AND 2009 WORLD CUP DOWNHILL CHAMPION*

RAIL A BERM

If you went to the circus as a kid, you probably remember the Cage of Death, where a team of motorcycle riders would zoom around the inside of a metal sphere just inches from a brave—and, of course, scantily clad—female assistant. Thanks to speed, the motorcycles stayed glued to the sides of the cage.

High-banked turns bring the same basic principle to mountain biking—though in most cases, without the assistant. If you have the right form and adequate speed, inertia will push your tires into the dirt so forcefully that the bike doesn't slide out, even when you lean way into the turn. Here's how to get started.

LOOK, THEN LEAN. Study the berm's graceful arc before hitting it at speed. First, check the angle and height of the bank: The steeper it is, the more you can lean—your bike should be perpendicular to the bank—and the faster you can go. Next, find the grooved track where experienced riders have ridden the fastest line; that's the one you want to hit. Note how that line winds through the berm (a constant arc, low entrance/high exit or high entrance/low exit) so you know where to go.

MOVE YOUR FINGERS. With your body in a ready-to-attack position (standing on the pedals with cranks level, knees slightly bent; arms bent, elbows up and out; eyes looking ahead), enter the berm. Force yourself to move your fingers off the brake levers and onto your bar, and keep them there until you exit.

LEAD WITH YOUR ELBOW. Don't stare at your front wheel or even at the apex of the turn—look ahead to the exit and you'll find it easier to stay on course. At the same time, be sure to keep your outside elbow (if it's a left turn, this is your right elbow) up and out. Focus on leading with that elbow as you lean into the berm. If the berm isn't as smooth as you thought, drop your outside pedal and put more weight into it to dig your tires in even more.

STEP ON THE GAS. Berms are all about speed. Go slowly and you'll be forced to the bottom of the berm, where you can't make use of the bank. Go faster, however, and your tires will drive into the more-vertical surface as you lean in— you'll have phenomenal traction, and you'll gain speed because the berm will do the work of turning. On well-groomed, high-banked berms, you can ride ridiculously fast and still have an insane amount of traction.

PUMP IT UP. Once you get the hang of railing a berm with sheer speed, try pumping your bike through the turn to go even faster. As you approach the apex, lean forward and get lower on the bike. As you go through the apex, push the bar down and into your palms and extend your legs slightly. You'll move back on the bike somewhat as it scoots ahead to the exit. Zoom!

Fun Fact

There are two indoor mountain bike parks in the U.S.: Boulder Indoor Cycling (boulderindoorcycling.com) in Boulder, Colorado, and Ray's Indoor Mountain Bike Park (raysmtb.com) in Cleveland, Ohio.

DESCEND TRICKY SWITCHBACKS

Speed is second nature to rider Ryan Trebon: The 6-foot-5 Oregonian wore a stars-and-stripes National Champion's jersey three years in a row (in '06, it was for XC and cyclocross; in '07, short track; in '08, cyclocross). What may not be obvious is the amount of thought that goes into that speed, especially on tight, technical downhill switchbacks. "They're probably the most challenging thing for me to ride, simply because of my size," Trebon says. "My center of gravity is so high and the bike is so long that it makes negotiating them more difficult." The good news is that Trebon has spent plenty of time figuring out the best way to twist through those problem corners—and he's willing to share his hard-won knowledge. Here's his advice for tackling tight, tricky downhill turns.

PREPARE TO TURN. As you approach the turn, stand, level the cranks and move your weight behind the seat. If you need to brake, now's the time—during the turn, hard braking means less control overall. As for speed: "There's a fine line between going too slow and going too fast," says Trebon. "Many people, if they're apprehensive, make the mistake of going too slow. It's better to have a little speed."

AIM WIDE. Shoot for the outside line as you get closer to the turn, and ride that edge as you make the turn; as you exit, head back toward the center of the trail. "If you use the whole trail as you head into the turn," Trebon explains, "you basically make the turn longer and straighten it out a little more." He compares it to a semi truck making a 90-degree turn—cut it too soon, and the semi bangs into the curb

and all sorts of bad things happen. But ride the outside edge of the turn to its midpoint, and you get through with no problems.

KEEP YOUR EYE ON THE PRIZE. It's important to look where you want to go and not focus solely on what your front tire is encountering at every instant. But the outside edge of a switchback turn tends to collect a lot of debris, so you need to keep track of where you're rolling, too. Plus, Trebon explains, looking ahead will keep your front tire rolling along the outside edge of the trail, instead of rolling off the trail completely.

USE YOUR BODY. If things are especially tight and technical, a little body English might help you get through. "If there isn't much space on the trail, give your bike a hip check to slide the rear wheel around," Trebon explains. "I know this isn't what IMBA would want you to do, but it works—especially when you're racing." Sometimes the truth hurts, even if it helps.

Two Shifting Tips for Mountain Bikers

The Situation: A moderately steep, twisty, rocky descent on your mountain bike; the trail ends smoothly before transitioning to a long climb.

The Shift: This is a heavy shifting situation. On the way down the slope, you'll want to shift around to stay on the harder-geared side of your comfort zone, so you can power out of corners and over most obstacles. (But don't stray too far—if you get hung up on something, you'll want to be in a gear you can manage at a slower pace.) During the transition, soft pedal and shift to the lower gear you'll need to start the climb—you want to be in your comfort zone at the beginning of the uphill.

The Situation: You face a rock-strewn technical climb on your mountain bike.

The Shift: Use too low a gear on a loose, technical climb and you'll spin the rear wheel, lose momentum, and come to a halt. To avoid that, climb in a slightly higher-than-comfort-level gear, which helps the rear tire grip the terrain and gives you leeway for the short power bursts needed to ascend larger rocks or log step-ups. Don't expect to reach the top of the climb without feeling your muscles burn—in a good way, of course.

HOW TO FALL—OR NOT

Cyclists crash. We endo on logs, lose control in gravel and tip over while peering at steep descents, much to the amusement of our riding friends. Here's how to bail safely—and prevent such incidents in the first place.

LOOK AHEAD. If you focus on a rock or tree you'd like to avoid, chances are you'll hit it. Instead, look where you want to go. If you're threading the needle between rocks, look directly where you want your wheels to be.

STAY LOOSE. You don't want to tense up and lock your joints. Go with the flow as the bike hops and jerks. You might just ride it out. If not, you'll be relaxed and ready to curl up fast before touchdown.

PREP THE PEDALS. If you're riding a challenging trail, set clipless pedals loose (if possible), mostly so you won't stress about your escape. It's a natural reaction to swing your feet out when you're falling, so disengagement won't be a problem as long as you anticipate your crash and commit to it, rather than try to hang on too long.

STAY STABLE. For a slow-speed or uphill bail, stand to separate your body from the bike and click out a foot (on slanted slopes, use your uphill foot), planting it wide, so that your leg and the bike's two wheels form a stable tripod.

HANG ON. Often when falling, you'll want to push the bike away from you with your hands and feet, preferably in the opposite direction of where your body is going. But for sideways falls, hang on to the handlebar and try to let the bar end hit first to absorb some force, and round your body as you roll.

HEAL THY FRIEND

The last thing we want to think about is an injured riding buddy, but better to do so now than to try and figure out what to do after an accident happens. "It's a preparation issue," says Patrick Brighton, MD, a surgeon, author of *Mountain Bikers' Guide for Treating Medical Emergencies*, and former EcoChallenge competitor. "Know what to do, carry a few supplies, and you'll be able to help." Here's Brighton's advice for handling a trifecta of common cycling injuries—plus what to do if things get serious.

Broken Wrist

Your wrists are fragile, so sticking your hands out when you get pitched often results in a break. "It's obvious when a wrist is broken," says Brighton. "It hurts like the dickens, swells immediately and you lose hand function—you can wiggle your fingers, but not much else."

What to Do: Wrap a minipump in a jersey or some socks, place it against the forearm so it extends from the middle of the palm across the injured wrist and up the arm, and duct tape it into place. Gently stuff the injured arm into the rider's zipped-down jersey to keep it from moving. "Don't wrap the wrist too tight," warns Brighton, "or the tape could cut off the circulation as the wrist swells." Another option: Empty

The Mountain Biker's Med Kit

Make your own first-aid kit. Wrap 10 to 12 feet of duct tape around the outside of a 12-ounce MiniGrip Nalgene bottle with loop-top closure (fold the end of the tape over so it's easy to unroll when you need it), and put the following into the bottle: topical antibiotic or cleansing solution (such as betadyne; also available in handy swabs), gauze pads, gauze wrap (such as Curlex or Kling), a small container of hand sanitizer (such as Purell) and ibuprofen. Carry this with you, along with a cell phone, whenever you ride.

a hydration pack of its contents, wrap the pack around the injured part, and tape it into place. Then get to a doctor.

Broken Collarbone

The same force that snaps your wrist can also break your collarbone. Obvious signs of a clavicle fracture: swelling at the site of the break, and pain when the arm is moved.

What to Do: Stabilize the arm. Fashion a jersey into a sling, or use duct tape: Bend the elbow at 90 degrees, place the arm against the body, then tape it into place so it doesn't move. Wrap the tape diagonally from the hip, over the forearm, across the body in back, then underneath and back in front. Always stick the tape to itself; if you use small pieces on sweaty skin, the tape will slide off eventually. If you have enough tape, wrap the upper arm also, or do another loop around the body closer to the wrist. Wrap until you run out of tape.

Dislocated Shoulder

The force of a fall can wrench your shoulder out of joint, particularly if you've dislocated it before. Signs of a dislocation: searing pain and a grotesque bump where the ball at the top of your humerus (the upper arm bone) is out of place.

What to Do: If help is far away, make at least one attempt to pop the sucker back into place. Have your friend lie facedown on a big rock, "so his injured arm hangs freely," says Brighton. "Then pull down on the arm with gentle but incremental pressure." Be warned: "If it's a muscular guy, it could take a lot of pressure," says Brighton, "and the sound of it popping back into place is sickening." Once the shoulder is back in place (or if you can't get it back in), stabilize the arm the same way as for a clavicle fracture, and walk to where you can get help.

The Big Kahuna

If someone is knocked unconscious or complains of neck or back pain after a crash, do not move him—he could have a serious spine injury. After you stop any bleeding and make sure the injured rider is breathing, make him comfortable—drape extra clothing over him to keep him warm, offer some water—but do not allow him to move. "You need to call in the cavalry," says Brighton. Use your cell phone to call

9-1-1. No reception? If it's just the two of you, you'll have to leave your friend and get help. "All you do by waiting is worsen the victim's chances," says Brighton. "Make him comfortable, then get your butt to a phone as fast as you can."

Reader **Tip**

"NEVER UNDERESTIMATE THE BUNGEE CORD ON YOUR HYDRATION PACK. AFTER CRASHING IN THE WOODS AND BREAKING BOTH BONES IN MY LOWER LEG, I USED IT AND TWO BRANCHES TO MAKE A SPLINT. I WAS ABLE TO GET OUT AND FIND HELP ON MY OWN."—*PAUL PORTNOY, MASSACHUSETTS*

RIDE AT NIGHT

Be willing to take your mountain bike out when it's dark, and you'll gain hours of riding time. You'll be ready if your friends ask you to join their team for a 24-hour race. And riding at night might even make you braver: It's hard to fear an obstacle you can't see.

To help you navigate the murkiness, we turned to Mark Hendershot. He's a man of many talents: organic farmer, floor-covering expert, pedicab business owner. But where the 46-year-old Grand Rapids, Michigan, native truly excels is on the racecourse—especially the 24-hour kind. Over the past decade, Hendershot's been a consistent podium finisher in the World and National Solo 24 Hour Championships, effectively scratching out a place among the elite of the endurance world. His secrets? Confidence—and quality lights.

"When I first started, the equipment was junk," he says. "It was a common occurrence for your lights to go out on the trail." Today's high-end lights have all but relegated sudden darkness to the history books. The key to successful night rides now, Hendershot says, is knowing how to use your lights—and your head.

SET YOUR LIGHT RIGHT. The ideal light setup combines a helmet-mounted spotlight and a bar-mounted unit with a broad-coverage beam. But if you can afford only one, a helmet-mounted light is better because it directs the light where you are looking. Mount it close to the center-top of your helmet. "The higher you put it, the more stable it's going to be," says Hendershot, "which means it won't fatigue your neck as much over the course of the ride."

LOOK WHERE YOU WANT TO GO. Your light—like your bike—is going to follow your eyes, so look ahead, not down. "Your helmet light should be aimed at least eight feet ahead," says Hendershot. The final adjustments depend on the condition of the trail you're riding—which you should plan for well in advance. A first-timer? Stick to a trail you know like the back of your hand so you can test your night vision on known obstacles and corners.

LIGHTS AND ARM WARMERS GO TOGETHER. A good cold-weather rule: If you need lights to ride, wear arm warmers. "Temperatures can fall rapidly at night," says Hendershot. "And when you're shivering you burn more calories—and on a ride every calorie counts." Hendershot sticks with arm warmers because they're easy to remove, but in the fall, leg warmers and a vest aren't a bad idea, either.

KEEP YOUR PERSPECTIVE. Artificial light sources create shadows that skew your perspective on obstacles. Two keys to success in technical situations: knowing about the weird shadows, and saving your highest light-output setting for when things get rough. "The switch to high will give you more confidence," says Hendershot. "You'll think, 'This is great!' even if the difference is minimal."

BE CONFIDENT—AND DAYDREAM. Night-riding success comes down to confidence and a good attitude. "If you think you can do it, then you'll do it," says Hendershot. "That's the most important thing. You need to stay positive and think about fun things. I think about sex and tattoo designs. For me, that just works."

GIVING BACK: ORGANIZING A SUCCESSFUL TRAIL DAY

Once you've got the mountain biking bug, consider helping spruce up the trails that got you hooked. Showing that you're invested in taking care of the local singletrack goes a long way toward helping keep trails open—and getting permission for new ones.

As a veteran of the International Mountain Bicycling Association (IMBA)'s Trail Care Crew and the association's current field programs manager, Ryan Schutz knows something about planning a successful trail-maintenance day. So what's the secret? "You've got to make it sound fun," he says. "That's just good marketing."

Of course, there's more to trail maintenance than smart PR. Being a member of a local club is key: Joining those like-minded folks will give you the resources to back up your desire. Already a member? Here's how to make sure your next trail day is a hit.

PLAN WAY, WAY AHEAD. Picking a project is the easy part. The hard part is keeping people busy and happy. To do that, you need to plan for all kinds of contingencies: How will the day go if five people show up? What if 50 show up? How will you keep them all busy? Are there enough tools? Who will help you oversee the work? Who's bringing the food, water, entertainment and postwork beverages? Remember, your job isn't just to get the work done. It's also to make people feel welcome, appreciated and rewarded. And you need a plan for doing all of these before you set a date for the trail day.

REACH NEW PEOPLE. Inviting club members is a no-brainer. But you can expand your work crew, and potentially your club's membership, by plastering the local bike shops and biker hangout spots (coffee joints are a good choice) with fliers that tout the fun part of your plans as much as, if not more than, the work.

KNOW YOUR TOOLS. Bare-minimum requirements: handsaws, a Pulaski (an axe/wide pickaxe combo) and a McLeod (a rake/hoe combo). These tools can be hard to find. Look online or at a local hardware store that carries backcountry-firefighter supplies. Other tools to bring: metal leaf rakes, loppers and a peavey if you anticipate needing to move large logs. Bring as many tools as you can, and make sure everything's sharp. "Sharp tools make work easier," says Schutz.

KEEP IT SHORT. Keep your workday to four hours or less, so that you're done before people get tired and grouchy. And make sure everyone moves out together. "There's always the 'trail cult' few who want to do more," Schutz says. "And they should be able to go back, but not until everybody has left. If they just keep working,

other people either stay with them when they really don't want to, and never return—or they'll leave and feel guilty and never come back. You need to avoid creating that pressure."

PUBLICIZE YOUR WORK. Take some before and after photos, then post them on the club's website, along with a short write-up of the group's achievements. "That gets people excited about the club," Schutz explains. "And that's how you get even more people involved."

RIDER **RESOURCES**

IMBA (imba.org) works insanely hard to make sure that we'll always have places to mountain bike.

The Trek Dirt Series (dirtseries.com) offers co-ed and women's weekend-long mountain biking camps in Canada and the western United States.

Trips for Kids (tripsforkids.org) has helped more than 60,000 disadvantaged children in the United States, Canada and Israel get on two wheels, through earn-a-bike programs and organized mountain bike rides.

Cyclocross Magazine (cxmagazine.com) is a great source for all things related to the skinny-knobby sport.

XI

How to Raise a Cyclist

BY NOW, SURELY YOU'VE HEARD THE WARNINGS: KIDS are fatter than ever before. The rate of diabetes is skyrocketing. Some experts speculate that the current generation of children could be the first not to outlive their parents.

As a parent, you probably can't stop your kids from trading their carrots for cupcakes in the cafeteria. But you can make sure they get enough exercise. Also, riding bikes around town is a great opportunity to educate kids on the rules of the road long before they're eligible for a driver's license. And it's simply a ton of fun—for the entire family.

CHAPTER 31

It Starts with a Bike

Buying a kid a bike can be tricky—kids grow; bikes don't. And even ardent cyclists can be confounded by the world of junior bicycles, where size refers to wheel diameter instead of frame dimensions, and choosing the right bike often means measuring a child's enthusiasm and coordination along with his or her inseam. Fortunately, with some guidance it's easy to pick the bike that will get your kid hooked on cycling.

GET THE RIGHT BIKE. "Fit" is a broader concept on a kid's bike than it is on an adult bike, but it's still critical. Unless your shop offers a "swap it if it doesn't fit" guarantee, you're better off bringing the kid along to try out a few machines. Sure, this takes away the element of surprise, but you'll get to hear firsthand which bike is coolest, and you won't end up surprising him with a bike he doesn't like.

FIND A REPUTABLE SHOP. Buy at a big-box store or a neighbor's yard sale, and your inner voice will say, "Boy, I saved a boatload of dough." But you walk away with no guarantees, and you may end up spending more money in the long run to fix an unsafe and poorly built or maintained bike. Buy at a bike shop, and your inner voice will say, "I'm glad she's safe and that the bike is put together well." Because you bought at a shop, you get professional help, someone to turn to if you have questions—even if it's a year later—and, most important, peace of mind.

SIZE UP YOUR KID. Though there are guidelines for proper fit, remember that these are kids, and the rules must be bent slightly for each individual child. For example, if your three-year-old is bigger and more coordinated than her friends, she'll likely do better on a larger bike. But if your six-year-old is small, uncoordinated or timid, opt for a smaller bike that he can easily control. Kids' bikes are measured by wheel size: 14-, 16-, 20- and 24-inch. Choose one that allows plenty of stand-over room without forcing your child to be too stretched or hunched.

DON'T GROW INTO IT. It's tempting to buy a bike that's too big so the child can grow into it. With adjustable handlebars and saddles, it can work (within reason), especially on bikes smaller than the 20-inch size. But here's the problem:

Celeb Cyclist

"The first bike I ever bought—with my babysitting money—was a bright orange Schwinn."—FASHION DESIGNER CYNTHIA ROWLEY, WHO'S CREATED HER OWN LINE OF BEACH CRUISERS

Too-big bikes are hard to control, making it more likely that Junior will crash. Always remember the keys to small-fry fit: being able to easily put both feet on the ground, and being able to turn without reaching uncomfortably far. If the larger bike lets your child accomplish both, then go for it. If not, the bike is too big.

BUY QUALITY. Most kids' bikes are inexpensive, but some are cheap and prone to breaking. Quality bikes have serviceable bearings instead of bushings; wheels with spokes and nipples instead of one-piece wheels; plastic, not sharp metal, fenders; and at least a rear hand brake—it will come in handy when his feet slip off the pedals and he still needs to stop.

DON'T FORGET THE HELMET. Choose a CPSC-, ASTM-, or Snell-certified helmet for your child to wear. (To help get them excited about wearing it, let them pick the color.) A proper noggin-saver sits level, covering the forehead, straps lying flat and tight enough that you can fit just one finger between strap and chin. The helmet shouldn't tilt back to expose the forehead or slip forward to cover the eyes. If your child will be riding in a baby seat or trailer, choose a round profile—the tail of an aero-shaped helmet can hit the back of the seat and force your child's head down, leading to discomfort and meltdowns.

CHAPTER 32

Teaching Your Child to Ride

Like most cyclists, you probably remember the exhilaration and freedom of hopping on a two-wheeler and speeding off down the block as one of the most powerful and enduring memories of your childhood. Pass that glorious feeling on to your kids with these age-appropriate tips and techniques. After all, it's about more than taking off the training wheels.

1 TO 3 YEARS

If your child is old enough to support his head while wearing a helmet (at least a year old) but not coordinated enough to pedal, he can still enjoy cycling as a passenger in a trailer or baby seat.

What You Should Teach: Before the ride, put your helmet on, then help your child. Tell her she looks very grown-up, just like Mommy and Daddy. Resist the urge to extend the ride your first few times out. You want to familiarize your child with the process, not make him feel like he's being toted around. Ask him where he wants to go, and point out trees, birds and squirrels. On your first longer ride together, 90 minutes max (with stops), go to a cool destination—the park, the zoo, an ice cream stand. Build the connection that bikes take you to places that are fun.

2 TO 4 YEARS

Between the ages of two and three, kids typically start to explore riding on a tricycle. By the time they hit the halfway point of their third year, many young ones will be eager to hop on a small two-wheeler outfitted with training wheels.

What You Should Teach: Most children this age have an intuitive understanding of how to pedal, but they still need to develop their balance and body position, and the ability to steer and stop the bike. Driveway games make great skill sessions: Challenge your child to steer around small rocks, or to stop before hitting a chalk line. It's a great idea to get together with neighborhood parents and kids for a morning of fun riding at a local playground. Kids tend to learn best when simply following the example of others their size.

Talk about how everybody wrecks sometimes. Teach your kid to step over the top tube if the bike falls over (training wheels make rear dismounts tricky), as well as to tuck a shoulder and roll through a fall without sticking an arm out. Single best boo-boo saver: a pair of child-size cycling gloves.

4 TO 6 YEARS

By this age, most kids have a good sense of balance, a smooth pedaling motion and can steer with some precision. The most difficult challenges from ages four to six are mastering hand brakes and transitioning from trainers to two wheels.

What You Should Teach: Make sure your child knows how to use both coaster and hand brakes. For hand braking, show him how to squeeze the lever while keeping his eyes on the road. At first, it will take all his strength to get the brake pads to move toward the rim. As he graduates to a bike with two hand brakes, explain that the front brake provides about 75 percent of the bike's total stopping power, and should be used with greater finesse than the rear.

To wean your kid from training wheels, use this method, developed by *Bicycling*, that in our experience helps children learn to ride on their own in less time and with fewer spills than the run-beside-the-bike method most of us learned with.

Unbolt the training wheels and pedals from your child's bike and lower the saddle so that it is easy for her to sit on the saddle with both feet flat on the ground. Head to a smooth, grassy field that has a gentle downslope 30 to 50 yards in length. Be sure that it's not too steep, is wide enough to allow for unplanned weaving, and has grass short enough to allow the bike to roll freely. Before setting your young one off, walk the hill looking for holes, debris or other unexpected hazards.

Stand halfway up the hill and have your child straddle the bike with her feet on the ground while you place one hand on the handlebar and one on the back of the saddle. After a final pep talk to remind her what the brakes are for, where she should try to steer, and how to fall, have her lift her feet a few inches off the ground. Once she's ready, give her a slight push and let the bike coast down the hill. Because she's on grass, the bike isn't likely to pick up too much speed or feel out of control. If you can't resist running along, stay behind, not beside, so she can accomplish this feat on her own without distraction.

Have your child roll down the hill until she doesn't waver or fall, then replace the pedals. Have her roll down the hill with her feet on the pedals, making sure to keep them parallel to the ground. When she can coast with her feet on the pedals, have her begin to pedal slowly as she rolls down the hill, so she feels the sensation of balancing while pedaling. You'll also be able to raise her saddle to a height at which her leg is extended to roughly 80 percent of its overall length. Then try turning. And braking. And then go for a celebratory ride together. It's been a big day for both of you.

Celeb Cyclist

"When I first tried to ride a bike, my dad took me out in Riverside Park in New York City. I kept shouting, 'Hang on, Dad!' I started doing fine and he did what any dad does—and let go. I looked at him like, 'Oh, you have betrayed me.'"—JON CRYER, EMMY AWARD–WINNING ACTOR AND ENTHUSIAST TRIATHLETE

6 TO 8 YEARS

At this age, most children have developed strength, balance and fine motor skills to the point where they are capable of using hand brakes and shifting gears. They have the tools and are hungry for adventure.

What You Should Teach: Now's the time to emphasize safety and basic handling.

SAFETY FIRST. Tell your child that safety starts with a helmet, appropriate clothing—including shoes—and a well-tuned bike. Once you're rolling, safety means constantly assessing the situation, looking out for danger, and knowing the path away from it. Tell him that being safe on a bike is a process that never ends.

GET GOING. For a smooth start, have your child sit with one foot planted on the ground and the other on a pedal that is pointed toward the handlebar, roughly at the 2 o'clock position. Then he should step hard on the pedal, pull up slightly with the opposite hand, and bring his other foot up. Tell him: The key to a solid start is to keep your upper body relaxed. It keeps you from swerving as you build speed.

FLY STRAIGHT. Once your young rider is cranking down the block, the best thing for him to do is, again, relax his upper body and let the bike's gyroscopic effect help to keep it moving in a direct line.

CORNER WITH EASE. The technique is the same you use: brake first, then turn. Tell your child to slow down before the curve to the point that, once he's turning the bike, he can take pressure off the brakes completely.

Kids move in bursts and make up the rules as they go. Your rides should follow suit. But as your kids get older, you'll be able to take trail rides (Yay, jumps!) or shorter-distance charity rides. They'll enjoy the distance if they're riding for a purpose—and you'll get to share in the fun.

Pro **Tip**

"IF YOUR CHILDREN HAVE A COMPETITIVE SPIRIT, BMX RACING IS A GREAT WAY TO LET THEM LOOSE. THE SKILLS KIDS LEARN ON A BMX TRACK WILL DIRECTLY TRANSLATE TO ALL OTHER FACETS OF THE SPORT AS THEY GROW OLDER. THERE ARE RACES FOR ALL ABILITY LEVELS—CHECK WITH YOUR LOCAL BIKE STORE FOR MORE INFO."—*ALEX STIEDA*

8 TO 12 YEARS

Think back to when you were eight years old. As a third-grader, you were concerned with playground time, not with honing lifelong skills in a sport. And you turned out okay, right? Keep that in mind when it comes to cycling and your preteen child—he's focused on fun, ideally riding around with his friends. But that doesn't mean you can't help him have fun safely.

What You Should Teach: While you likely have taught your child the rules of the road by now, you should at this age hammer them home to ensure he forms safe street habits as he begins to venture on rides without you. The best advice to give: "Act like a car, but remember that cars can't see you." This will remind him to ride predictably, stay on the right side of the right-hand lane, give the right-of-way to pedestrians, always signal and obey signs and traffic lights.

As your child's sense of independence grows, you can also teach her to care for her bike by checking these areas before every ride; if something seems wrong, she should ask you for help.

BRAKES. Give the brakes a squeeze. Tell her: The levers should move freely and pop back when she lets go. She shouldn't be able to pull them all the way to the handlebar, either.

SADDLE. Check that the seat is straight and set at the right height. Make sure the seatpost is held tightly in the frame.

QUICK-RELEASES. Check that the quick-releases are closed and snug.

Fun Fact

The first Saturday in October is the International Mountain Bicycling Association's Take a Kid Mountain Biking Day.

TIRES. Give the tires a squeeze with your thumb and forefinger—they should feel solid. If one is soft, it needs air. Then give the wheel a slow spin. Check the tire for cuts or missing tread, and be sure that the brakes don't rub any part of the rim.

Here are two fun skill-building techniques for preteens.

BALANCE BEAM. Lay a 10-foot 2x6 or 2x8 flat on a grassy surface. Have your child practice pulling up on the handlebar and giving the pedals a quick stab as he leans back slightly and lofts the front tire onto the board. (The piece of wood isn't thick enough to cause any problems if your child misjudges the lift.) Then have him slowly ride the length of the board—the goal is to stay on top of the board for its entire length and then ride off the other end. As this gets easier, swap to a narrower piece of wood, or add another board at the end to double the distance.

CONE CORNERING. Tight cornering requires that you lean the bike over a bit. To help your child practice, have her weave through a line of four or five safety cones or similar objects, each spaced about 8 feet apart. As her skill improves, encourage her to go faster, or move the cones out of a straight line so that they are staggered, and she has to turn more to get around each cone.

TEEN YEARS

Teenagers and bikes were meant for each other. Teenagers have an abundance of energy, which bikes help them burn off healthfully. And bikes can give a teenager a sense of independence, especially before the appearance of a driver's license. Bikes mean freedom, and that can be hard for parents—it can be tough to accept that your teen will be doing serious rides without you.

What You Should Teach: In addition to reinforcing rules of the road, helmet safety, and other lessons you've taught, encourage your teen to go on a local shop ride, or to join a club. Organized rides are a great way for your teenager to feel some independence, yet still be influenced by other responsible cyclists. It might take a few tries before you find the right ride, but don't let your child give up. When a group clicks, it's magic. Plus, local shops and clubs are the best ways to find out about charity rides, races, mountain bike festivals or cycling-focused camps in your area.

It's also the ideal time to educate your high school or college student, for whom discretionary income may very well consist of just enough cash to buy a few boxes of macaroni and cheese, that a bike can be an effective form of transportation and a money-saving tool. The average cost of owning and operating a car is $9,369 per year, according to AAA. The average cost of owning a bicycle is just $120 per year, according to the Pedestrian and Bicycle Information Center. Also, 25 percent of all trips by car in the U.S. are less than 1 mile; 40 percent are less than 2 miles. So it's important for your young adult to have an inexpensive city bike complete with fenders, lights and some kind of rack. The most thoughtful gift a cycling parent can give? A care package of the bike's most wear-prone parts—tubes, tires, chains, lube, etc.—so your student can keep her precious bike in good riding condition.

Pro **Tip**

"MAKE IT ABOUT THE RIDE, NOT ABOUT THE LESSON. THE WORST THING YOU CAN HEAR FROM A KID IS THAT LEARNING ABOUT BIKES IS LIKE SCHOOL."—*DOUG DETWILLER, FOUNDER OF THE SPROCKIDS MOUNTAIN BIKE PROGRAM*

READING, WRITING, AND RIDING

In 1969, nearly 50 percent of students in the United States walked or biked to school, according to the advocacy group Safe Routes to School. By 2001, that figure had plummeted to 15 percent. (Is it any surprise kids are getting fatter?) While riding to school isn't always feasible, you can make your kids' journey much safer by joining them for the ride.

PEDAL TOGETHER. If your schedule allows or you can strike a deal with your boss to start early and leave early, ride with your child to school. After the drop-off, ride on to work, or ride home and drive to work. After school, if you can't pick up your child on two wheels, toss the bike into the trunk.

Why I Ride

"I can use my bike whenever I want, to go wherever I want . . . my cello case has backpack straps so I can ride my bike to lessons. Luckily, I have never wiped out because of the cello."
—KATHY KIMBALL, TEENAGE CYCLIST AND 2006 BIKETOWNER

FIND FRIENDS. Split responsibilities with other parents: One drops off, another picks up, or you can divide the days of the week. This not only shares the load, but it also creates a larger group of kids on bikes. Safety in numbers, after all.

RIDER **RESOURCES**

The National Center for Safe Routes to Schools (saferoutesinfo.org) can help you start and sustain an SRTS program in your community.

The Boltage program (boltage.org), which operates in more than a dozen schools in the U.S. and Canada, helps kids keep track of the number of times they ride to school—and offers prizes for racking up the miles.

Even the most avowed helmet-hater won't be able to resist the fun designs from Nutcase (nutcasehelmets.com).

Credits

Chapter 1: The Greatest Sport in the World
"It Helps You Have More (And Better) Sex" reprinted from "In the Mood," by Brian Fiske. Copyright 2005 by Brian Fiske.
"Okay You've Convinced Me . . . But Where Do I Find the Time?" includes material from "Find More Daylight to Ride" by Selene Yeager. Copyright 2005 by Selene Yeager.

Chapter 2: How to Buy a Bike
"The Burning Questions" reprinted from "The Burning Questions" by Brian Fiske. Copyright 2006 by Brian Fiske.
"How to Buy a Bike" reprinted from "How to Buy a Bike" by Brian Fiske. Copyright 2007 by Brian Fiske.
Pro Tip (Peter Mooney) reprinted from "Smart Shopper" by Alan Coté. Copyright 2009 by Alan Coté.

Chapter 3: Find Your Perfect Fit
"Make Your Bike Fit Your Body" reprinted from "If the Bike Fits, Buy It" and "Make Your Bike Fit Your Body" by Joe Lindsey. Copyright 2006 and 2007 by Joe Lindsey.

Chapter 4: Everything But the Bike
"The Hard Truth About Saddles" reprinted from "The Hard Truth" by Joe Lindsey. Copyright 2005 by Joe Lindsey.
"How To: Wash Your Cycling Duds" reprinted from "How To: Wash Your Cycling Duds" by Brian Fiske. Copyright 2007 by Brian Fiske.

Chapter 6: The Fundamentals
"Advanced Balance: The Trackstand" reprinted from "How To . . . Trackstand" by Lee McCormack. Copyright 2007 by Lee McCormack.

Chapter 7: Up, Down, and All Around
"Smart Shifting" reprinted from "Smart Shifting" by Brian Fiske. Copyright 2008 by Brian Fiske.
"Descending" reprinted from "Descend Like a Rocket" by Brian Fiske. Copyright 2007 by Brian Fiske.

Chapter 9: Stopping—Intentionally or Otherwise
"Better Braking" and Pro Tip (Chris Wherry) include material from "Stop Safely" by Brian Fiske. Copyright 2007 by Brian Fiske.
"Road Rash Rx" reprinted from "Don't Be Rash" by Alan Coté. Copyright 2009 by Alan Coté.

Chapter 10: The Real World
"Break Wind" reprinted from "Break Wind" by Alan Coté. Copyright 2009 by Alan Coté.

Chapter 12: Do It Yourself
"Tune Your Suspension to Match Your Riding Style" reprinted from "Tune Your Suspension to Match Your Riding Style" by Joe Lindsey. Copyright 2007 by Joe Lindsey.

Chapter 13: Never Walk Home
"More Mid-Ride Fixes", "Myth Busters", "Impromptu Fixes Anyone Can Do", "The Kludge That Won the Tour de France" and "Avoiding Our Advice" reprinted from "Never Walk Home" by Alan Coté. Copyright 2005 by Alan Coté.

Chapter 16: Be Careful Out There
"Lock Your Bike" reprinted from "Lock Your Bike" by Joe Lindsey. Copyright 2007 by Joe Lindsey.

Chapter 18: Training Tips and Workouts Galore
"Plan #1: Build Your Base in Four Weeks" reprinted from "Build Your Base Fast" by Selene Yeager. Copyright 2007 by Selene Yeager.
"Find Your Threshold" reprinted from "Lactate Threshold 101" by Selene Yeager. Copyright 2005 by Selene Yeager.
"The Midday Stress-Buster" reprinted from "The Power Lunch" by Chris Carmichael. Copyright 2008 by Chris Carmichael.
"Workouts for Weight Loss" reprinted from "Pedal Away Your Spare Tire" by Selene Yeager. Copyright 2006 by Selene Yeager.
"Plan #2: Race the Clock" and "Plan #3: Win a Sprint" reprinted from "New Year, New You" by Chris Carmichael. Copyright 2006 by Chris Carmichael.
"Should You Ride While Sick?" reprinted from "Should You Ride While Sick?" by Selene Yeager. Copyright 2006 by Selene Yeager.
"How to . . . Blast the Flats" reprinted fro "Ride Flats Without Fatigue" by Selene Yeager. Copyright 2005 by Selene Yeager.
"The Ideal Dog Day Workout" reprinted from "Keep It Cool" by Chris Carmichael. Copyright 2007 by Chris Carmichael.
"Pimp Your Indoor Ride" reprinted from "Pimp Your Indoor Ride" by Selene Yeager. Copyright 2006 by Selene Yeager.
"Mix It Up: Your Guide to Cross-Training" reprinted from "Take a Vacation From Your Bike" by Selene Yeager. Copyright 2006 by Selene Yeager.
Pro Tip (Jamey Driscoll) reprinted from "Off-Season Fitness" by Alan Coté. Copyright 2010 by Alan Coté.

Chapter 19: Get Strong
"Support Your Supporters" reprinted from "Your Whole Body Tune-Up" by Selene Yeager. Copyright 2007 by Selene Yeager.
"Power Up With Plyometrics" reprinted from "Peak Now" by Selene Yeager. Copyright 2007 by Selene Yeager.

Index

Also available

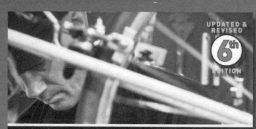
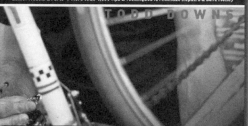
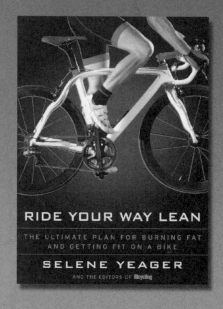
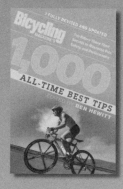
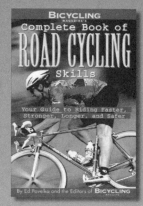
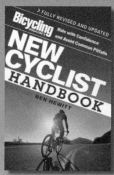
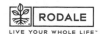